T0259506

# Congenital Vascular Lesions of the Head and Neck

*Editors*

TERESA M. O
MILTON WANER

# OTOLARYNGOLOGIC CLINICS OF NORTH AMERICA

www.oto.theclinics.com

*Consulting Editor*
SUJANA S. CHANDRASEKHAR

FEBRUARY 2018 • Volume 51 • Number 1

**ELSEVIER**

1600 John F. Kennedy Boulevard • Suite 1800 • Philadelphia, Pennsylvania, 19103-2899

http://www.oto.theclinics.com

**OTOLARYNGOLOGIC CLINICS OF NORTH AMERICA Volume 51, Number 1**
**February 2018 ISSN 0030-6665, ISBN-13: 978-0-323-55288-2**

Editor: Jessica McCool
Developmental Editor: Sara Watkins



*Otolaryngologic Clinics of North America* (ISSN 0030-6665) is published bimonthly by Elsevier, Inc., 360 Park Avenue South, New York, NY 10010-1710. Months of issue are February, April, June, August, October, and December. Business and Editorial Offices: 1600 John F. Kennedy Blvd., Suite 1800, Philadelphia, PA 19103-2899. Customer Service Office: 6277 Sea Harbor Drive, Orlando, FL 32887-4800. Periodicals postage paid at New York, NY and additional mailing offices. Subscription prices are $396.00 per year (US individuals), $835.00 per year (US institutions), $100.00 per year (US student/resident), $519.00 per year (Canadian individuals), $1058.00 per year (Canadian institutions), $556.00 per year (international individuals), $1058.00 per year (international institutions), $270.00 per year (international & Canadian student/resident). Foreign air speed delivery is included in all *Clinics*' subscription prices. All prices are subject to change without notice. **POSTMASTER:** Send address changes to *Otolaryngologic Clinics of North America*, Elsevier Health Sciences Division, Subscription Customer Service, 3251 Riverport Lane, Maryland Heights, MO 63043. **Telephone: 1-800-654-2452 (U.S. and Canada); 314-447-8871 (outside U.S. and Canada). Fax: 314-447-8029. E-mail: journalscustomerservice-usa@elsevier.com (for print support); journalsonlinesupport-usa@elsevier.com (for online support).**

*Reprints*. For copies of 100 or more of articles in this publication, please contact the Commercial Reprints Department, Elsevier Inc., 360 Park Avenue South, New York, NY 10010-1710. Tel.: 212-633-3874; Fax: 212-633-3820; E-mail: reprints@elsevier.com.

*Otolaryngologic Clinics of North America* is also published in Spanish by McGraw-Hill Interamericana Editores S.A., P.O. Box 5-237, 06500 Mexico D.F., Mexico.

*Otolaryngologic Clinics of North America* is covered in *MEDLINE/PubMed (Index Medicus), Current Contents/Clinical Medicine, Excerpta Medica, BIOSIS, Science Citation Index,* and *ISI/BIOMED.*

## PROGRAM OBJECTIVE

The goal of the *Otolaryngologic Clinics of North America* is to provide information on the latest trends in patient management, the newest advances; and provide a sound basis for choosing treatment options in the field of otolaryngology.

## LEARNING OBJECTIVES

Upon completion of this activity, participants will be able to:

1. Review the classification and etiology of congenital vascular abnormalities of the head and neck.
2. Discuss surgical management of congenital vascular abnormalities of the head and neck.
3. Recognize management and outcome measures for congenital vascular abnormalities of the head and neck.

## ACCREDITATION

The Elsevier Office of Continuing Medical Education (EOCME) is accredited by the Accreditation Council for Continuing Medical Education (ACCME) to provide continuing medical education for physicians.

The EOCME designates this enduring material for a maximum of 15 *AMA PRA Category 1 Credit*(s)™. Physicians should claim only the credit commensurate with the extent of their participation in the activity.

All other healthcare professionals requesting continuing education credit for this enduring material will be issued a certificate of participation.

## DISCLOSURE OF CONFLICTS OF INTEREST

The EOCME assesses conflict of interest with its instructors, faculty, planners, and other individuals who are in a position to control the content of CME activities. All relevant conflicts of interest that are identified are thoroughly vetted by EOCME for fair balance, scientific objectivity, and patient care recommendations. EOCME is committed to providing its learners with CME activities that promote improvements or quality in healthcare and not a specific proprietary business or a commercial interest.

**The planning committee, staff, authors and editors listed below have identified no financial relationships or relationships to products or devices they or their spouse/life partner have with commercial interest related to the content of this CME activity:**

Denise M. Adams, MD; Nancy M. Bauman, MD, FACS, FAAP; Laurence M. Boon, MD, PhD; Sujana S. Chandrasekhar, MD; Ajay Chavan, MD; Ho Yun Chung, MD, PhD; David H. Darrow, MD, DDS; Luis Delgado, DMD; Alexandra G. Espinel, MD; Katja Evert, MD; Anjali Fortna; Jeremy A. Goss, MD; Arin K. Greene, MD, MMSc; Kristen Helm; Marcelo Hochman, MD; Sophie E.R. Horbach, MD; Tristan Klosterman, MD; Thomas Kühnel, MD; Jessica McCool; Teresa M. O, MD, MArch, FACS; Jonathan A. Perkins, DO; Mark Persky, MD; Angela Queisser, PhD; Kiersten W. Ricci, MD, FACS, FAAP; Gresham T. Richter, MD; A.P.M. Rongen; Tara L. Rosenberg, MD; Emmanuel Seront, MD, PhD; Deborah R. Shatzkes, MD; Jared M. Steinklein, MD; James Y. Suen, MD; Jeyanthi Surendrakumar; Stuart Super, DMD; Theresa Tran, MD; Chantal M.A.M. Van Der Horst, MD, PhD; Avanti Verma, MD; Veronika Vielsmeier, MD; Miikka Vikkula, MD, PhD; Milton Waner, MBBCh(Wits), FCS(SA), MD; Kornelia Wirsching, MD; Walter Wohlgemuth, MD.

**The planning committee, staff, authors and editors listed below have identified financial relationships or relationships to products or devices they or their spouse/life partner have with commercial interest related to the content of this CME activity:**

**Jeong Woo Lee, MD, PhD** has research support from sanofi-aventis and Allakos, Inc.

**Paula E. North, MD, PhD** is a consultant/advisor for, with stock ownership in, and and employment affiliation with, TAI Diagnostics.

## UNAPPROVED/OFF-LABEL USE DISCLOSURE

The EOCME requires CME faculty to disclose to the participants:

1. When products or procedures being discussed are off-label, unlabelled, experimental, and/or investigational (not US Food and Drug Administration [FDA] approved); and
2. Any limitations on the information presented, such as data that are preliminary or that represent ongoing research, interim analyses, and/or unsupported opinions. Faculty may discuss information about pharmaceutical agents that is outside of FDA-approved labelling. This information is intended solely for CME and is not intended to promote off-label use of these medications. If you have any questions, contact the medical affairs department of the manufacturer for the most recent prescribing information.

## TO ENROLL

To enroll in the *Otolaryngologic Clinics of North America* Continuing Medical Education program, call customer service at 1-800-654-2452 or sign up online at http://www.theclinics.com/home/cme. The CME program is available to subscribers for an additional annual fee of USD 260.

## METHOD OF PARTICIPATION

In order to claim credit, participants must complete the following:

1. Complete enrolment as indicated above.
2. Read the activity.
3. Complete the CME Test and Evaluation. Participants must achieve a score of 70% on the test. All CME Tests and Evaluations must be completed online.

## CME INQUIRIES/SPECIAL NEEDS

For all CME inquiries or special needs, please contact elsevierCME@elsevier.com.

# Contributors

## CONSULTING EDITOR

**SUJANA S. CHANDRASEKHAR, MD**
Director, New York Otology; Clinical Professor of Otolaryngology-HNS, Hofstra-Northwell School of Medicine, Hempstead, New York, USA; Clinical Associate Professor of Otolaryngology-HNS, Mount Sinai School of Medicine, New York, New York, USA

## EDITORS

**TERESA M. O, MD, MArch, FACS**
Co-Director, Department of Otolaryngology-Head and Neck Surgery, Facial Plastic and Reconstructive Surgery, Facial Nerve Center, Vascular Birthmark Institute of New York, Manhattan Eye, Ear, and Throat Hospital, Lenox Hill Hospital, New York, New York, USA

**MILTON WANER, MBBCh(Wits), FCS(SA), MD**
Director, Department of Otolaryngology–Head and Neck Surgery, Vascular Birthmark Institute of New York, Manhattan Eye, Ear, and Throat Hospital, Lenox Hill Hospital, New York, New York, USA

## AUTHORS

**DENISE M. ADAMS, MD**
Vascular Anomalies Center, Cancer and Blood Disorders Center, Boston Children's Hospital, Boston, Massachusetts, USA

**NANCY M. BAUMAN, MD, FACS, FAAP**
Professor, Otolaryngology–Head and Neck Surgery, Children's National Health System, The George Washington University, Washington, DC, USA

**LAURENCE M. BOON, MD, PhD**
Human Molecular Genetics, de Duve Institute, University of Louvain, Division of Plastic Surgery, Center for Vascular Anomalies, Cliniques Universitaires Saint Luc, University of Louvain, Brussels, Belgium

**AJAY CHAVAN, MD**
Professor, Head of Department of Radiology, University of Oldenburg, Germany

**HO YUN CHUNG, MD, PhD**
Department of Plastic and Reconstructive Surgery, Kyungpook National University School of Medicine, Daegu, Republic of Korea

**DAVID H. DARROW, MD, DDS**
Professor of Otolaryngology and Pediatrics, Eastern Virginia Medical School, Attending Physician, Children's Hospital of The King's Daughters, Norfolk, Virginia, USA

**LUIS DELGADO, DMD**
Department of Oral and Maxillofacial Surgery, Lenox Hill Hospital, New York, New York, USA

**ALEXANDRA G. ESPINEL, MD**
Assistant Professor, Otolaryngology–Head and Neck Surgery, Children's National Health System, The George Washington University, Washington, DC, USA

**KATJA EVERT, MD**
Department of Pathology, University Hospital Regensburg, Regensburg, Germany

**JEREMY A. GOSS, MD**
Research Fellow, Department of Plastic and Oral Surgery, Boston Children's Hospital, Harvard Medical School, Boston, Massachusetts, USA

**ARIN K. GREENE, MD, MMSc**
Associate Professor, Department of Plastic and Oral Surgery, Vascular Anomalies Center, Boston Children's Hospital, Harvard Medical School, Boston, Massachusetts, USA

**MARCELO HOCHMAN, MD**
Hemangioma and Malformation Treatment Center, Charleston, South Carolina, USA

**SOPHIE E.R. HORBACH, MD**
Department of Plastic, Reconstructive and Hand Surgery, Academic Medical Center, University of Amsterdam, Amsterdam, The Netherlands; Department of Head and Neck Surgery, Vascular Birthmark Institute of New York, Manhattan Eye, Ear, and Throat and Lenox Hill Hospitals, New York, New York, USA

**TRISTAN KLOSTERMAN, MD**
Vascular Birthmark Institute of New York, Head and Neck Institute, Lenox Hill Hospital, New York, New York, USA

**THOMAS KÜHNEL, MD**
Professor, Department of Otorhinolaryngology, University Hospital Regensburg, Regensburg, Germany

**JEONG WOO LEE, MD, PhD**
Department of Plastic and Reconstructive Surgery, Kyungpook National University School of Medicine, Daegu, Republic of Korea

**PAULA E. NORTH, MD, PhD**
Professor, Department of Pathology, Medical College of Wisconsin, Milwaukee, Wisconsin, USA

**TERESA M. O, MD, MArch, FACS**
Co-Director, Department of Otolaryngology-Head and Neck Surgery, Facial Plastic and Reconstructive Surgery, Facial Nerve Center, Vascular Birthmark Institute of New York, Manhattan Eye, Ear, and Throat Hospital, Lenox Hill Hospital, New York, New York, USA

**JONATHAN A. PERKINS, DO**
Professor, Otolaryngology–Head and Neck Surgery, UW School of Medicine, Director, Vascular Anomalies Program, Division of Pediatric Otolaryngology, Department of Surgery, Seattle Children's Hospital, Seattle, Washington, USA

**MARK PERSKY, MD**
Department of Otolaryngology–Head and Neck Surgery, NYU School of Medicine, New York, New York, USA

**ANGELA QUEISSER, PhD**
Human Molecular Genetics, de Duve Institute, University of Louvain, Brussels, Belgium

**KIERSTEN W. RICCI, MD**
Division of Hematology, Hemangioma and Vascular Malformation Center, Cancer and Blood Diseases Institute, Cincinnati Children's Hospital Medical Center, Cincinnati, Ohio, USA

**GRESHAM T. RICHTER, MD, FACS, FAAP**
Professor and Chief of Pediatric Otolaryngology, Benjamin and Milton Waner Endowed Chair, Vascular Anomalies Clinic and Research Director, Department of Otolaryngology–Head and Neck Surgery, University of Arkansas for Medical Sciences, Arkansas Children's Hospital, Little Rock, Arkansas, USA

**AMBER P.M. RONGEN, MD**
Department of Plastic, Reconstructive and Hand Surgery, Academic Medical Center, University of Amsterdam, Amsterdam, The Netherlands

**TARA L. ROSENBERG, MD**
Assistant Professor, Department of Otolaryngology–Head and Neck Surgery, Baylor College of Medicine, Surgical Director, Vascular Anomalies Center, Texas Children's Hospital, Houston, Texas, USA

**EMMANUEL SERONT, MD, PhD**
Department of Medical Oncology, Institut Roi Albert II, Cliniques Universitaires Saint Luc, University of Louvain, Brussels, Belgium

**DEBORAH R. SHATZKES, MD**
Department of Radiology, Lenox Hill Hospital, New York, New York, USA

**JARED M. STEINKLEIN, MD**
Department of Radiology, Lenox Hill Hospital, New York, New York, USA

**JAMES Y. SUEN, MD**
Professor and Chair, Department of Otolaryngology–Head and Neck Surgery, University of Arkansas for Medical Sciences, Little Rock, Arkansas, USA

**STUART SUPER, DMD**
Director Emeritus, Department of Oral and Maxillofacial Surgery, Lenox Hill Hospital, New York, New York, USA

**THERESA TRAN, MD**
Department of Otolaryngology–Head and Neck Surgery, NYU School of Medicine, New York, New York, USA

**CHANTAL M.A.M. VAN DER HORST, MD, PhD**
Department of Plastic, Reconstructive and Hand Surgery, Academic Medical Center, University of Amsterdam, Amsterdam, The Netherlands

**AVANTI VERMA, MD**
Department of Otolaryngology–Head and Neck Surgery, Vascular Birthmark Institute of New York, Manhattan Eye, Ear, and Throat Hospital, New York, New York, USA

**VERONIKA VIELSMEIER, MD**
Department of Otorhinolaryngology, University Hospital Regensburg, Regensburg, Germany

**MIIKKA VIKKULA, MD, PhD**
Human Molecular Genetics, de Duve Institute, University of Louvain, Brussels, Belgium

**MILTON WANER, MBBCh(Wits), FCS(SA), MD**
Director, Vascular Birthmark Institute of New York, Co-Director, Otolaryngology–Head and Neck Surgery, Manhattan Eye, Ear, and Throat Hospital, Lenox Hill Hospital, New York, New York, USA

**KORNELIA WIRSCHING, MD**
Department of Otorhinolaryngology, University Hospital Regensburg, Regensburg, Germany

**WALTER WOHLGEMUTH, MD**
Professor, Head of Department of Radiology, University of Halle, Germany

# Contents

**Foreword: Multidisciplinary Approach to Vascular Anomalies Maximizes Outcomes** **xv**

Sujana S. Chandrasekhar

**Preface: Congenital Vascular Lesions of the Head and Neck** **xvii**

Teresa M. O and Milton Waner

**Classification and Pathology of Congenital and Perinatal Vascular Anomalies of the Head and Neck** **1**

Paula E. North

Accurate histopathologic description in correlation with clinical and radiologic evaluation is required for the treatment of vascular anomalies, both neoplastic and malformative. It is important to examine current clinical, histologic, and immunophenotypical features that distinguish the major types of congenital and perinatal vascular anomalies affecting the head and neck. General discussions of pathogenesis and molecular diagnosis must also be taken into account. This article provides an overview of the features that distinguish the major types of congenital and perinatal vascular anomalies affecting the head and neck and summarizes the diagnostic histopathologic criteria and nomenclature currently applied to these lesions.

**Etiology and Genetics of Congenital Vascular Lesions** **41**

Angela Queisser, Laurence M. Boon, and Miikka Vikkula

The detection of somatic, activating genetic mutations that underlie the development of vascular tumors and malformations led to a better understanding of their pathophysiology. Proteins encoded by the detected mutated genes activate the two major signaling pathways, also involved in cancer: the RAS/MAPK/ERK pathway and/or the PI3K/AKT/mTOR pathway. This gives a strong basis for studies to repurpose cancer therapeutics to patients with vascular tumors and malformations.

**Imaging of Vascular Lesions of the Head and Neck** **55**

Jared M. Steinklein and Deborah R. Shatzkes

This article provides an overview of imaging findings of common and uncommon vascular lesions in the head and neck and showcases images highlighting imaging findings. Both hemangiomas and vascular malformations are covered.

**Infantile Hemangiomas in the Head and Neck Region** **77**

Denise M. Adams and Kiersten W. Ricci

Infantile hemangiomas (IHs) are benign vascular tumors of infancy most common in the region of the head and neck. Infantile hemangiomas are common, but they are extremely heterogeneous and cause a range of complications depending on their morphology, size, or location. Medical interventions for high-risk patients include topical and systemic therapies, including oral propranolol, which has revolutionized the management of IHs over the past years. In this article, the authors provide a review of the natural history, pathology, complications, syndromes, and medical management of infantile hemangioma.

**Congenital Vascular Tumors** **89**

Jeremy A. Goss and Arin K. Greene

Vascular tumors are benign neoplasms, which result from proliferating endothelial cells. These lesions present during infancy or childhood, may affect any location, and exhibit postnatal growth. Local complications include bleeding, tissue destruction, and pain, whereas systemic sequelae include thrombocytopenia, congestive heart failure, and death. Vascular tumors should be differentiated from vascular malformations, which present at birth, have a quiescent endothelium, and grow in proportion to the child. Together, vascular tumors and malformations comprise the field of vascular anomalies.

**Psychosocial Impact of Vascular Anomalies on Children and Their Families** **99**

Alexandra G. Espinel and Nancy M. Bauman

Vascular anomalies are divided into tumors and malformations based on their clinical and cytologic attributes. Vascular malformations are further subcategorized as low-flow lymphatic, venous, capillary, or mixed lesions and as high-flow arteriovenous malformations. Treatment is reserved for vascular anomalies that are symptomatic or cosmetically disfiguring, and surgical and nonsurgical treatment options are widely varied with variable outcomes.

**Outcome Measurement for Vascular Malformations of the Head and Neck** **111**

Sophie E.R. Horbach, Amber P.M. Rongen, Teresa M. O, Milton Waner, and Chantal M.A.M. van der Horst

Vascular malformations are congenital anomalies of the vascular and/or lymphatic system that affect the head and neck region. The most common treatment options are sclerotherapy, laser therapy, surgery, and embolization. Because vascular malformations are variable in type, size, extent, and location, it is a challenge to select methods for evaluation of treatment outcome. Without standardized outcome reporting, it is difficult to compare and combine scientific evidence to support therapeutic decision making. Standardized collection and reporting of outcome data are the first steps toward a fair comparison between treatments. This article describes outcome measurements for vascular malformations and initiatives to improve outcome reporting.

**The Role of Surgery in the Management of Infantile Hemangiomas: What is the Best Timing?** **119**

Marcelo Hochman

Surgery for the management of infantile hemangiomas has become commonplace. Surgical technique articles are plentiful; however, little has been written about the timing of surgery. Knowledge of the biology of the tumors, data from developmental psychology, and the utility of facial reconstruction provide guidelines for timing of surgical intervention.

**The Surgical Management of Infantile Hemangiomas** **125**

Milton Waner

The surgical management of facial infantile hemangiomas presents a unique challenge. The aim of the surgeon should be to remove the hemangioma and to restore normal facial features. Each of the facial zones has its own special features and challenges. The surgeon should remember that the child started out with normal anatomy and that as the hemangioma proliferated, it displaced and thinned these normal structures and, in many cases, expanded adjacent tissue. Hemangiomas do not as a rule invade adjacent tissues as they proliferate. These facts will help in planning the various surgical approaches.

**Management of Infantile Hemangiomas of the Airway** **133**

David H. Darrow

Infantile hemangiomas (IHs) of the airway are far less common than their cutaneous counterparts, and their symptoms mimic those of viral croup. As a result, by the time these lesions are diagnosed, they are often advanced and causing airway compromise. Fortunately, the evolution of propranolol as an effective and safe pharmacotherapy has simplified management of IH and reduced the likelihood of complications previously seen with steroid therapy and surgery. Nevertheless, the otolaryngologist must be prepared with an alternate plan to manage lesions refractory to pharmacotherapy. This article reviews the clinical presentation and current management of IHs of the airway.

**New Frontiers in Our Understanding of Lymphatic Malformations of the Head and Neck: Natural History and Basic Research** **147**

Jonathan A. Perkins

The future of head and neck lymphatic malformation (HNLM) evaluation and treatment is changing because of 2 decades of clinical research and recent basic science investigation. Basic science investigation using cellular biology and molecular genetics has revealed the genetic cause of some HNLMs, which has created the possibility of medical treatment specific to HNLM. This article summarizes the clinical and basic science research that will likely influence the future of HNLM assessment and treatment.

**Multidisciplinary Approach to the Management of Lymphatic Malformations of the Head and Neck** **159**

Milton Waner and Teresa M. O

Lymphatic malformations (LMs) occur in 2.8 to 5 per 100,000 live births. Most involve the head and neck, and they are equally common in men and women. They are developmental anomalies of unknown cause, although recent evidence suggests that an upregulation of the mammalian

strategies. Physicians treating these entities should have a high level of suspicion to consider airway evaluation even in the absence of overt symptoms. However, cutaneous head and neck venous malformations or other lesions affecting the lips, oral cavity, or tongue can herald the presence of coexisting airway lesions. A multidisciplinary approach is critical in achieving comprehensive treatment.

**Orthognathic Considerations of Vascular Malformations** **225**

Luis Delgado, Avanti Verma, Teresa M. O, and Stuart Super

Vascular malformations affect the craniofacial skeleton in many ways, depending on the type of the lesion and its location. The lesions may exert a mass effect and cause thinning or thickening of the bone or cause expansion from direct bony infiltration. Orthognathic surgery can be used to correct any malocclusion or open bite deformities after the soft tissues are addressed.

**Hereditary Hemorrhagic Telangiectasia** **237**

Thomas Kühnel, Kornelia Wirsching, Walter Wohlgemuth, Ajay Chavan, Katja Evert, and Veronika Vielsmeier

Hereditary hemorrhagic telangiectasia (HHT) describes the presenting manifestations of a disorder that is characterized by pathologic blood vessels. HHT is inherited as an autosomal dominant trait with variable penetrance. The abnormal vascular structures (dysplasias) can affect all the organs in the human body. The link between a physical stimulus and new lesion development has been established for mucosal trauma owing to nasal airflow turbulence, for ultraviolet exposure to the fingers, and for mechanical trauma to the dominant hand. The pressing question then is whether HHT treatment constitutes a stimulus that is sufficient to trigger new lesion development.

**Acquired Vascular Tumors of the Head and Neck** **255**

Mark Persky and Theresa Tran

Vascular neoplasms of the head and neck present with a wide spectrum of signs and symptoms. Diagnosis requires a high index of suspicion and is usually made after tumors are large enough to be visually apparent or cause symptoms. This article discusses the most common acquired benign and malignant vascular tumors, with an emphasis on their evaluation and treatment.

*Congenital Vascular Lesions of the Head and Neck*

# OTOLARYNGOLOGIC CLINICS OF NORTH AMERICA

**FORTHCOMING ISSUES**

***April 2018***
**Otosclerosis and Stapes Surgery**
Adrien A. Eshraghi and Fred F. Telischi, *Editors*

***June 2018***
**Global Health in Otolaryngology**
James E. Saunders, Susan R. Cordes, and Mark Zafereo, *Editors*

***August 2018***
**Geriatric Otolaryngology**
Natasha Mirza and Jennifer Lee, *Editors*

**RECENT ISSUES**

***December 2017***
**Allergy for the Otolaryngologist**
Murugappan Ramanathan, Jr, and James Whitman Mims, *Editors*

***October 2017***
**Simulation in Otolaryngology**
Sonya Malekzadeh, *Editor*

***August 2017***
**Multidisciplinary Approach to Head and Neck Cancer**
Maie A. St. John, *Editor*

**ISSUE OF RELATED INTEREST**

*Skull Base Imaging*, January 2017 (Vol. 55, No. 1)
**Radiologic Clinics of North America**
Nafi Aygun, *Editor*
Available at: http://www.radiologic.theclinics.com/

# Foreword

# Multidisciplinary Approach to Vascular Anomalies Maximizes Outcomes

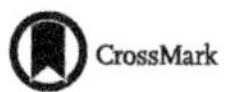

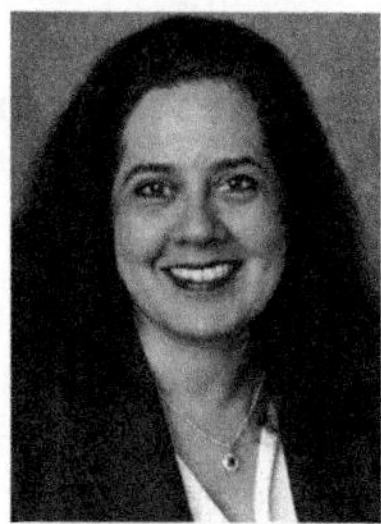

Sujana S. Chandrasekhar, MD
*Consulting Editor*

The birth of a child is a glorious and simultaneously nerve-wracking event in every family. If this is the 1 in 22 children born with a vascular lesion of the head and neck (which is visible in every picture and to every visitor), the parents' concerns multiply. Will my baby bleed? Will my baby stay deformed by this lesion? Is this the tip of the iceberg of other problems? Will my baby be forced to enter chronic medical/surgical care? These are some of the questions that race through the parents' brains, even as they marvel at the wondrousness of new life.

Managing the child with a congenital vascular lesion involves interaction from a number of disciplines.[1] Drs O and Waner have assembled a comprehensive series of articles by authorities in each of these disciplines. The reader of this issue of *Otolaryngologic Clinics of North America* will be able to organize their thoughts so as to approach the patient and their family with a systematic method of evaluation and treatment options, when called to the patient's bedside.

A strong system of classification takes into account the underlying pathology and helps families understand prognosis, etiology, and whether there is a genetic predisposition. Minimizing radiation exposure and sedation/anesthetic medications in order to obtain the most helpful radiographic images at the right timing is very important, as physicians and families become more cognizant of attendant risks. Otolaryngologists are not psychiatrists, but remaining attuned to the psychosocial aspects of visible abnormalities in children is vitally important. We are healers, after all, and helping a family through this process is as important as performing the appropriate intervention.

Various vascular anomalies act differently. A hemangioma is not a lymphangioma. A high-flow vascular malformation is different from one of low flow. The reader of this *Otolaryngologic Clinics of North America* will know the difference, and know when

Otolaryngol Clin N Am 51 (2018) xv–xvi
https://doi.org/10.1016/j.otc.2017.09.023

and how to intervene, and when to offer support and observation for involution. Airway management with potential for bleeding necessitates thorough consultation between otolaryngologist and anesthesiologist. A vascular lesion that may affect maxillary or mandibular growth will affect dentition and bite, and early discussion between otolaryngologist and oral-maxillofacial surgeon is likewise warranted. This *Otolaryngologic Clinics of North America* rounds out the discussion with articles dedicated to understanding and management of hereditary hemorrhagic telangiectasia and acquired vascular tumors of the head and neck, which are encountered in adults and children.

I congratulate Drs O and Waner on the comprehensiveness of this issue of *Otolaryngologic Clinics of North America.* Otolaryngologists are at the head of the multidisciplinary team that is needed for care of patients with vascular malformations. You, the reader, will find that perusing the comprehensive articles that have been assembled here in a logical flow fashion will enable you to assess, counsel, and intervene with confidence.

Sujana S. Chandrasekhar, MD
Director, New York Otology
Clinical Professor of Otolaryngology-HNS
Hofstra-Northwell School of Medicine
Clinical Associate Professor of Otolaryngolgy-HNS
Mount Sinai School of Medicine
210 East 64th Street, 3rd Floor
New York, NY 10065, USA

*E-mail address:*
ssc@nyotology.com

## REFERENCE

1. Mahady K, Thust S, Berkeley R, et al. Vascular anomalies of the head and neck in children. Quant Imaging Med Surg 2015;5(6):886–97.

# Preface

# Congenital Vascular Lesions of the Head and Neck

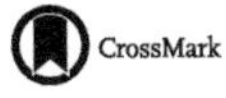

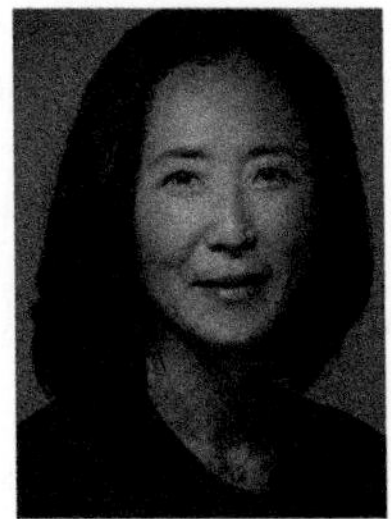

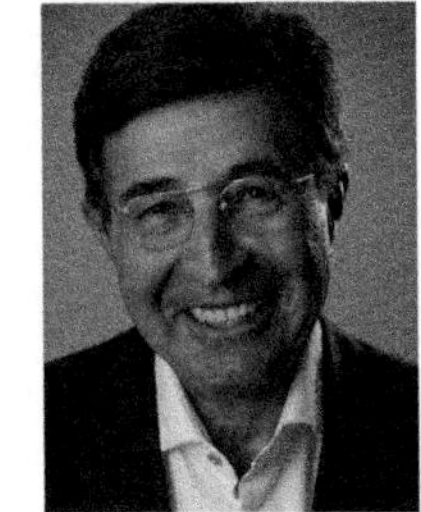

Teresa M. O, MD, MArch, FACS Milton Waner, MBBCh(Wits), FCS(SA), MD

*Editors*

The number of physicians interested in the treatment of vascular anomalies has grown exponentially over the last several decades from a mere handful in the mid 1980s to several thousand today. Every year, hundreds of peer-reviewed articles are published in this field. Some of the most interesting articles have shed light on the underlying genetic and molecular bases of some of these conditions. This has led to the development of at least one group of medical therapies for some vascular lesions.

Ongoing research will no doubt offer many more alternatives for the management of these complex problems. Despite these advances, there is still much to be done, especially in the field of clinical outcomes analysis. It has become evident that several modalities may be used to treat some of these conditions. Good research comparing and contrasting the outcomes will enable us to choose the most appropriate therapy for a particular lesion.

In this issue, we introduce the relevant basic science as well as the diagnostic and clinical aspects of these diseases. Since so many physicians from multiple specialties have a stake in this field, we have invited experts from a wide range of disciplines to contribute articles. By so doing, we hope that this review is comprehensive and will

Otolaryngol Clin N Am 51 (2018) xvii–xviii
https://doi.org/10.1016/j.otc.2017.09.021
0030-6665/18/© 2017 Published by Elsevier Inc. 

give an overview and understanding of vascular lesions to our specialty. Otolaryngology is a core specialty involved in the management of vascular lesions of the head and neck, and a comprehensive review of the subject is timely.

Teresa M. O, MD, MArch, FACS
Department of Otolaryngology–Head and Neck Surgery
Facial Plastic and Reconstructive Surgery
Facial Nerve Center
Vascular Birthmark Institute of New York
Manhattan Eye, Ear, and Throat Hospital
Lenox Hill Hospital
210 East 64th Street
7 Floor
New York, NY 10065, USA

Milton Waner, MBBCh(Wits), FCS(SA), MD
Department of Otolaryngology–Head and Neck Surgery
Vascular Birthmark Institute of New York
Manhattan Eye, Ear and Throat Hospital
Lenox Hill Hospital
210 East 64th Street
7 Floor
New York, NY 10065, USA

*E-mail addresses:*
to@vbiny.org (T.M. O)
Mwmd01@gmail.com (M. Waner)

# Classification and Pathology of Congenital and Perinatal Vascular Anomalies of the Head and Neck

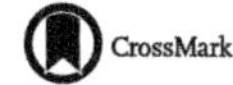

Paula E. North, MD, PhD*

KEYWORDS

• Congenital • Perinatal • Vascular anomalies • Head • Neck

## KEY POINTS

- Accurate histopathologic description in correlation with clinical and radiological evaluation is often required for diagnosis and treatment of vascular anomalies, both neoplastic and malformative.
- It is important to examine current clinical, histologic, and immunophenotypical features that distinguish the major types of congenital and perinatal vascular anomalies affecting the head and neck.
- General discussions of pathogenesis and molecular diagnosis must also be taken into account.

## INTRODUCTION

This article provides an overview of the current clinical, histologic, and immunophenotypical features that distinguish the major types of congenital and perinatal vascular anomalies affecting the head and neck, and summarizes the diagnostic histopathologic criteria and nomenclature currently applied to these lesions in most major vascular anomalies centers globally. General discussions of pathogenesis and molecular diagnosis are also included, providing an overview of correlations between clinical, epidemiologic, histoimmunophenotypic, and (where applicable) genetic features. Pathogenic considerations, along with radiological evaluation and clinical management strategies for the major entities, are presented in depth in subsequent articles. Congenital vascular anomalies that do not, or only rarely, affect the head and neck are not included, nor are

Disclosure: P.E. North has nothing to disclose.
* Department of Pathology, Medical College of Wisconsin, Milwaukee, WI 53202.
*E-mail address:* pnorth@mcw.edu

Otolaryngol Clin N Am 51 (2018) 1–39
https://doi.org/10.1016/j.otc.2017.09.020
oto.theclinics.com

vascular tumors acquired beyond the immediate postnatal period (clinical aspects of the latter are presented in Mark Persky and Theresa Tran's article, "Acquired Vascular Tumors of the Head and Neck," in this issue).

Accurate histopathologic description in correlation with clinical and radiological evaluation is often required for diagnosis and treatment of vascular anomalies, both neoplastic and malformative. However, traditional overgeneric use of the term hemangioma has caused inappropriate grouping of entities that are now known to be both biologically as well as clinically dissimilar. This persistent problem was recognized more than 2 decades ago by the multidisciplinary International Society for the Study of Vascular Anomalies (ISSVA), which produced a landmark general framework of a biologically based classification system derived in part from that proposed by Mulliken and Glowacki[1] in which vascular anomalies, based on presence or absence of endothelial mitotic activity, were divided into tumors and malformations. According to this simplified scheme, the suffix angioma (as in hemangioma) should be reserved for benign vascular tumors that arise by cellular hyperplasia. In contrast, the term vascular malformation should designate true errors in vascular morphogenesis, usually clinically evident at birth and showing growth proportional (±) to that of the patient and little endothelial mitotic activity (eg, arteriovenous malformation [AVM]). Accumulated experience has shown that endothelial mitotic activity alone is not sufficient to separate vascular tumors from malformations, because of secondary effects such as ischemia and turbulence that may stimulate mitotic activity. Nevertheless, when considered in combination with other histologic features and clinical behavior, endothelial mitotic activity remains a useful consideration in the approach to these diagnostically challenging lesions.

The ISSVA-sanctioned classification is now widely adopted and has been incrementally refined and expanded over the years, leading to a major published and online update[2] in 2014, cross-referenced to clinical characteristics, associated syndromes, and genetics accrue findings. A synopsis of the basic framework of this classification provided in **Table 1**. This approach has proved itself in practice as an increasingly useful, biology-based diagnostic system, although continuing updates to the classification will be necessary as lesions that defy classification based on current criteria are revisited and discoveries in vascular biology and genetics accrue.

The ISSVA-encouraged distinction between vascular tumors (angiomas) and malformations represents a significant departure from the traditional, and still often applied, nomenclature in which the term hemangioma was overapplied without regard to cause or clinical behavior, at best modified by clinically or histologically based morphologic descriptors such as cavernous and capillary. As an example, even now it is common for clinicians and experienced pathologists to refer to venous malformations (VMs), which consist of mitotically quiescent collections of developmentally abnormal veins, as cavernous hemangiomas. Similarly, developmental abnormalities of lymphatic vessel beds (lymphatic malformations [LMs] by the current classification), are often still referred to as lymphangiomas, and AVMs as arteriovenous (AV) hemangiomas. Continued use of this poor traditional terminology, rooted in previous lack of etiologic clarity, perpetuates past misconceptions even in the face of new understanding. With the biology-based, ISSVA-sanctioned classification, jointly applied and revised by consensus in a multidisciplinary fashion, clinicians are more prepared to recognize biologically distinct entities and improve patient outcomes through better targeted therapies. The histopathologic classification of congenital vascular anomalies presented here is congruent with the latest ISSVA consensus statement.[2]

**Table 1**
**ISSVA Classification (2014)[2], basic framework**

| Vascular Anomalies[a] | | | | |
|---|---|---|---|---|
| **Vascular Tumors** | **Vascular Malformations** | | | |
| Benign<br>• Infantile hemangioma<br>• Congenital hemangioma (RICH, NICH, PICH)[b]<br>• Tufted angioma[c]<br>• Spindle cell hemangioma<br>• Epithelioid hemangioma<br>• Pyogenic granuloma<br>• Others<br>Locally aggressive or borderline<br>• Kaposiform hemangioendothelioma[c]<br>• Papillary intralymphatic angioendothelioma (PILA), Dabska tumor<br>• Kaposi sarcoma<br>• Retiform hemangioendothelioma<br>• Composite hemangioendothelioma<br>• Others<br>Malignant<br>• Angiosarcoma<br>• Epithelioid hemangioendothelioma<br>• Others | Simple | Combined | Of major named vessels (aka, channel/truncal-type | Associated with other anomalies |
| | Capillary malformations (CM)<br>Lymphatic malformations (LM)<br>Primary lymphedema<br>Venous malformations (VM)<br>Glomuvenous malformations (GVM)<br>Arteriovenous malformations (AVM)<br>Arteriovenous fistulas (AVF) | CM + VM<br>CM + LM<br>CM + AVM<br>LM + VM<br>CM + LM + VM<br>CM + LM + AVM<br>CM + VM + AVM<br>CM + LM + VM + AVM | See details on ISSVA website | See list and known genetic associations on ISSVA website |

[a] Vascular anomalies are divided in the ISSVA classification (2014)[2] into two primary groups: vascular tumors and vascular malformations. Entities for which this distinction has not yet been made are listed separately as "provisionally unclassified" and include verrucous venulocapillary malformation (aka, verrucous "hemangioma"), multifocal lymphangio endotheliomatosis with thrombocytopenia /cutaneovisceral angiomatosis with thrombocytopenia (MLT/CAT), kaposiform lymphangiomatosis (KLA), and PTEN (type) hamartoma of soft tissue.
[b] The rapidly involuting, partially involuting, and noninvoluting variants of congenital hemangioma are considered clinical variants of the same biological entity. Although currently classified as a tumor, recent research favors classification as a vascular malformation (see text).
[c] Most consider tufted angioma to be a more superficial form of kaposiform hemangioendothelioma (see text).

*Data from* International Society for the Study of Vascular Anomalies (ISSVA). ISSVA classification for vascular anomalies. Melbourne, Australia; 2014. Available at: http://www.issva.org/classification.

## VASCULAR TUMORS AND TUMORLIKE LESIONS

Classically, vascular tumors, as originally defined by ISSVA, arise by cellular hyperplasia and show disproportionate growth compared with the child. In contrast, vascular malformations develop in utero as errors in vascular morphogenesis and typically grow in proportion to the child's growth. However, this is a controversial division. For instance, some vascular tumors per the latest ISSVA classification[2] are congenitally fully formed and typically do not show disproportionate postnatal growth; these are the congenital nonprogressive hemangiomas subcategorized by the anachronisms rapidly involuting congenital hemangioma (RICH), noninvoluting congenital hemangioma (NICH), and partially involuting congenital hemangioma (PICH). Until there is a better understanding of the pathogenesis of these lesions, which share features of vascular malformations, they are perhaps best discussed provisionally as tumorlike lesions, as in this article. Note that many vascular tumorlike lesions of major clinical importance, including congenital nonprogressive hemangiomas, are not included in the current World Health Organization (WHO) classification of soft tissue tumors,[3] although this is likely to change in the next revision. Histopathologic features of the major categories of congenital and perinatally presenting vascular tumors and tumorlike lesions that commonly affect the head and neck are discussed later, accompanied by brief clinical and pathogenic information for orientation. Discussion begins with infantile hemangioma (IH), the most common type of vascular tumor and the most common tumor of infancy. Several other histologically and clinically distinct types of vascular tumors and tumorlike lesions that typically present in early childhood or during gestation are then addressed. Some of these are life threatening and all are important to diagnose precisely so that appropriate therapies can be applied. Those with established infectious cause, including Kaposi sarcoma, bacillary angiomatosis, and verruga peruana, and those commonly thought to be reactive vascular proliferations, including so-called pyogenic granuloma, glomeruloid hemangioma, microvenular hemangioma, and reactive angioendotheliomatosis, are omitted.

### *Infantile Hemangioma*

#### *Clinical features*

IH is the most common tumor of infancy, affecting approximately 4% of children, with a 3-fold female to male ratio. Previously used synonyms include juvenile hemangioma and cellular hemangioma of infancy. IHs of this type display a remarkably predictable natural course: they present shortly after birth, sometimes with a fairly subtle nascent lesion congenitally evident, grow rapidly in the first year of life, then spontaneously involute slowly over a period of years. Low-birth-weight and fair-skinned infants are at increased risk, although all races are affected.[4,5]

Although all IHs spontaneously involute to variable degrees and with variable speed over the course of years, significant cosmetic or functional residua are common.[6,7] Complications during the proliferative phase may include airway compromise; cutaneous ulceration; bleeding; infection; and, with large/multiple lesions, congestive heart failure. Periorbital lesions may cause amblyopia by blocking the visual axis. Diffuse hepatic involvement by IH may cause severe hypothyroidism because of tumoral expression of type 3 iodothyronine deiodinase.[8]

IHs show several anatomic predilections and patterns of tissue involvement that suggest pathogenic clues. Approximately 60% occur on the head and neck, although they also occur on the extremities, trunk, genitals, and in viscera, notably including the liver, intestine, and less often the lung. Skin and subcutis seem to be most commonly affected, even considering the more obvious presentation. Deep skeletal muscle and brain parenchyma are spared. True IH can involve the tissues investing leptomeningeal vessels and thus can be intracranial. Most present as solitary cutaneous and/or subcutaneous lesions, but a significant percentage of patients (about 15%) have multiple skin lesions, in some cases accompanied by multiple visceral hemangiomas, usually hepatic, intuitively suggesting dissemination. Although most cutaneous and subcutaneous IHs appear as focal masses, others show a distinctly segmental distribution.[9] Segmental facial IH may occur in association with 1 or more of the abnormalities in the syndrome with the acronym PHACE (posterior fossa brain malformations, arterial cerebrovascular anomalies, cardiovascular anomalies, and eye anomalies), or PHACES syndrome when accompanied by supraumbilical raphe and/or defects of the sternum.[10] The cause of this association is not understood, but it seems likely that the IH represents a secondary occurrence in a developmentally altered segment. Patients with PHACE with cerebrovascular anomalies are at risk for progressive vasculopathy that results in stenotic and occlusive changes with rare risk of ischemic stroke.[11] Similarly, lower body cutaneous segmental IHs on the lower body have been described in association with regional congenital anomalies under the suggested acronym of LUMBAR syndrome.[12–14]

Large involuted tumors may be excised for cosmetic reasons. For some clinically problematic proliferative phase IHs (eg, those obscuring the visual axis), surgical excision is preferable to medical therapy[15] (treatment options are more extensively described in the article [See Denise M. Adams and Kiersten W. Ricci article, "Infantile Hemangiomas in the Head and Neck Region" and Milton Waner's article, "The Surgical Management of Infantile Hemangiomas", in this issue]).

#### *Histology*

Proliferative phase IHs consist of cellular masses of densely packed capillaries with small rounded lumina, lined by plump endothelial cells rimmed by equally plump pericytes (**Fig. 1**). Lesional endothelial cells and pericytes both show occasional mitoses. Interspersed pericapillary immature dendritic-type cells are moderately abundant, and the capillary basement membrane becomes multilaminated over time. The proliferating capillaries are arranged in variably well-defined lobules, which are separated by delicate fibrous septae or normal intervening tissue (**Fig. 2**). Lesional capillaries interdigitate nondestructively with normal structures (salivary glands, superficial skeletal muscle fibers, adipocytes, skin adnexae, and peripheral nerves). Draining veins become enlarged and develop thickened asymmetrical walls. IHs do not show necrosis, intravascular thrombosis, or hemosiderin deposition, unless secondary to ulceration or presurgical embolization.

In the involuting phase of IH, lesional capillaries gradually disappear, basement membranes thicken and show embedded apoptotic dust, and pericapillary masts cells increase in number (**Fig. 3**). As in the proliferative phase, thrombosis and significant inflammation are not typically present. Near the end stage of involution, lobules are replaced by loose fibrous or fibrofatty stroma, with only few residual vessels, which remarkably preserve their immunophenotype. So-called ghost vessels show thickened multilayered rinds of basement membrane material, with apoptotic debris and little or no intact cellular lining (**Fig. 4**). Lesions that have previously ulcerated show epidermal atrophy and fibrous scarring. Large arteries and draining veins do not completely regress. This phenomenon, paired with loss of mitotic activity, may lead to mistaken histologic diagnosis of the lesion as a vascular malformation (**Fig. 5**). This misinterpretation can usually be avoided by consideration of clinical history and overall histologic appearance.

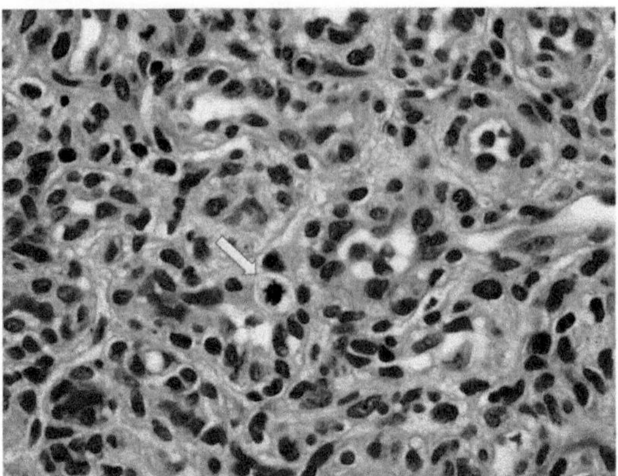

**Fig. 1.** Infantile hemangioma, proliferative phase. Endothelial cells and pericytes form plump, tightly packed capillaries. Note the mitotic figure (*arrow*).

Immunohistochemical studies of IH (**Fig. 6**) have revealed a unique and complex endothelial phenotype, shared only by placental capillaries, which includes strong expression of glucose transporter isoform 1 (GLUT1), Lewis Y antigen, Fc gamma receptor II, CD15, CCR6, indoleamine 2,3-dioxygenase (IDO), and insulin-like growth factor 2 (IGF2).[16–20] The IH capillary basement membrane is strongly enriched in merosin, also characteristic of placental capillary basement membranes.[19] This membrane is a committed vascular phenotype for which most of the component placenta-associated markers persist throughout the natural course of IH. Consequently, GLUT1 immunohistochemistry, in particular, has become extremely useful for diagnostic confirmation of IH and is widely considered the international gold standard for that purpose. Caution is warranted in differentiating strongly GLUT1-positive circulating erythrocytes, or their degeneration products, from endothelial positivity (or the lack of it.) Lesional capillaries of IH are also positive for normal blood vascular endothelial markers (including CD31, CD34, von Willebrand factor [vWF], *Ulex*

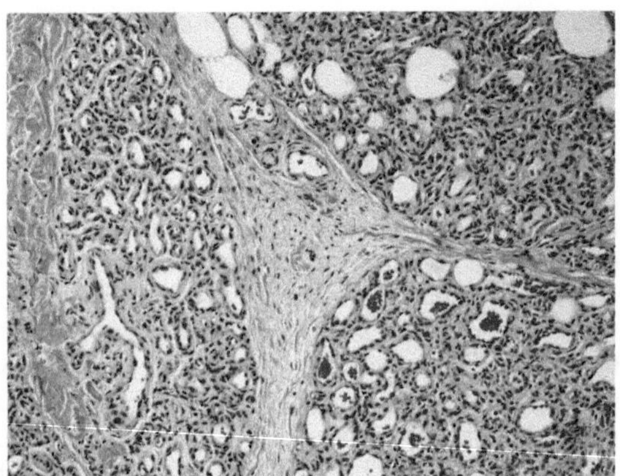

**Fig. 2.** Infantile hemangioma, proliferative phase, typical lobularity. Capillary lobules in this cutaneous example are separated by normal intervening dermal stroma.

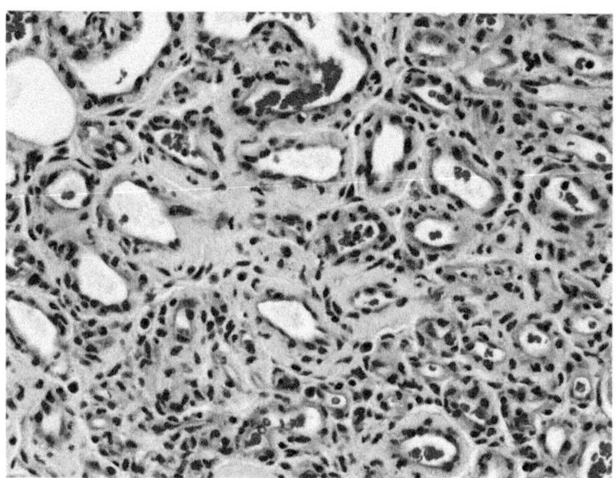

**Fig. 3.** Infantile hemangioma, actively involuting phase. Note the thickened capillary basement membranes containing apoptotic debris. Pericapillary mast cells are numerous.

*europaeus* lectin I, friend leukemia virus integration 1 (Fli-1), endothelial transcription factor ETS-related gene (ERG), and vascular endothelial cadherin).

***Pathogenesis***

Rare families with increased incidence of IH have shown linkage to chromosome 5q31-33, suggesting potential influential mutations.[21,22] However, IHs are extremely common and almost all are sporadic, making it unlikely that IH is intrinsically a genetic disease. IHs are notably more common in low-birth-weight infants and twins, but there is a lack of concordance in twin studies, further arguing against strongly predisposing inherited factors.[23] Although all races are affected by IH, being white, female, or fair haired seems to lower the threshold for development of these lesions, the mechanisms for which remain obscure.

Independent of consideration of potential genetic determinants/modulators of IH, which seem likely to be weak at best, the unusual molecular signature that is shared only by IH capillaries and the fetal capillaries of placental villi has elicited much etiologic discussion but is difficult to investigate experimentally because of the lack of

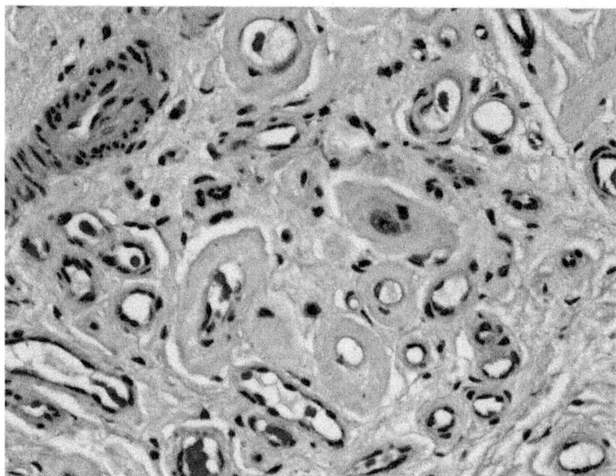

**Fig. 4.** Infantile hemangioma, late involuting stage. Basement membranes of residual capillaries are thick and hyalinized. Some of the residual endothelial cells have enlarged, senescent nuclei.

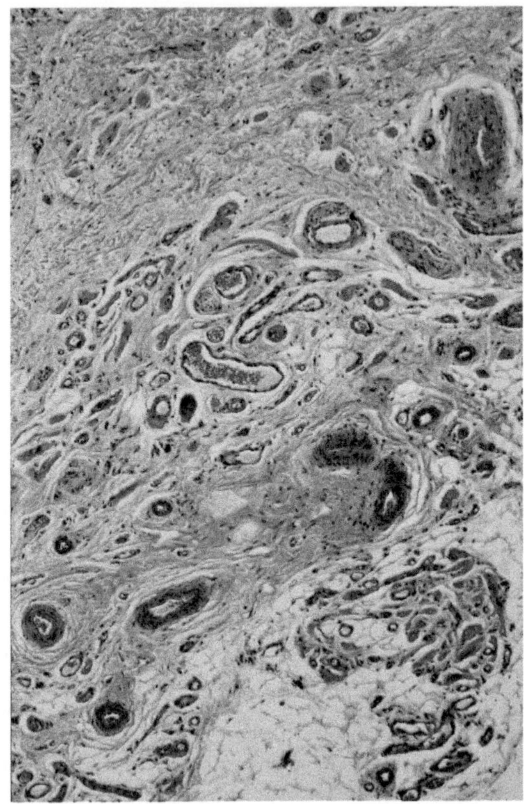

**Fig. 5.** Infantile hemangioma, end stage. Residual feeding and draining vessels persist after capillaries drop out, lending an appearance resembling vascular malformation.

appropriate animal models. Current evidence favors the hypothesis that IH arises from multipotent vascular precursor cells, which may originate from the placenta.[16,18,19,24–29] It is also noteworthy that the phenotype of placental and IH endothelial cells, exemplified by CD31, CD34, GLUT1, Lewis Y antigen, IDO, CD15, CCR6, and Fc$\gamma$RII coexpression, shows great overlap with that of early hematopoietic and vasculogenic cells, and in part with mature cells of the myelomonocytic lineage.[16,19] These shared patterns of expression emphasize the close ontological relation between hematopoietic and vascular development that begins in the yolk sac and continues into the adult bone marrow and support the supposition that the endothelial cells of both IH and placenta are arrested (presumably by evolutionary plan in the case of placenta), in a specialized, intermediate state of vascular/hematopoietic differentiation that must have selective advantage in the case of the placenta.[19,26,30] A recent study by Jinnin and colleagues[31] reported low vascular endothelial growth factor receptor 1 expression in cultured endothelial cells from IH, compared with various controls, with resultant activation of VEGRF2 and its downstream targets. This low expression may have significant therapeutic implications, as yet uninvestigated. It is probable that extraneous systemic factors affect the behavior of IH; a recent study reported recurrence of IH in late childhood in 2 patients on exogenous growth hormone therapy.[32]

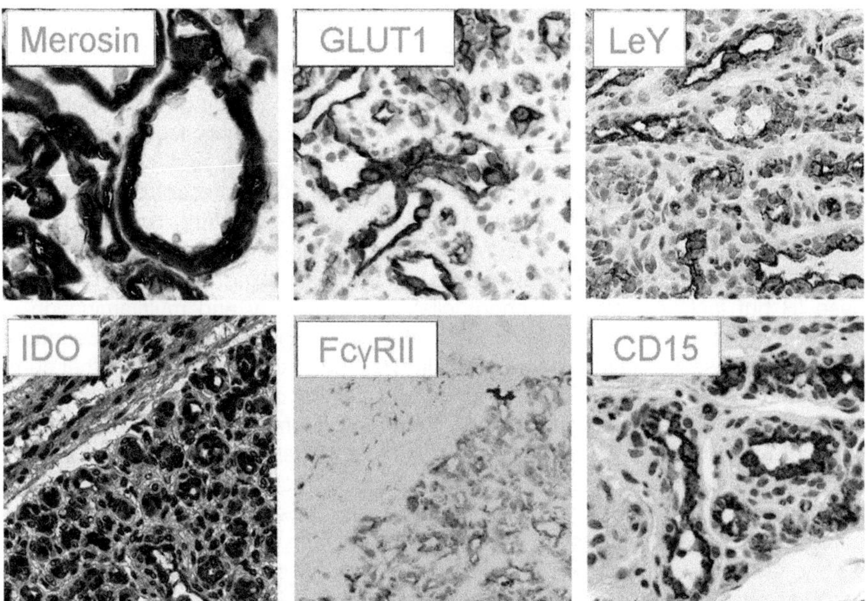


**Fig. 6.** Infantile hemangioma, unique capillary immunophenotype shared by placental capillaries.

### *Congenital Nonprogressive Hemangiomas: Rapidly Involuting Congenital Hemangioma and Noninvoluting Congenital Hemangioma*

#### *Clinical*

Congenital nonprogressive hemangiomas: Rapidly involuting congenital hemangioma (RICH) and Noninvoluting congenital hemangioma (NICH) are congenital vascular lesions that, unlike IH, are typically fully formed at birth and then follow either a static clinical course (NICH) or very rapidly regress in 3 to 5 months because of central infarction (RICH).[33–35] Only rare examples show limited progressive postnatal clinical growth, and they occur with equal sex predilection (like vascular malformations). There is considerable histologic overlap between the NICH and RICH clinical subtypes; current opinion favors that they are biologically synonymous entities that vary primarily in propensity for infarction and thus regression. Some lesions of this type only partially regress and have been dubbed PICH.[36] Most are cutaneous and/or subcutaneous. Visceral lesions are typically solitary and centrally necrotic, primarily located in the liver, and occasionally in the brain. Reportedly multifocal visceral lesions have been poorly documented histologically. MRI reveals well-circumscribed masses with large flow voids reminiscent of AVM. Regressing stages of RICH show central necrosis, often with superimposed calcification. Complications are influenced by location and size and include hemorrhage; scarring; atrophy; and, for large lesions, high-output heart failure.[37] During central infarction and lesional regression, large RICHs may be complicated by transient mild to moderate thrombocytopenia and consumptive coagulopathy.

#### *Histology*

Histologic features of RICH and NICH vary along an evolving spectrum, dictated largely by the degree of infarction, with PICH as an intermediate state. To emphasize this spectrum, it is good practice for pathologists to provide a diagnosis of congenital nonprogressive hemangioma, modified as either the rapidly involuting (RICH) or noninvoluting (NICH) clinical variant. The term PICH is not often applied.

Whether rapidly involuting or noninvoluting, congenital nonprogressive hemangiomas are typically composed of variably circumscribed capillary lobules separated by abnormally dense fibrous tissue, with frequent atrophy and loss of dermal adnexal appendages in involved and overlying skin (**Fig. 7**). This condition contrasts with IH, in which tumor lobules are typically separated by normal-appearing tissue elements (see **Fig. 2**). Endothelial cells and pericytes of the component capillaries within the lobules are in some cases moderately plump, focally resembling those of proliferative phase IH but lacking increased endothelial mitotic activity and multilamination of basement membranes (**Fig. 8**). The lobules often show stellate, thin-walled, centrilobular, draining vessels and may be peripherally or globally sclerotic (**Fig. 9**). Other common features are thrombosis, hemosiderin deposition, and foci of calcification and/or extramedullary hematopoiesis. Typically, there is a prominent interlobular vascular network of arterial, venous, and often lymphatic channels that are more prominent than the more cellular capillary lobules in some cases, requiring careful differentiation from AV or capillary LM (**Fig. 10**). In regressing RICH, grossly evident areas of central depression and scarring correlate with a central core with large central draining channels and few capillary lobules. Features more commonly seen in NICH than RICH are hobnailed endothelium, large and loosely defined capillary lobules, and AV fistulae (AVFs).[33,35] The residual lesion of RICH of peripheral soft tissues shows cutaneous and subcutaneous collapse with variable loss of dermal and adipose tissue that may extend down to the muscle fascia. In both RICH and NICH, the lesional endothelial cells are negative for GLUT1 and the other distinctive markers of IH (**Fig. 11**).[33]

#### *Pathogenesis*

The pathogenesis of this family of lesions (RICH, NICH, and PICH) is biologically unrelated to classic IH, based on strongly differing histologic features and immunophenotype as well as clinical presentation and behavior. The histology of the capillary lobules of these lesions resembles so-called pyogenic granulomas, acquired lesions sometimes associated with precedent trauma, which suggests the possibility of contribution by focal intrauterine vascular accident or tissue injury that spawns a local reparative vascular process in utero. Recently, somatic activating mutations in the

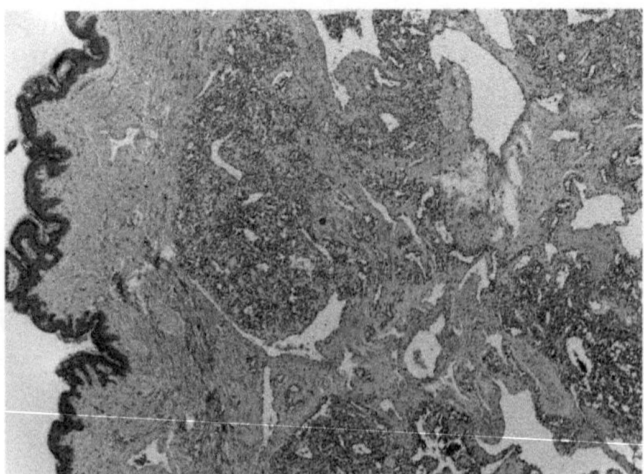

**Fig. 7.** Congenital nonprogressive hemangioma, cutaneous. Capillary lobules are separated by fibrotic dermal stroma, with loss of skin appendages and epidermal atrophy.

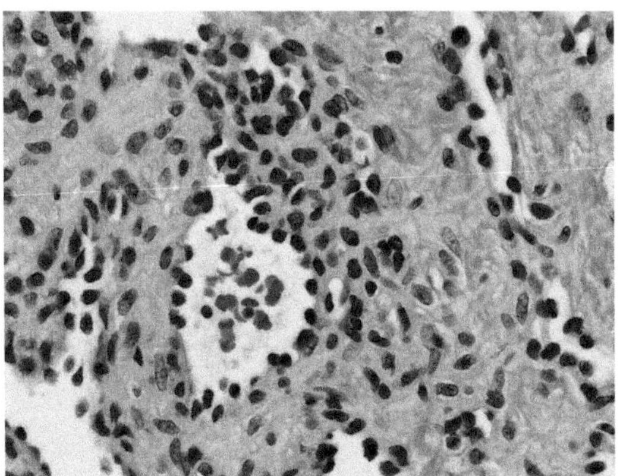

**Fig. 8.** Congenital nonprogressive hemangioma, high magnification. Endothelial cells have generally small, buttonlike nuclei that lack significant mitotic activity.

GNAQ and GNA11 genes have been reported in RICH and NICH.[38] Because the same GNAQ or GNA11 mutation was found in both RICH-type and NICH-type lesions, other factors must be presumed to cause the differing postnatal behaviors of these clinical variants, confirming the histologic similarity of these clinical variants within the parent category of congenital nonprogressive hemangioma.

### *Kaposiform Hemangioendothelioma and Tufted Angioma*

#### *Clinical*

Kasabach-Merritt phenomenon (KMP) was first defined in 1940 as life-threatening thrombocytopenic purpura occurring in the setting of an enlarging hemangioma, long before the many clinically and biologically distinct categories of vascular anomalies were grouped under the term hemangioma. KMP is characterized by profound sustained thrombocytopenia, sometimes accompanied by microangiopathic hemolytic anemia and secondary consumption of fibrinogen and coagulation factors. It differs from the chronic consumptive coagulopathy that may complicate large LMs or VMs in which platelet counts are normal or only slightly decreased, but fibrinogen

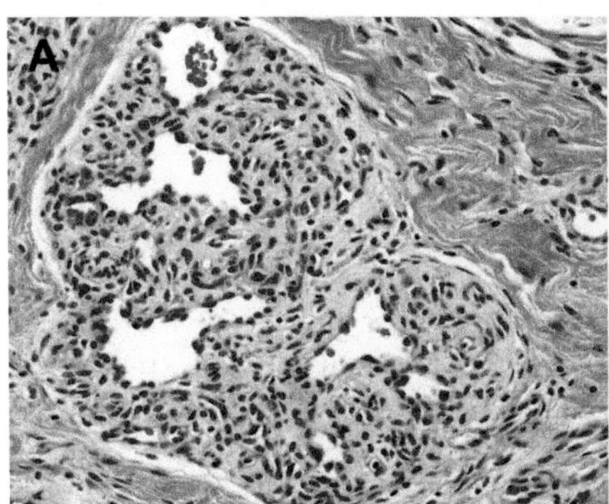



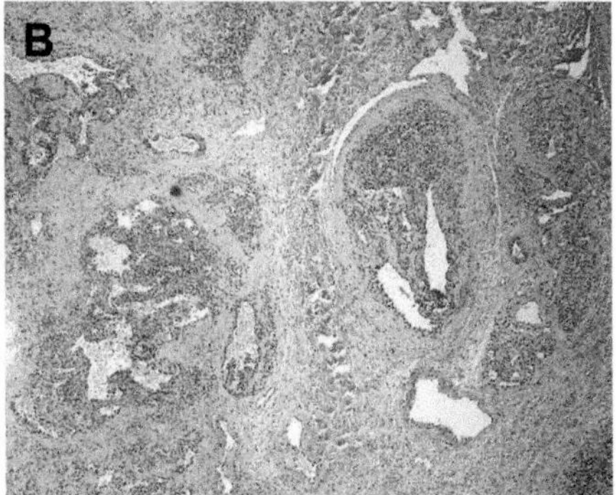



**Fig. 9.** Congenital nonprogressive hemangioma, lobules. (*A*) Many have stellate draining vessels. (*B*) Lobular sclerosis is common.

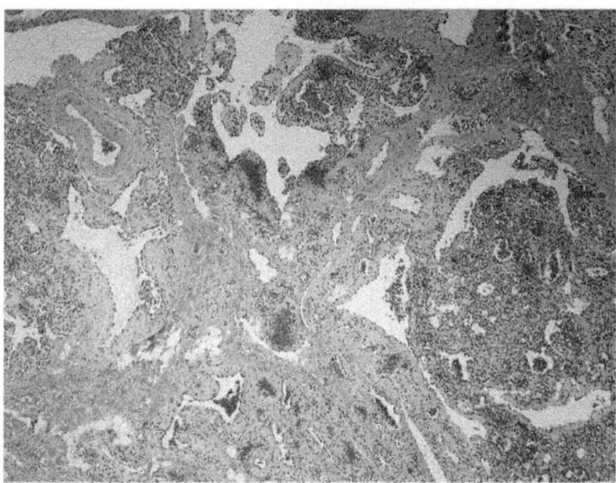

**Fig. 10.** Congenital nonprogressive hemangioma, prominent septal vasculature.

and clotting factor levels are low. It is now realized that KMP is not caused by the common IH, even when very large, but is a complication of 2, likely synonymous, vascular tumors that histologically overlap: tufted angioma (TA) and kaposiform hemangioendothelioma (KHE).[39,40] The histologic resemblance of KHE and TA, with resection specimens of KHE often showing cutaneous changes that would have been interpreted in small biopsy specimens as tufted angioma, and the virtually exclusive association of these two entities with KMP, support the now prevalent opinion[39–42] that KHE and TA are variants of the same clinicopathologic entity, with the term TA historically used to describe superficial, often less aggressive, examples of KHE. Unlike IH, which shows significant female predilection, KHE and TA are equally prevalent in men and women. Preferred tissue distributions of the KHE/TA spectrum include skin and subcutis, deep soft tissues, bone, and spleen. Also unlike IH, involvement of the liver is absent to rare.

Some KHE/TA are congenital, and most are reported in infants and young children less than 5 years of age. Rarely, they present in older children and adults. KMP is seen

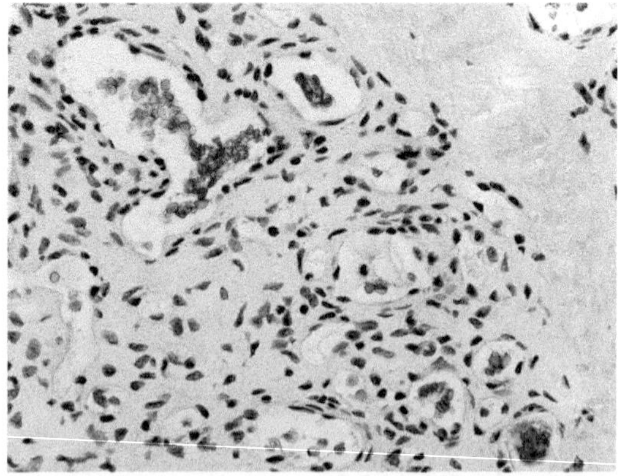

**Fig. 11.** Congenital nonprogressive hemangioma, GLUT1 immunoreaction. Lesional capillary endothelial cells are negative for GLUT1, unlike those of infantile hemangioma (see **Fig. 6**). Note that intraluminal erythrocytes are GLUT1 positive, a useful internal positive control.

only in congenital/early infantile cases, and not always in those. Lesions range from locally infiltrative stains and plaques of the skin and subcutis to large masses in deep soft tissues. Typical locations include the head and neck, extremities, and trunk. They occasionally present as bulky body cavity or retroperitoneal masses and more rarely in bone and spleen. On MRI they are usually diffusely enhancing, T2 hyperintense, with ill-defined margins that cross tissue planes.

Rarely, KMP has been reported in patients with congenital fibrosarcoma or congenital hemangiopericytoma, but almost all cases are associated with KHE/TA, caused at least in large part by platelet trapping within the tumor. Untreated lesions do not permanently regress, although they may wax and wane. KHE is categorized as an intermediate (locally aggressive) soft tissue tumor by the WHO[3] in light of rare reports of spread along (or perhaps multifocal involvement of) local lymphatic chains. True metastasis is unlikely, with no distant metastases reported.

Treatment options (described in more detail in Jeremy A. Goss and Arin K. Greene's article, "Congenital Vascular Tumors," in this issue) include wide local excision, which can be curative when feasible, although recurrences are common.[43,44]

### *Histology*

As indicated earlier, the histologic features of KHE and TA overlap and often coexist in the same lesion, with the more subtle features of TA commonly seen in cutaneous aspects of a large mass in which fully developed features of KHE are seen more deeply. Classic KHEs are infiltrative, ill-defined lesions composed of often coalescing nodules of spindled endothelial cells that form elongated slitlike lumina containing erythrocytes and curve around epithelioid nests enriched in pericytes surrounding entrapped platelet-rich microthrombi (**Fig. 12**A). There are also focal areas of more typical capillary formation (**Fig. 12**B). Lesional endothelial cells show infrequent, normally configured mitoses and are moderately plump, with eosinophilic to clear cytoplasm and bland nuclei. Hemosiderin deposition, red cell extravasation and fragmentation, and hyaline globules may be prominent. Dilated crescentic lymphatic vessels surround and intermingle with nodules, most prominently at margins of the lesion. Residual KHE lesions following successful medical treatment appear as dormant, often sclerotic, versions of the original disease process.

TAs, as originally described in the dermatology literature, are composed of discrete lobules of capillaries scattered within dermis and subcutis in a cannonball pattern. The

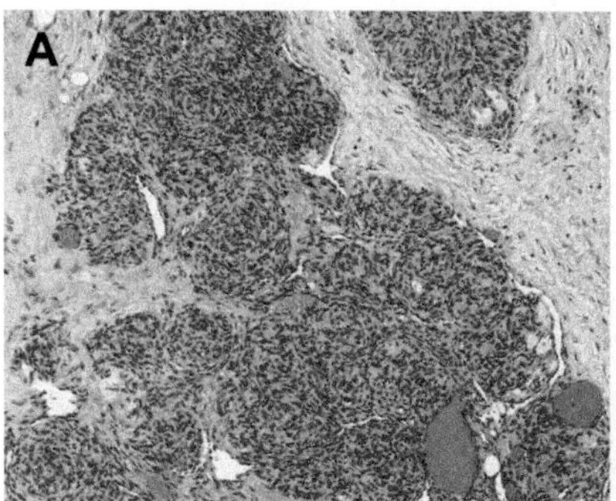


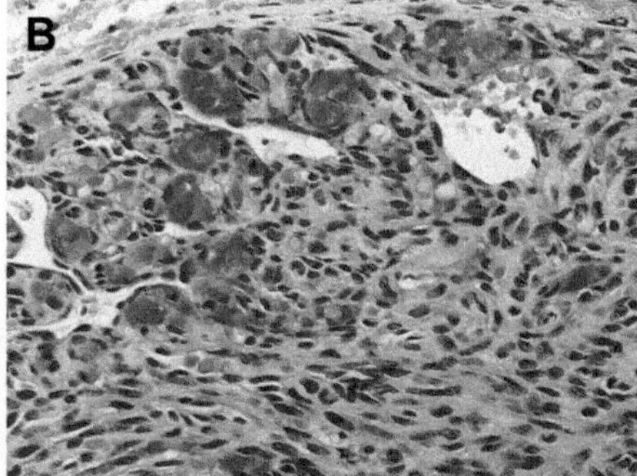


**Fig. 12.** KHE. (*A*) Infiltrative coalescing nodules of spindled endothelial cell fascicles curve around pericyte-rich epithelioid nests often containing a central platelet-rich microthrombus. (*B*) Some areas show more typically capillarylike formation.

intervening dermal stroma and subcutis may be normal but are often desmoplastic. The cannonball appearance is imparted by tightly packed tumoral capillaries, often bulging into peripheral crescentic, thin-walled vessels. Capillary pinpoint lumina may contain platelet microthrombi. Endothelial cells may be focally spindled but typically less prominently than in KHE; sweeping spindled cell fascicles and epithelioid nodules are absent.

By immunohistochemistry, spindled endothelial cells in classic KHE are positive for CD31 and CD34, variably weakly positive for vWF, and strongly positive for the lymphatic endothelial markers podoplanin, lymphatic vessel endothelial hyaluronan receptor-1 (LYVE-1), and prospero-related homeobox 1 (Prox1) (**Fig. 13**). They are negative for GLUT1. Endothelial cells of TA may focally be positive for podoplanin, LYVE-1, and Prox1, but less extensively than in KHE, seemingly correlated with the relative absence of endothelial spindling.[42] They, too, are negative for GLUT1 and other distinctive markers of IH. Platelet-rich microthrombi can be highlighted by immunostains for CD31 or CD61 (**Fig. 14**).

### *Pathogenesis*

The selective thrombocytopenia characteristic of KMP can be attributed at least in part to platelet trapping within KHE/TA vascular beds. Endothelial expression of lymphatic-associated antigens (Prox1 and LYVE-1) and the blood vascular marker CD34 displayed by KHE/TA supports the concept that these tumors, like Kaposi sarcoma and many angiosarcomas, have a partial lymphatic endothelial phenotype. This abnormal, mixed lymphatic-blood vascular phenotype may explain the observed propensity for platelet trapping because podoplanin is the natural ligand of C-type lectin-like receptor CLEC-2, a platelet-bound receptor.[45] Platelet transfusions, although sometimes clinically necessary, have in some cases worsened KMP, suggesting that platelet activation within the tumor may stimulate its vascular proliferation,[39] presumably through release of platelet-associated angiogenic agonists. A self-sustaining cycle of platelet trapping and tumor growth thus hypothetically may drive progression of these lesions and development of KMP. Human herpes virus 8 sequences, characteristically detected in Kaposi sarcoma, have not been identified in KHE or TA; neither has been linked to HIV infection.[41] No genetic causes or influences have been discovered.

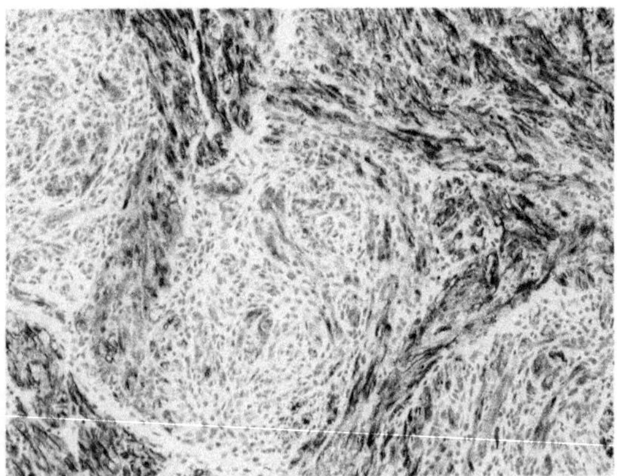

**Fig. 13.** KHE. The spindled endothelial cells are strongly positive for lymphatic endothelial markers such as podoplanin (shown) as well as LYVE-1, and PROX1.

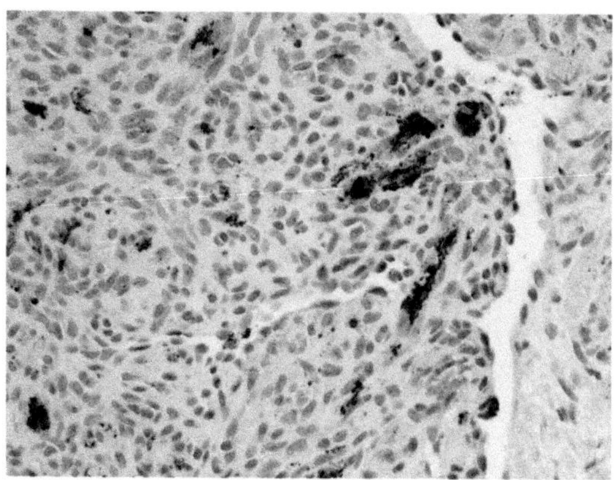

**Fig. 14.** KHE. CD61 immunostaining highlights abundant platelet trapping within the tumor.

## *Multifocal Lymphangioendotheliomatosis with Thrombocytopenia*

### *Clinical*

Multifocal lymphangioendotheliomatosis with thrombocytopenia (MLT) is a sporadic, newly described and still poorly understood, clinically and histologically distinctive vascular anomaly complicated by chronic mild to profound fluctuating thrombocytopenia and clinically significant gastrointestinal (GI) bleeding and/or pulmonary hemorrhage, particularly in infancy.[45] This entity has alternatively been termed congenital cutaneovisceral angiomatosis with thrombocytopenia.[46] It is not complicated by the more severe degree of thrombocytopenia seen in congenital KHE/TA. It occurs sporadically without clear racial or sexual predilection as multiple congenital vascular lesions, with appearance of new lesions, slow progression of individual lesion, and no evidence of regression. Lesions are widely distributed in the skin, often with hundreds present at birth, and in the viscera and GI system, lungs, liver, spleen, and kidney, and in some cases in bone, synovium, or muscle.[47] Skin lesions are flat or indurated, red-brown to burgundy, plaques or papules, often with central pallor or scaling, measuring up to a few centimeters in diameter. Clinically significant GI bleeding is near universally present, and may be life threatening in infancy. Partial GI resection may be required to control bleeding. Medical treatment options have been reported to be of possible value in some, but not all, cases.

### *Histology*

Lesions are composed of delicate vessels scattered throughout the tissue and lined by a monolayer of slightly hobnailed endothelial cells. Focally, endothelial cells line complex papillary projections that appear to float in the luminal plane of section (**Fig. 15**). Mitotic figures are rare to absent, although Ki-67 expression is positive in approximately 15% of cells. By immunohistochemical studies, lesional endothelial cells are strongly positive for CD31, CD34, and LYVE-1, with light to absent positivity for podoplanin; they are negative for GLUT1.

### *Pathogenesis*

The pathogenesis of MLT is unknown; whether it represents a multifocal tumor or a multifocal vascular malformation is debatable. Its abnormal endothelial phenotype, with coexpression of lymphatic and blood vascular markers, suggests possible

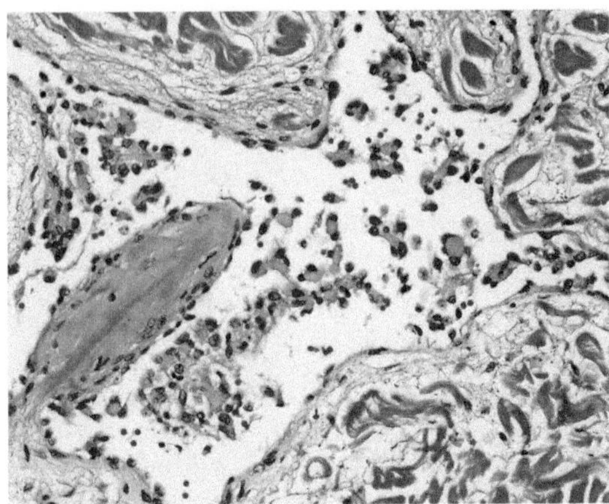

**Fig. 15.** MLT. Intraluminal endothelial-lined papillae appear to float in the plane of section.

linkage to the associated selective thrombocytopenia, analogous to the association between KHE/TA and KMP, but this remains purely speculative. Intuitively, it seems consistent with a multifocal vascular malformation syndrome. It is currently not included in the WHO soft tissue tumor classification[3] and is listed in the current ISSVA classification as a "provisionally unclassified vascular anomaly."[2]

## VASCULAR MALFORMATIONS

Vascular malformations, as congenital abnormalities in embryonic vascular morphogenesis, have limited postnatal endothelial mitotic activity. They are by definition present at birth (although may be hidden by deep location) and grow slowly and, in general, proportionately to the growth of the child. They persist throughout life in continued relative mitotic quiescence. Like vascular tumors, the malformations are a heterogeneous group of clinicopathologically distinct entities with diverse, increasingly unveiled causes.

Histopathologic distinction of vascular malformations from vascular tumors can at times be difficult, largely because the gross and microscopic appearances of vascular malformations tend to evolve postnatally and may include areas of vascular proliferation. Factors causing this evolution include progressive or intermittent vascular ectasia, recruitment of collateral vessels, thrombosis, hormonal modulation, infection, scarring, and reactive neovascularization in response to abnormal intralesional hemodynamics or tissue ischemia. Despite these challenges, vascular malformations can usually be recognized as such. Correlation with clinical and radiological information is always wise, and often essential.

Recent advances in the understanding of underlying pathogenetic mechanisms of several categories of familial and sporadic vascular malformations have empowered precise classification and development of more specifically targeted therapies. Vascular malformations may contain venous, capillary, lymphatic, or arterial components in any combination. Some forms are highly distinctive and easily recognized. Others are more diagnostically challenging. Accurate histopathologic diagnosis is often required to guide effective therapy and meaningful research, complementing clinical and radiological evaluation. The pathologist's task is not only to subclassify these lesions per constituent vessel types and presence or absence of increased endothelial mitotic activity but to confirm or dispute the clinical and radiological impression; recognize patterns indicative or suggestive of specific subtypes that may have known genetic associations or predictable clinical behaviors; assess (for blood vascular malformations) histologic evidence for stasis, high flow, or AV shunting; and advise the clinician regarding any indicated additional clinical laboratory and/or genetic testing. At a minimum, it can be helpful to indicate what the lesion is not, and what remains in the histologic differential.

The current ISSVA-sanctioned classification of vascular anomalies, also downloadable in an interactive form at www.issva.org, stratifies vascular malformations first as simple or combined.[2] The simple malformations include (1) capillary malformations (CMs), (2) lymphatic malformations (LMs), (3) venous malformations (VMs), and (4) arteriovenous malformations (AVMs), and congenital arteriovenous fistulas (AVFs). Subgroups to each of these groups are added, typically as genetic variants associated with specific types of lesions within each broader category become recognized. The combined malformations, not surprisingly, comprise various clinically relevant mixtures of 2 or more simple malformations, specifically of CM, LM, VM, or AVM. The ISSVA classification is an important resource for the field; – first, because it was formulated and approved by a large multidisciplinary group of specialists in vascular anomalies, and, second, because the current WHO classifications and most current textbooks do not yet adequately or accurately reflect the current state of knowledge and nosology in this field, certainly not for the malformations.

The key clinical features and current histopathologic diagnostic criteria for each of the major categories of vascular malformations (CM, VM, AVM, and LM) that affect the head and neck are summarized later. Histologic features of syndromic mixed VM-LM malformations and a short list of rare distinctive malformations with recently recognized genetic determinants are provided. Omitted from discussion are malformations of major named conducting vessels of the head and neck, as well as the telangiectasias.

### *Capillary/Venulocapillary Malformations*

The term CM encompasses several distinct clinicopathologic entities but still, in this era of heightened nosologic awareness, is used alone freely by pathologists and clinicians alike, often creating considerable confusion that reflects still limited understanding. Care must be taken to provide, whenever possible, appropriate modifications of this term in order to clearly convey which type of CM is intended. Clinicians often use the term to refer to any clinically evident cutaneous vascular discoloration or stain, a nonspecific phenomenon that can be associated with telangiectasias and AVMs, VMs, and LMs, with or without a true capillary malformative component. CMs (or often more properly venulocapillary malformations), as histologically well-characterized components, also occur as part of several complex syndromes, for many of which causative gene defects have recently been identified. The most common and well characterized of the capillary/venulocapillary malformations that affect the head and neck is the clinically and histologically distinctive cutaneous and sometimes deeper venulocapillary malformation known as facial port-wine stain (PWS), caused by GNAQ somatic mutation[48] and discussed at length later. This specific cutaneous vascular malformation, when combined with ipsilateral leptomeningeal and/or choroidal involvement, comprises Sturge-Weber syndrome.[49]

Other types of capillary/venulocapillary malformations not further discussed here include macrocephaly-CM syndrome,[50] diffuse CM with overgrowth,[51] and verrucous venulocapillary malformation (historically termed verrucous hemangioma, associated with MAP3K3 mutations, and typically involving the extremities).[52] Note that the current (2014) ISSVA classification of so-called CMs is still all-inclusive and clinically oriented, and without clear histologic grounds, including, for instance, true capillary/venulocapillary malformations such as PWS and Sturge-Weber syndrome, RASA1-mutation associated CM-AVM (micro-AVMs with cutaneous involvement imparting focal cutaneous staining without histologically documented CM), telangiectasias, cutis marmorata telangiectasia congenital, and nevus simplex (a likely functional disorder affecting local vascular flow). Rozas-Munoz and colleagues[53] recently sought to address this problem via a clinical classification scheme for vascular stains to help guide diagnosis and continuing management.

### *Cutaneous Capillary/Venulocapillary Malformations Caused by GNAQ Mutation (Port-wine Stains)*

#### *Clinical*

The focus here is on a sporadic, clinically distinctive, and well-recognized type of cutaneous venulocapillary malformation traditionally referred to by clinicians as port-wine stain (PWS). PWSs are congenital, nonproliferative, noninvoluting lesions but often become thickened, cobble-stoned, and grossly nodular over many years. Although primarily affecting dermis, some extend deeply into the subcutis. Generalized soft tissue and/or bone hypertrophy is common in affected areas and may be extreme (See Ho Yun Chung's article, "Capillary Malformations (Portwine Stains) of the Head and Neck: Natural History, Investigations, Laser, and Surgical Management", in this issue for further details). Gingival hypertrophy with subsequent dental abnormalities may also be present.[54] PWSs occur with equal sex predilection, in 0.3% of all newborns, and usually affect the head and neck region. Most are unilateral and segmental, but they may be bilateral and/or multisegmental. Those affecting the area innervated by the first branch of the trigeminal nerve (V1), especially when large or bilateral, are at risk for similar venulocapillary abnormalities and malformations of the ipsilateral leptomeninges of the brain and choroid of the eye, producing the neurocutaneous disorder known as Sturge-Weber syndrome.[55–57] Waelchli and colleagues[58] recently reported that the best predictor of Sturge-Weber syndrome is a PWS involving a line of vascular development of the face extending from the midline of the forehead to a line joining the outer canthus of the eye to the top of the ear and including the upper eyelid. Complications of Sturge-Weber syndrome are often significant, including seizures, glaucoma, cerebral atrophy and focal calcification, focal neurologic deficits, headaches, and cognitive difficulties.[59–62]

#### *Histology*

PWSs are composed of dilated vessels of mature capillary or venular type. Vascular ectasia may not become histologically evident until about 10 years of age, despite clinically obvious red skin discoloration at birth. Dermal vessels of venulocapillary size progressively acquire a rounded dilated contour and are filled with blood, lined by thin endothelia associated with pericytes and occasionally a few well-differentiated smooth muscle cells, with no evidence of increased mitotic activity (**Fig. 16**A). The vascular wall becomes thickened and fibrotic over time. With development of generalized soft tissue hypertrophy in the region of the cutaneous stain, vessels may develop loosely organized thick coats of plump smooth muscle fibers (**Fig. 16**B).[63] Cobble-stoning of the skin surface in adulthood is caused by progressive dermal vascular ectasia within a weakened collagen framework that begins superficially and extends to deeper vessels over time. Gross nodule formation, sometimes seen

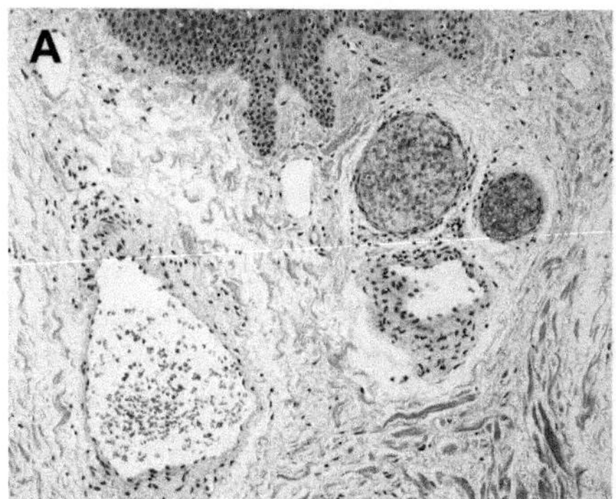


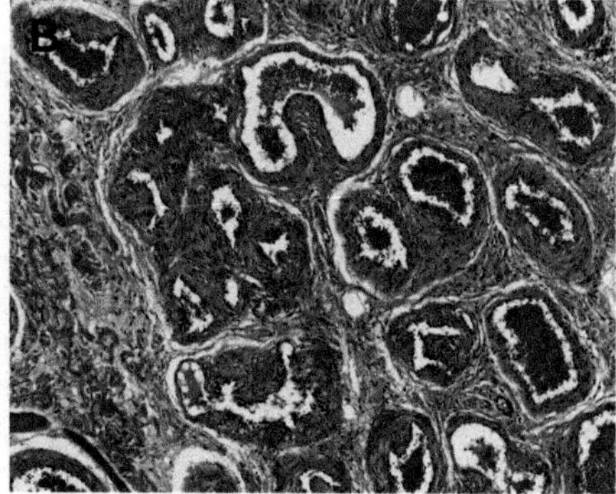


**Fig. 16.** Cutaneous PWS, caused by somatic GNAQ mutation. (*A*) Dermal vessels of venulocapillary size slowly dilate over years without evidence of increased mitotic activity and little, if any, well-differentiated mural smooth muscle. (*B*) Particularly in cases complicated by soft tissue hypertrophy, vessels may develop thick coats of unusually plump smooth muscle.

in older lesions, reflects focally exaggerated vascular ectasia and/or late development of complex epithelial, mesenchymal, and neural hamartomatous changes.[64]

The vascular malformations affecting the brain of patients with Sturge-Weber syndrome are largely manifest in the leptomeninges ipsilateral to an associated cutaneous facial PWS and have been less rigorously studied than their cutaneous counterparts. As in the skin, the predominant vessels are dilated capillaries and venules (**Fig. 17**). Occasional dilated vessels may also be seen focally within the underlying cortex, typically accompanied by multiple foci of calcification and other reactive changes presumably secondary to chronic seizure activity and altered blood flow.

***Pathogenesis***

Immunohistochemical evaluation of PWS for general endothelial and pericytic markers, basement membrane proteins, and fibronectin have not shown differences between normal skin and PWS.[65] Although controversy remains as to whether dermal vessels are increased in number in PWS compared with normal skin,[66,67] there is no clear evidence that lesional vessel numbers change with time. Studies using S-100

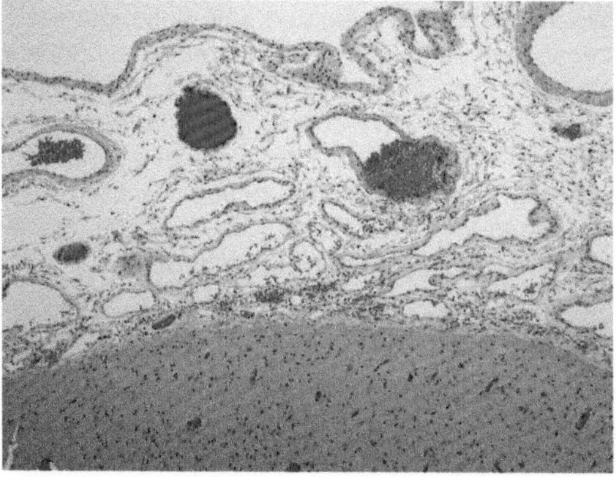

**Fig. 17.** Leptomeningeal venulocapillary malformation of Sturge-Weber syndrome (GNAQ mutation).

immunostaining have reported a decrease in perivascular nerve density in PWS, suggesting that the progressive vascular dilatation characteristic of these lesions may be influenced by inadequate innervation,[67,68] although this has not been confirmed by other studies. Observations of development of complex epithelial, mesenchymal, and neural hamartomatous changes in aged PWS have suggested genetically determined, multilineage developmental field defect in the pathogenesis of this lesion.[64] The strongly segmental pattern of PWS and Sturge-Weber syndrome has long suggested the probability of mosaicism caused by somatic mutation of otherwise lethal genes. Very recently, the causative somatic mutation of almost all cases of Sturge-Weber syndrome and nonsyndromic PWSs of the head and neck region was discovered: an activating nonsynonymous single nucleotide variant (c.548G→A, p.Arg183Gln) in the GNAQ gene.[48] Follow-up studies have confirmed this causative association and have also revealed rare linkages to somatic mutations at other nucleotides within the GNAQ gene sequence.[69] GNAQ encodes Gαq, a member of the q class of G-protein alpha subunits that mediates signals between G-protein–coupled receptors and downstream effectors.[48] Shirley and colleagues[48] also showed that the somatic mosaic GNAQ encoding p.Arg183Gln amino acid substitutions in skin and brain tissue from patients with the Sturge-Weber syndrome and in skin tissue with nonsyndromic PWSs activates downstream mitogen-activated protein kinase signaling. Activating mutations in genes encoding Gα subunits have previously been shown to be associated with several clinically important phenotypes, including the McCune-Albright syndrome,[70] blue nevi and nevi of Ota,[71] and uveal melanoma.[71]

Recently, somatic activating Gln209 mutations in GNAQ and GNA11 have specifically been associated with congenital nonprogressive hemangiomas (NICH and RICH).[38] It is reasonable to conclude that the phenotypic effects of activating somatic GNAQ mutations would be determined by the specific cell lineages harboring or indirectly affected by the mutation as well as by the timing of the mutation during development and the degree of gene activation.

## *Venous Malformations*

### *Clinical*

VMs are usually solitary lesions, localized or segmental, superficial or deep. Approximately 40% occur in the head and heck region.[72] Most are sporadic, but some occur in association with complex syndromes and some are familial and multiple. Combination with LMs is common. By MRI, VMs are slow-flow lesions, with low vascular resistance and bright hypersignal on T2-weighted spin-echo images. Superficial lesions enlarge over time because of venous pressure increased by dependency or exertion. Common complications include ulceration, bleeding, compression of adjacent structures, chronic low-grade consumptive coagulopathy in large/extensive lesions, and pain of unclear origin. In the head and neck region, these complications may severely affect speech, swallowing, and respiratory function. Clinical presentation and treatment options are described in (See Miikka Vikkula's article, "Venous Malformations of the Head and Neck", in this issue for further details).[73]

### *Histology*

Endothelia of VMs are flattened and mitotically inactive. The vessel walls have fragmented or no elastic internae and contain a variable number of well-differentiated, sometimes disorganized smooth muscle cells (usually scant relative to luminal diameter) (**Fig. 18**A). Vessels of capillary or venular proportions are usually also present within the lesion. Dilated lumina contain red blood cells and are often collapsed and undulating in tissue sections; luminal thrombi in various stages of organization, including calcified phleboliths, are often present, reflective of stasis (**Fig. 18**B). Presence of organizing thrombi helps distinguish these low-flow lesions from high-flow AVMs, which is often helpful in small biopsies. Recanalizing thrombi may show intravascular papillary endothelial hyperplasia (Masson lesion). In early lesions, endothelial sprouts extend into loosely fibrinous thrombus material, forming papillary fronds lined by a single layer of plump endothelial cells with no significant cytologic atypia. In later states, fibrin cores become collagenized and hyalinized and endothelia attenuate. Fusion of the papillary fronds results in an anastomosing meshwork of vessels, mimicking angiosarcoma, but without pleomorphism, necrosis, or high mitotic activity (**Fig. 19**).

***Pathogenesis***

Although most VMs occur sporadically, multiple mucocutaneous venous malformations (VMCMs) (OMIM [Online Mendelian Inheritance In Man] 600195) are inherited as an autosomal dominant trait linked to a locus (*VMCM1*) on chromosome 9p21 carrying germline activating missense mutation in the *TEK* gene that encodes the endothelial cell–specific tyrosine kinase receptor TIE2, which binds angiopoietin-1 and angiopoietin-2.[74,75] These mutations cause ligand-independent phosphorylation of the TIE2 receptor, resulting in aberrant downstream signaling.[76] Formation of a VMCM lesion requires a second-hit mutation in the second allele by somatic mutation, and an example of 1 such second hit has been identified.[77] This need for a second hit could explain why many inherited VMCM lesions appear in adolescence rather than at birth.

In more than half of inherited VMs, the TEK (TIE2) mutation is an Arg849 to tryptophan (R849W) substitution.[75,76] More recent studies have also identified somatic *TEK/TIE2* mutations in 85% of sporadic VMs, although in these cases the mutation (L914F) leads to substitution of a leucine to a phenylalanine, producing a stronger TIE2-hyperphosphorylation effect than the inherited R849W mutation of VMCM.[77,78] The L914F mutation of TIE2 in sporadic VM has not been identified in inherited cases, and is likely lethal in germline. Sporadic VMs are present at birth and are typically solitary; new lesions do not appear over time. In vitro studies have shown that the mutated TIE2 receptors of inherited and sporadic VMs

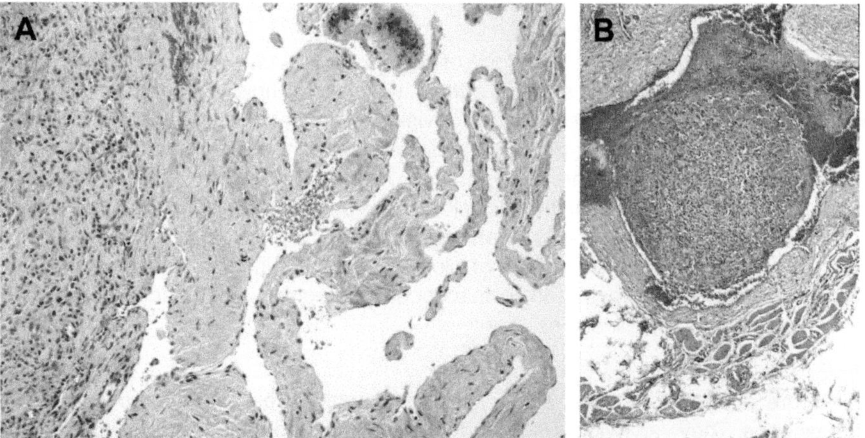


**Fig. 18.** VM. (*A*) Lesional veins have scant mural smooth muscle and are widely dilated or collapsed. (*B*) Because of stasis in the low-flow vessels, organizing luminal thrombi are frequently seen.

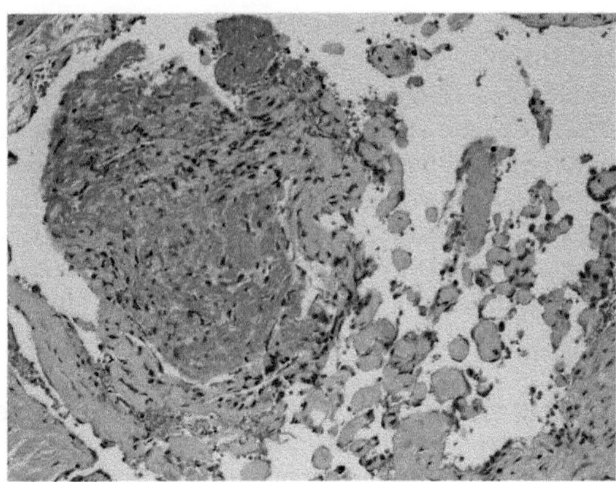

**Fig. 19.** Venous malformation, intravascular papillary endothelial hyperplasia (Masson lesion). Organizing, recanalizing thrombus may form complex papillary networks of stromal cores lined by endothelial cells.

upregulate Akt signaling and signal transducer and activator of transcription 1 (STAT1) phosphorylation and cause decreased platelet-derived growth factor-B (PDGFB) production and secretion.[79,80] Because PDGFB is an important recruiter of mural cells and a mesenchymal mitogen, this may explain in part why the smooth muscle coats of VMs are irregular and attenuated.[79]

Multiple VMs also occur in the poorly understood dysmorphic syndrome first described in 1958 by Bean[81] as blue rubber bleb nevus syndrome (BRBNS). BRBNS comprises an association between multiple VMs of skin and the GI tract, complicated by anemia from GI bleeding. Some cases are sporadic, others autosomal dominant. Somatic *TIE2* mutations have also been identified in most patients with BRBNS but differ from the causative mutations of VMCM and common sporadic VM in that they occur as double cis-mutations on the same TIE2/TEK allele (See Angela Queisser's article, "Etiology and Genetics of Congenital Vascular Lesions", in this issue for further details).[82]

### *Glomuvenous Malformations*

Lesions characterized by the presence of benign glomus cells historically have been subclassified into categories such as diffuse, solitary, multiple, solid, adult, and pediatric types. Current evidence supports division of these lesions into 2 major categories: (1) the glomus tumor proper, a cellular neoplasm usually occurring in adults that tends to be well circumscribed, solitary, and subungual; and (2) the so-called glomangioma, a frequently multifocal lesion, more properly termed glomuvenous malformation (GVM), which presents in infants or children. On histology, GVMs resemble VMs but with the addition of layers of glomus cells rimming the lesional veins. The following discussion is restricted to this second category, which accounts for 10% to 20% of all glomus cell lesions.

#### *Clinical*

GVMs are superficial lesions either present at birth or appearing in childhood or adolescence. They vary widely in phenotype from single punctate lesions to multiple, widely distributed to confluent, soft red to blue nodules to large pink to deep blue plaques. Although clinically resembling VMs to a degree, GVMs tend to be bluer and more nodular or cobble-stone–like in appearance, are less compressible, and do not swell with exercise or dependency.[83–85] There is no significant sex preponderance. Lesions typically thicken and become more blue over time. Although less painful than the glomus tumor, GVMs may be tender to palpation, with attacks of pain sometimes occurring during menstruation or pregnancy. All reported cases have behaved in a benign fashion. Laser surgery using $CO_2$, KTP, neodymium-doped yttrium aluminum garnet, and pulsed dye lasers may also be helpful.

#### *Histology*

GVMs consist of dilated, thin-walled veins in the dermis and subcutis, often distributed as discreet nodules. The component vessels histologically resemble those of VMs but are surrounded by 1 or more layers of cuboidal glomus cells (**Fig. 20**). The glomus cell component can be variable from region to region and vessel to vessel, making adequate sampling important to allow distinction from VMs. Like VMs without glomus cells, many GVMs contain organizing thrombi or phleboliths.

#### *Pathogenesis*

Some GVMs are sporadic and in this case are always present at birth. However, at least 68% of GVMs show an autosomal dominant pattern of inheritance.[86,87] The inherited forms tend to be multiple and continue to appear later in life.[88] Based on linkage disequilibrium studies of families with inherited GVM, a locus for GVM (termed GLMN) has been mapped to chromosome 1p21-p22 and codes for a protein of still uncertain function termed glomulin.[89–91] The wide phenotypic variation in GVM, and variability of penetrance in affected families, has suggested possible important genotype-phenotype relationships. A recent study by Brouillard and colleagues[92] of 162 families with GLMN mutation found 40 different mutations within the GLMN gene, the most frequent one of which is present in about 45% of the families, without specific genotype-phenotype correlation and with a penetrance of 90%.

The high but incomplete penetrance, frequent multifocality, and delayed development of autosomal dominant inherited GVM has suggested the likelihood of second-hit somatic mutations in the pathogenesis of GVM. Amyere and colleagues[93] investigated this possibility in a recent study of 28 cases of familial GVM and found 16 hits in 16 lesions, most of which were not intragenic but were incidences of acquired

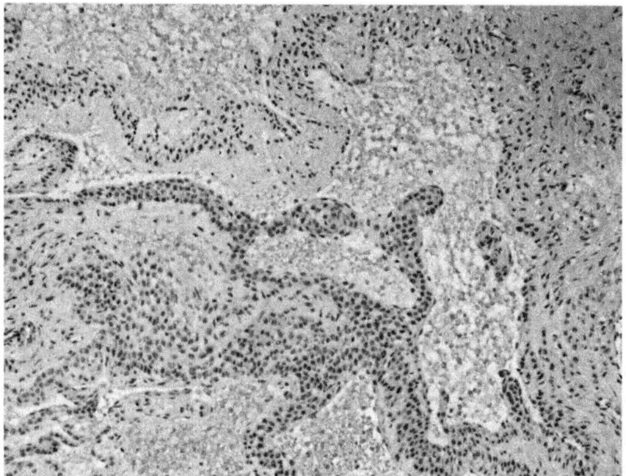

**Fig. 20.** Glomuvenous malformation. Component vessels are veins rimmed by 1 to several layers of bland, rounded glomus cells.

uniparental isodisomy with breakpoints at 1p13.1-1p12, leading to duplication of the germline GLMN mutation at 1p22.1 without causing quantitative loss at other genes. Thus, as with inherited VMCM, familial GVM is inherited in a paradominant fashion, requiring a second-hit somatic mutation for lesion development. It is assumed that somatic mutations in or affecting GLMN are the cause of sporadic cases of GVM.

The normal function of glomulin, also called FAP68, is still poorly understood. Pathways by which loss of glomulin/FAP68 function might affect GVM development are myriad and have recently been reviewed.[82] These possibilities include suggested glomulin interactions with hepatocyte growth factor and transforming growth factor beta (TGFβ) signaling pathways[94,95] and established binding of glomulin to the Rbx1 RING domain, leading to inhibition of the E3 ubiquitin ligase activity of the Cul1-RING1 ligase complex and thus affecting ubiquitination and degradation of various proteins such as cyclin E and c-Myc. Tron and colleagues[96] recently showed that glomulin deficiency is associated with increased levels of cyclin E and c-Myc. Knockout mouse studies have shown that glomulin is essential for the appropriate development and viability of the embryonic vasculature during vascular remodeling.[96] In the embryonic and adult mouse, glomulin is primarily expressed in vascular smooth muscle cells.[97]

## *Sporadic Arteriovenous Malformations*

### *Clinical*

Most AVMs occur sporadically as solitary lesions and may involve skin and subcutis, soft tissue, viscera, or bone. Roughly half are obvious at birth, whereas most others become evident during early childhood as clinically significant AV shunting develops. Deep or intracranial lesions may not be apparent until later childhood or adulthood, particularly if shunting is low grade. AVMs progress over time, usually beginning in adolescence,[98] as collateral arterial flow is increasingly recruited into the low-resistance vascular bed. Those with superficial extension may increase the skin temperature and produce a palpable thrill or pulsation caused by shunting. Common major complications include clinically significant, sometimes life-threatening, hemorrhage, and local tissue ischemia secondary to arterial steal. AVMs often recur aggressively if incompletely excised or inadequately embolized. See Gresham T. Richter's article, “Arteriovenous Malformations of the Head and Neck” in this issue for further clinical details and treatment options.

### *Histology*

Unlike AVFs, which are typically acquired lesions characterized by 1 or a few large AV shunts, sporadic AVMs are more complex developmental anomalies with potentially millions of small abnormal AV connections that bypass a normally controlled, high-resistance vascular bed. Microscopic features vary widely from one area to another in the same lesion and between different lesions. Most histologic sections show beds of arterioles, capillaries, and venules within a densely fibrous or fibromyxomatous background, intermixed with numerous larger-caliber arteries and thick-walled veins (**Figs. 21**A). In well-developed examples with high-grade shunting, the arteries are characteristically irregular in caliber and tortuous in contour, with thickened and fragmented mural elastic laminae. Component veins show changes reflective of increased local venous pressure and turbulence, including irregular intimal and adventitial fibrosis with irregularly thickened, focally fibrotic smooth muscle coats, often with intimal bumpers at points of venous tortuosity. AVMs early in their evolution or with inherently lower-grade shunting show more subtle findings. There is no evidence of thrombosis or intravascular papillary endothelial hyperplasia (which are typical of

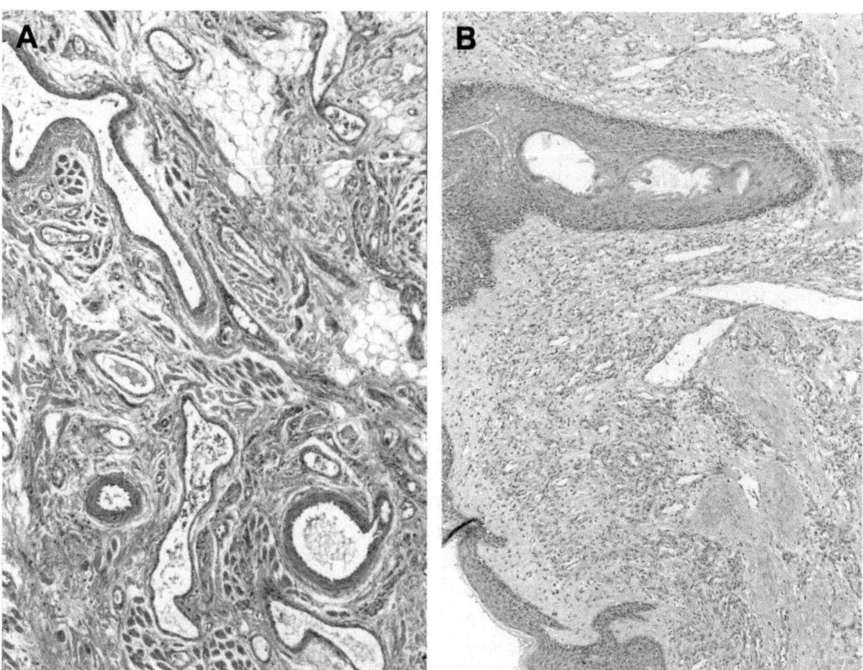


**Fig. 21.** Sporadic AVM, histology. (*A*) A complex combination of arterioles, capillaries, and venules are set within fibromyxoid stroma intermingled with larger, often tortuous, arteries and thick-walled veins with walls remodeled by high flow. (*B*) Involved skin may show a ragged small vessel proliferation that lacks the delicate lobularity of IH.

low-flow VM), consistent with the abnormally high venous flow and pressure of AVM. The AV shunts are difficult to impossible to find without extensive histologic sectioning or special techniques.

Small vessel collections are a diagnostically important and variably prominent, sometimes dominant component of AVM, varying widely in architecture between different lesions and within individual lesions. Many of these small vessel components are proliferatively active and enriched in plump capillaries that mimic, in some ways, a vascular tumor such as IH or pyogenic granuloma. To be clear, these proliferations are negative for GLUT1 and in no way consistent with IH.[16,18] Scattered among larger-caliber arterial and venous components, these cellular small vessel proliferations are particularly prominent in ulcerated skin overlying and/or involved by AVM, producing a ragged pseudokaposiform proliferation of small vessels that lack the delicate lobularity of IH (**Fig. 21**B). This cutaneous phenomenon has traditionally been termed Stewart-Bluefarb syndrome[99] and is probably caused, at least in part, by tissue ischemia caused by bypass of the normal capillary bed caused by shunting.

Small vessel–rich AVMs centered deep in skeletal muscle tend to have low-grade shunting and be more well circumscribed and therefore amenable to complete surgical resection compare to typical large vessel AVMs (**Fig. 22**).[100] The tongue is a common location of small vessel–rich AVMs in the head and neck region. The cellularity of these lesions and frequent presentation near puberty, likely under hormonal influence, has led to historical use of the term intramuscular hemangioma to describe them.

Although still controversially considered a vascular tumor by some clinicians, histologically these appear most consistent with a vascular malformation, and they are negative for GLUT1.[16–18,100]

### *Syndromic Arteriovenous Malformations*

Almost all AVMs are sporadically occurring single lesions of unknown cause.

Rare AVMs and other high-flow vascular lesions are associated with inherited syndromes and recently identified genetic defects. These conditions, which include capillary malformation-arteriovenous malformation (CM-AVM) and Parkes Weber syndrome,[101] PTEN hamartoma tumor syndrome (PHTS),[102] and hereditary hemorrhagic telangiectasia (HHT; Rendu-Osler-Weber syndrome),[103,104] overlap in histology with the much more common sporadic AVMs but show some distinctive features.

CM-AVM (OMIM 608354) is an inherited condition caused by germline RASA1 mutations and characterized clinically by multiple small cutaneous vascular stains associated with AVMs/AVFs.[101,105] The cutaneous stains of CM-AVM are small and both histologically and clinically unlike other more common cutaneous CMs. Grossly, they are often surrounded by a halo of pale skin and they increase in number with age. Biopsies of these are so rare that few pathologists, even those specializing in vascular anomalies, have seen more than a few. The histology has been described as minimally dilated capillaries in the dermis,[106] and as subtle dilatation of the superficial dermal microvasculature, with increase in small arteries and veins in the subcutis.[107] Given that these small cutaneous stains often show high flow on Doppler examination, it has been suggested that these are a manifestation of an underlying AVM and not of a CM.[106] The term CM-AVM is therefore a misnomer. The AVMs of CM-AVM are histologically similar to sporadic AVM (see **Fig. 23**), although less well documented. Reported examples have been located on the face or an extremity, intracranially, on intraspinally.[105]

Approximately a third of patients with CM-AVM with the cutaneous CMs and pathognomonic heterozygous germline RASA1 mutations of this disorder also have fast-flow vascular lesions, either AVMs or AVFs.[105] These patients include approximately one-half of those with Parkes Weber syndrome, a condition that combines AVM, cutaneous CM, limb overgrowth, and sometimes LM.[105] More than 100 different RASA1 mutations have been identified in 132 CM-AVM families.[101,105,108–110] Most of these reported mutations result in premature stop codons, likely causing loss of

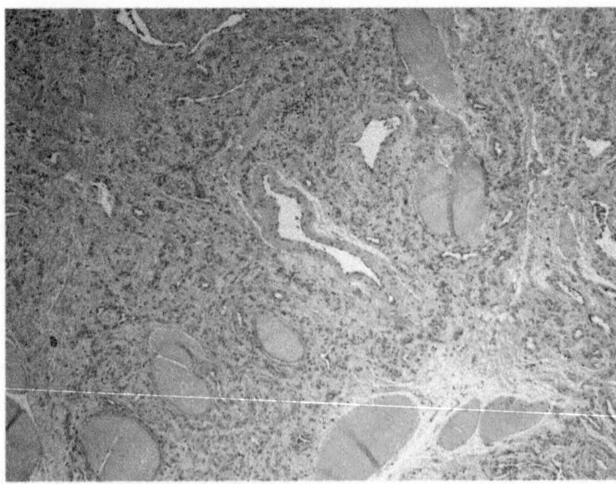

**Fig. 22.** Intramuscular small vessel–rich AVM.

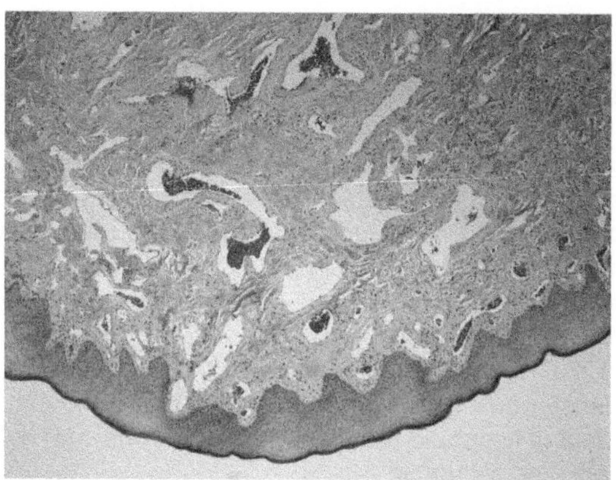

**Fig. 23.** AVM of CM-AVM, caused by RASA1 mutation.

function.[101,105] In approximately one-third of patients with phenotypic findings equivalent to CM-AVM, RASA1 mutation has not been detected by applied methodologies, and about 25% of cases are caused by de novo RASA1 mutations.[105]

Homozygous RASA1 knockout in mice is lethal at E9-9.5 because of severe vascular defects.[111] The multifocal nature and wide phenotypic variation of CM-AVM, with underlying germline RASA1 loss in 1 allele, could be explained by the need for a second-hit somatic mutation to complete local loss of RASA1 function, precipitating development of a focal vascular lesion. Evidence to support that possibility has been reported for 1 patient.[105] The specific mechanism by which RASA1 loss causes CM-AVM lesions is unclear. RASA1 codes for the small cytoplasmic molecule p120RasGAP, which negatively modulates the Ras signal transduction pathway by activating the Ras GTPase activity, thus helping convert Ras into its inactive ADP-bound form. Thus loss of RASA1 function through mutation would be expected to result in Ras signaling overactivity in response to stimulation by growth factors/hormones/cytokines that act through the Ras signaling pathway. Because the vascular lesions of CM-AVM are focal and likely require a second-hit mutation to cause lesion development, the timing of that second hit during vascular development, and the specific cell types that harbor the second hit, would be expected to be important variables in resultant phenotypic expression. RASA1 mutations have also been implicated in basal cell carcinoma,[112] and somatic mutations in RAS gene isoforms are frequent in cancer, but increased risk of malignancy in CM-AVM has not been observed.[105] Lymphatic abnormalities, in addition to CM-AVM, have been reported in human patients with germline RASA1 abnormities and in RASA1 knockout/knockin mice.[113,114] In mice, RASA1 maintains the lymphatic vasculature in a quiescent state.[115] Kawasaki and colleagues[116] presented evidence that RASA1 suppresses endothelial mTORC1 activity within the EPHB4 signaling pathway.

### *PTEN hamartoma tumor syndrome*

This uncommon autosomal dominant syndrome comprises a spectrum of inherited disorders, the best characterized of which are Bannayan-Riley-Ruvalcaba syndrome (BRRS) and Cowden syndrome, associated with germline mutations in the PTEN tumor suppressor gene on 10q23.3. BRRS (OMIM 153480) presents in childhood, most commonly as macrocephaly, developmental delay, penile lentigines, and benign lesions of primarily mesodermal origin, including historically poorly characterized vascular anomalies, primarily in soft tissue and skin but also in viscera, bone, and the central nervous system. These lesions most commonly affect the extremities, occasionally affect the head and neck, and rarely are congenitally evident. The vascular anomalies that arise in soft tissue as elements of PHTSs are histologically variable but often contain a high-flow component with characteristic and visually peculiar features, including clusters of bizarre, thick-walled veins with concentrically fibrotic, muscular walls, honeycomblike vascular complexes, tortuous small arteries, abundant fat and perivascular myxoid stroma, and hypertrophic nerves (**Fig. 24**). Kurek and colleagues[117] reported a distinctive soft tissue lesion highly associated with PHTS and termed it PTEN hamartoma of soft tissue, characterized by a peculiar overgrowth pattern of mingled soft tissue elements, including adipose tissue admixed variable combinations of dense and myxoid fibrous tissues, and abnormal blood vessels of various types with foci of lymphoid tissue, metaplastic bone, and hypertrophic nerves demonstrating onion-bulb formation.

The mechanisms by which germline PTEN mutations in PHTS produce vascular malformations is poorly understood. The tumor suppressor gene PTEN encodes for a dual-specificity phosphatase that antagonizes the phosphoinositol-3-kinase (PI3K)/Akt pathway, leading to G1 cell cycle arrest and/or apoptosis and also inhibits cell spreading via the focal adhesion kinase pathway.[118]

***Hereditary hemorrhagic telangiectasia***

Also known as Osler-Rendu-Weber syndrome, HHT is an autosomal dominant disorder characterized by multisystemic angiodysplasia leading to frequent epistaxis; telangiectasias; GI bleeding; and AV shunts in the liver, brain c Telangiectasia, and lung. It rarely becomes evident in infancy but more typically develops around the age of 12 years, as nasal bleeding. Clinical presentation and treatment options are focused upon by (See Thomas Kuhnel's article, "Hereditary Hemorrhagic Telangiectasia", in this issue for further details). The vascular lesions of HHT range from ectatic capillaries and venules in the skin and oral/nasal/GI mucosa to prominent AVMs and AVFs with dilated veins and arteries in the brain, liver, lung, and GI tract.[107] HHT has been linked to mutations in 2 genes and has therefore been designated HHT type 1 (HHT1: gene, *ENG*; chromosome 9q34.1) and HHT type 2 (HHT2: gene, *ACVRL1*, chromosome 12q11-q14).[119,120] HHT in association with juvenile polyposis has been linked to mutations in *SMAD4*.[121] ENG codes for endoglin, a coreceptor of the TGFβ family, whereas *ACVRL1* encodes ALK1, a type 1 receptor of the TGFβ

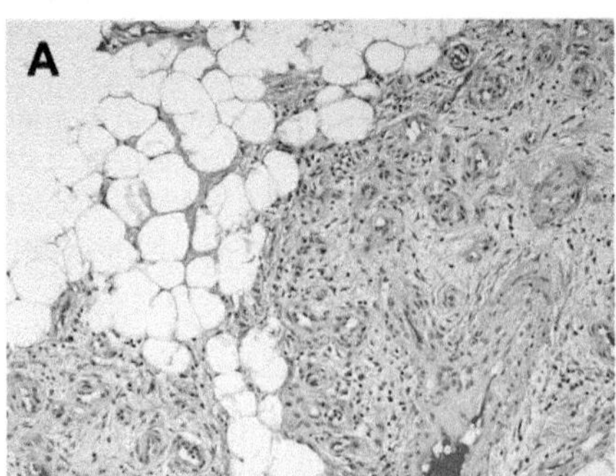


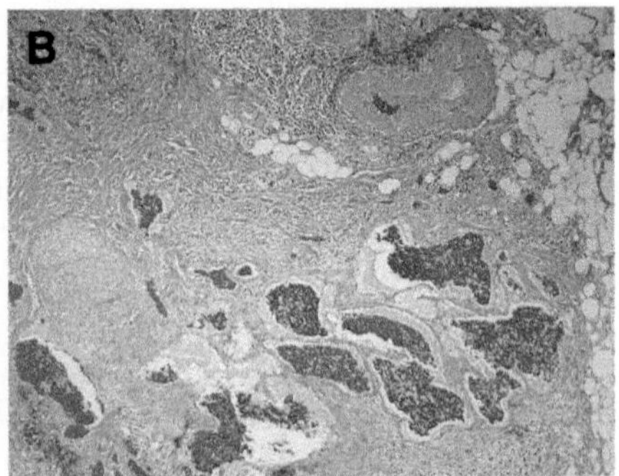


**Fig. 24.** PTEN-associated vascular hamartoma. Highly variable histology characteristically includes peculiar thick-walled veins with concentrically fibrotic walls and abundant perivascular myxoid stroma accompanying tortuous arteries (*A*). Other features include abundant fat and honeycomblike complexes of dilated thin-walled vessels (*B*).

family; SMAD4 encodes a transcription factor critical for TGFβ signaling.[122] Recently, bone morphogenetic protein (BMP) 9 loss of function mutations have been causally linked to a vascular anomaly syndrome with phenotypic overlap with HHT.[123] BMP9 and BMP10 are circulating growth factors of the TGFβ family that have been shown to bind directly with high affinity to ALK1 and endoglin; both are thought to help maintain endothelial cells in a quiescent state that depends on the level of ALK1/endoglin activation in endothelial cells. Tillet and Bailly[122] hypothesized that a deficient BMP9/BMP10/ALK1/endoglin pathway may lead to reactivation of angiogenesis or a greater sensitivity to an angiogenic stimulus, resulting in endothelial hyperproliferation and hypermigration that could lead to vasodilatation and generation of an AVM.

### *Lymphatic and Mixed Lymphatic-Venous Malformations*

#### *Clinical*

LMs have traditionally been referred to as lymphangiomas, despite general absence of significant endothelial mitotic activity. Just as blood vascular malformations are presumed to be developmental errors in morphogenesis of the blood vasculature, LMs are thought to be errors in morphogenesis of the lymphatic vascular system. Superficial LMs are usually evident at birth or within in the first year or two of life. In addition to the more common presentations in skin and subcutis, LMs may also involve deeper soft tissues, bone, or viscera and may not become evident until older childhood or later. They can be localized or regional and may diffusely involve many tissue planes or organ systems.

Historically, it has been found to be useful to subclassify LM as either macrocystic, microcystic, or combined. Macrocystic LM, defined arbitrarily by a cyst diameter of at least 2 cm, most commonly occurs in the loose connective tissue of the neck, axilla, chest wall, or groin and often changes in size because of progressive distention of the lymphatic spaces by lymph fluid. The microcystic pattern of LM is the most common and may develop anywhere lymphatic vessels occur. Microcystic and macrocystic patterns often coexist in individual lesions, both components often enlarging with systemic or local infection. Multimodal therapy including medical treatment, sclerotherapy, and surgery all play a role in management of LMs[124,125] and are described in Milton Waner's article, "Multidisciplinary Approach to the Management of Lymphatic Malformations of the Head and Neck", in this issue.

LMs are often associated with significant soft tissue (particularly fat) and bony overgrowth. LMs involving the superficial skin or mucosae typically form fragile, clear surface vesicles that may ulcerate, bleed, and become dark. Dermal or mucosal LMs often are associated with more deeply seated lesions composed of larger vessels, explaining the frequent recurrence of resected superficial lesions. Upper airway obstruction is a significant risk in LM involving the tongue or oropharynx. Chylous ascites/intestinal lymphangiectasia or pleural or pericardial effusions may complicate abdominal and thoracic LM.

Generalized lymphatic anomaly (GLA), historically termed lymphangiomatosis, is an extensive LM involving viscera and/or bone, often with coincident involvement of skin or soft tissues. Spleen, liver, lung, and intestine are commonly involved viscera. Clinical morbidity is high because of the lung involvement, effusions, and bone erosion and fracture.

The close relationship between the lymphatic and venous systems during embryonic development may explain why some low-flow malformations include both lymphatic and venous and/or capillary components. Lesions from patients with Klippel-Trénaunay syndrome (KTS) and related disorders most consistently exemplify this phenomenon, but solitary mixed malformations of lymphatic, venous, and capillary vessels are also commonly observed in nonsyndromic patients. KTS envelops a spectrum of complex, segmental congenital disorders characterized by a variable combination of lymphatic and capillary VMs associated with skeletal and adipose tissue overgrowth in the involved segment (See Jonathan A. Perkins's article "New Frontiers in Our Understanding of Lymphatic Malformations of the Head and Neck: Natural History and Basic Research", in this issue for further details).[7,126]

***Histology***

Primarily microcystic LMs are composed largely of dilated small vessels with angular to rounded contours lined by a monolayer of flattened to slightly hobnailed endothelial cells, rimmed by rare pericytes and little or no smooth muscle (**Fig. 25**A). These LMs contain clear fluid and sometimes a few lymphocytes and/or macrophages. Traumatized lymphatic vessels may contain abundant erythrocytes. In microcystic LMs involving skin or mucosa, the dilated lymphatic vessels often protrude into superficial vascular papillae, causing bleb formation and epidermal/mucosal hyperplasia. Overlying epidermis may appear hyperkeratotic and verrucous, and the surrounding stroma may be fibrotic and chronically or acutely inflamed. The vessels of diffusely infiltrative microcystic LMs tend to wrap extensively around tissue structures, producing the appearance of free-floating tissue elements and a complex anastomosing vasculature reminiscent of lymphangiosarcoma (**Fig. 25**B). Focal lymphoendothelial spindling and hyperplasia may be evident in some of the lesional vessels of these diffuse LMs, imparting a kaposiform appearance. A low but appreciable level of proliferative activity indicated by cell cycle markers such as Ki-67 may be present. Macrocystic vessels of LM tend to have thicker, irregular coats of smooth muscle and/or fibrous tissue and may have intraluminal valves. Vessel lumens usually contain proteinaceous material and a few lymphocytes and/or macrophages. Grossly dilated lymphatic channels may contain abundant blood or organizing myxoid thrombus material resulting from vessel wall injury or communication with the venous system, which

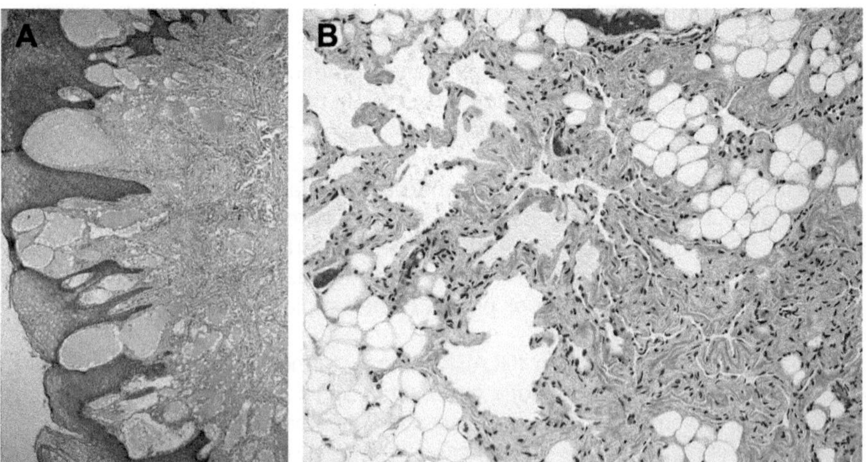


**Fig. 25.** LM, predominantly microcystic. (*A*) Component vessels are dilated and rounded to angular, filled with proteinaceous fluid and often a few lymphocytes and/or macrophages. Vessel walls are composed of flattened to slightly "hobnailed" endothelial cells associated with a few pericytes. (*B*) Some examples are more infiltrative, ramifying among and between tissue elements.

makes it difficult to distinguish veins from lymphatics and may suggest a venous or mixed VM-LM. This distinction can usually be made by immunoreaction for antigens such as podoplanin (with the D2-40 antibody) or PROX1 that are expressed by lymphatic endothelial, but not blood, vascular endothelial cells (**Fig. 26**). However, care must be taken in interpretation, because the attenuated endothelial cells of larger lymphatic vessels may show spotty or even absent staining for lymphatic endothelial markers. The surrounding stromata often show a lymphocytic infiltrate varying from a few scattered cells to striking, organoid aggregates containing lymphoid follicles.

Gorham-Stout disease, also called disappearing bone disease, is a form of GLA characterized by prominent, typically multifocal intraosseous LM. The affected bones undergo cystic cortical osteolysis, likely at least in part because of cortical remodeling caused by progressive dilatation by intraosseous lymphatic spaces. This process results in the apparent disappearance of bones in imaging studies, particularly plain film. On histology, dilated, extremely thin-walled lymphatic vessels that may be extremely difficult to appreciate in routine sections expand the marrow space, compressing against thinned cortical bone, sometimes thinned to the point of pathologic fracture. Immunohistochemistry for the panendothelial marker CD31 is useful to identify the endothelial lining of the cystically dilated spaces, and immunohistochemistry for podoplanin confirms lymphatic differentiation. In many patients with multifocal bony involvement by LM, viscera (especially spleen) is also affected by LM. Periosseous soft tissue extension is common. Rare cases of osteolysis with similar but localized clinical and radiological presentation may be associated with VM or AVF instead of LM.

Some spontaneously aborted fetuses with posterior cervical swellings traditionally referred to as cystic hygroma have been shown to have increased cutaneous lymphatics (eg, trisomy 13 and 21), whereas those with monosomy X (Turner syndrome) do not show increased or dilated lymphatics.[127]

The histology of KTS is generally typical of VM and LM, with variably distributed components of each. Overlying areas of cutaneous involvement compounded by reaction to expansion of dermal papillae by ectatic capillaries, venules, or lymphatics creates the clinical impression of a PWS-like surface stain punctuated by angiokeratomalike lesions. Eccrine glands are often notably enlarged and surrounded by expanded myxoid stroma. Veins may show striking mural smooth muscle disarray.

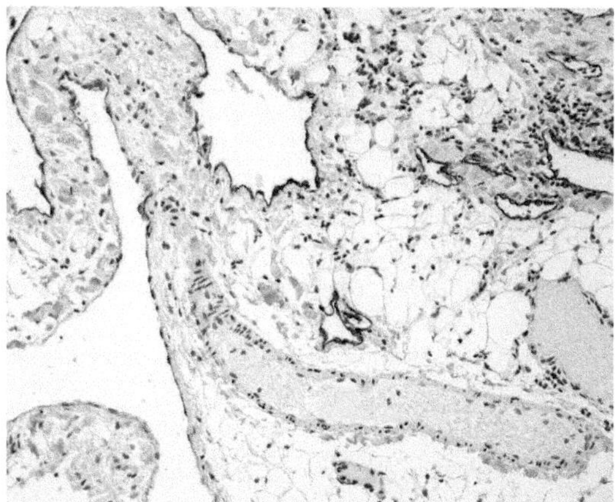

**Fig. 26.** Lymphatic malformation, podoplanin immunostaining. Endothelial immunopositivity for podoplanin is useful in distinguishing lymphatic from blood vascular vessels.

The malformations are largely cutaneous and subcutaneous but may also infiltrate deep skeletal muscle. Subcutaneous fat is increased.

***Pathogenesis***

Several malformative/overgrowth syndromes, including ones that often include LMs as a component, including CLOVES (Congenital Lipomatous asymmetric Overgrowth of the trunk with lymphatic, capillary, venous, and combined-type Vascular malformations, Epidermal naevi, Scoliosis/Skeletal and spinal anomalies, OMIM 612918) syndrome and KTS, have recently been linked to activating mutations in phosphatidylinositol-4,5-bisphosphate 3-kinase, catalytic subunit alpha (*PIK3CA*), which encodes the catalytic subunit of the enzyme PI3K.[128–131] Importantly, somatic *PIK3CA* mutations were also found in 16 out of 17 cases of isolated LM, occurring at low frequency (<10%) in the affected tissue, determined by highly sensitive droplet digital polymerase chain reaction for 5 common *PIK3CA* mutations.[128] This study did not include matched normal tissues (eg, blood) in the mutational analysis. Activating *PIK3CA* mutations also occur frequently in human cancer,[132] in which they enhance tumor growth in the setting of other oncogenic mutations.[133] It is not yet clear whether *PIK3CA* mutation alone can produce LM or whether additional genetic or environmental influences are necessary. Specific *PIK3CA* mutations have not correlated with the specific phenotype of the various disorders characterized by *PIK3CA* mutation.[128] As with somatic mutations in other genes and other groups of disorders, influential factors intuitively would include developmental stage at the time of somatic mutation, cell type and location within the embryo of the originally mutated cell, and pluripotent or multipotent potential of the mutated cell population.

## REFERENCES


1. Mulliken JB, Glowacki J. Hemangiomas and vascular malformations in infants and children: a classification based on endothelial characteristics. Plast Reconstr Surg 1982;69:412–22.
2. Wassef M, Blei F, Adams D, et al. Vascular anomalies classification: recommendations from the international society for the study of vascular anomalies. Pediatrics 2015. https://doi.org/10.1542/peds.2014-3673.
3. Fletcher CDM, Bridge JA, Hogendoorn PCW, et al. WHO classification of soft tissue tumours. In: Fletcher CDM, Unni KK, Mertens F, editors. WHO classification of tumours of soft tissue and bone. 4th edition. Lyon (France): IARC Press; 2013. p. 11.
4. Bowers RE, Graham EA, Thominson KM. The natural history of the strawberry nevus. Arch Dermatol 1960;82:667–70.
5. Powell TG, West CR, Pharoah PO, et al. Epidemiology of strawberry haemangioma in low birthweight infants. Br J Dermatol 1987;116:635–41.
6. Waner M, Suen JY. The natural history of hemangiomas. In: Waner M, Suen JY, editors. Hemangiomas and vascular malformations of the head and neck. New York: John Wiley-Liss; 1999. p. 13–45.
7. Mulliken JB, Fishman SJ, Burrows PE. Vascular anomalies. Curr Probl Surg 2000;37:519–84.
8. Huang SA, Tu HM, Harney JW, et al. Severe hypothyroidism caused by type 3 iodothyronine deiodinase in infantile hemangiomas. N Engl J Med 2000; 343(3):185–9.
9. Waner M, North PE, Scherer K, et al. The non-random distribution of facial hemangiomas. Arch Dermatol 2003;139:869–75.

10. Metry DW, Haggstrom AN, Drolet BA, et al. A prospective study of PHACE syndrome in infantile hemangiomas: demographic features, clinical findings, and complications. Am J Med Genet A 2006;140A:975–86.
11. Drolet BA, Dohil M, Golomb MR, et al. Early stroke and cerebral vasculopathy in children with facial hemangiomas and PHACE association. Pediatrics 2006; 117(3):959–64.
12. Iacobas I, Burrows PE, Frieden IJ, et al. LUMBAR: association between cutaneous infantile hemangiomas of the lower body and regional congenital anomalies. J Pediatr 2010;157(5):795–801.e1-7.
13. Leaute-Babreze C, Dumas de la Roque E, Hubiche T, et al. Propranolol for severe hemangiomas of infancy. N Engl J Med 2008;358(24):2649–51.
14. Drolet BA, Frommelt PC, Chamlin SL, et al. Initiation and use of propranolol for infantile hemangioma: report of a consensus conference. Pediatrics 2013; 131(1):128–40.
15. Mawn LA. Infantile hemangioma: treatment with surgery or steroids. Am Orthopt J 2013;63:6–13.
16. North PE, Waner M, Buckmiller L, et al. Vascular tumors of infancy and childhood: beyond capillary hemangioma. Cardiovasc Pathol 2006;15:303–17.
17. North PE. Vascular tumors and malformations of infancy and childhood. Pathol Case Rev 2008;13(6):213–35.
18. North PE, Waner M, Mizeracki A, et al. GLUT1: a newly discovered immunohistochemical marker for juvenile hemangiomas. Hum Pathol 2000;31:11–22.
19. North PE, Waner M, Mizeracki A, et al. A unique microvascular phenotype shared by juvenile hemangiomas and human placenta. Arch Dermatol 2001; 137:559–70.
20. Ritter MR, Dorrell MI, Edmonds J, et al. Insulin-like growth factor 2 and potential regulators of hemangioma growth and involution identified by large-scale expression analysis. Proc Natl Acad Sci U S A 2002;99:7455–60.
21. Blei F, Walter J, Orlow SJ, et al. Familial segregation of hemangiomas and vascular malformations as an autosomal dominant trait. Arch Dermatol 1998; 134:718–22.
22. Walter JW, Blei F, Anderson JL, et al. Genetic mapping of a novel familial form of infantile hemangioma. Am J Med Genet 1999;82:77–83.
23. Cheung DS, Warman ML, Mulliken JB. Hemangioma in twins. Ann Plast Surg 1997;38:269–74.
24. Barnes C, Huang S, Kaipainen A, et al. Evidence by molecular profiling for a placental origin of infantile hemangioma. Proc Natl Acad Sci U S A 2005;102: 19097–102.
25. Ritter MR, Butschek RA, Friedlander M, et al. Pathogenesis of infantile hemangioma: new molecular and cellular insights. Expert Rev Mol Med 2007;9:1–19.
26. North PE, Waner M, Brodsky MC. Are infantile hemangiomas of placental origin? Ophthalmology 2002;109:633–4.
27. Kleinman ME, Tepper OM, Capla JM, et al. Increased circulating AC133+ CD34+ endothelial progenitor cells in children with hemangioma. Lymphat Res Biol 2003;1(4):301–7.
28. Yu Y, Flint AF, Mulliken JB, et al. Endothelial progenitor cells in infantile hemangioma. Blood 2004;103(4):1373–5.
29. Khan ZA, Boscolo E, Picard A, et al. Multipotential stem cells recapitulate human infantile hemangioma in immunodeficient mice. J Clin Invest 2008;118(7): 2592–9.

30. Dadras SS, North PE, Bertoncini J, et al. Infantile hemangiomas are arrested in an early developmental vascular differentiation state. Mod Pathol 2004;17(9): 1068–79.
31. Jinnin M, Medici D, Park L, et al. Suppressed NFAT-dependent VEGFR1 expression and constitutive VEGFR2 signaling in infantile hemangioma. Nat Med 2008; 14(11):1236–46.
32. Munabi NC, Tan QK, Garzon MC, et al. Growth hormone induces recurrence of infantile hemangiomas after apparent involution: evidence of growth hormone receptors in infantile hemangioma. Pediatr Dermatol 2015;32(4):539–43.
33. North PE, Waner M, James CJ, et al. Congenital nonprogressive hemangioma: a distinct clinicopathological entity unlike infantile hemangioma. Arch Dermatol 2001;137:1607–20.
34. Enjolras O, Mulliken JB, Boon LM, et al. Noninvoluting congenital hemangioma: a rare cutaneous vascular anomaly. Plast Reconstr Surg 2001;107:1647–54.
35. Berenguer B, Mulliken JB, Enjolras O, et al. Rapidly involuting congenital hemangioma: clinical and histopathologic features. Pediatr Dev Pathol 2003;6: 495–510.
36. Nasseri E, Piram M, McCuaig CC, et al. Partially involuting congenital hemangiomas: a report of 8 cases and review of the literature. J Am Acad Dermatol 2014;70(1):75–9.
37. Gorincour G, Kokta V, Rypens F, et al. Imaging characteristics of two subtypes of congenital hemangiomas: rapidly involuting congenital hemangiomas and non-involuting congenital hemangiomas. Pediatr Radiol 2005;35(12):1178–85.
38. Ayturk UM, Couto JA, Hann S, et al. Somatic activating mutations in GNAQ and GNA11 are associated with congenital hemangioma. Am J Hum Genet 2016; 98(4):789–95.
39. Enjolras O, Wassef M, Mazoyer E, et al. Infants with Kasabach-Merritt syndrome do not have "true" hemangiomas. J Pediatr 1997;130:631–40.
40. Zukerberg LR, Nickoloff BJ, Weiss SW. Kaposiform hemangioendothelioma of infancy and childhood. An aggressive neoplasm associated with Kasabach-Merritt syndrome and lymphangiomatosis. Am J Surg Pathol 1993;17:321–8.
41. Lyons LL, North PE, Mac-Moune Lai F, et al. Kaposiform hemangioendothelioma: a study of 33 cases emphasizing its pathologic, immunophenotypic, and biologic uniqueness from juvenile hemangioma. Am J Surg Pathol 2004; 28(5):559–68.
42. Le Huu AR, Jokinen CH, Ruben BP, et al. Expression of Prox1, lymphatic endothelial nuclear transcription factor, in kaposiform hemangioendothelioma and tufted hemangioma. Am J Surg Pathol 2010;34(11):1563–73.
43. Fahrtash F, McCahon E, Arbuckle S. Successful treatment of kaposiform hemangioendothelioma and tufted angioma with vincristine. J Pediatr Hematol Oncol 2010;32:506–10.
44. Adams DM, Trenor CC, Hammill AM, et al. Efficacy and safety of sirolimus in the treatment of complicated vascular anomalies. Pediatrics 2016;137(2): e20153257.
45. North PE, Kahn T, Cordisco MR, et al. Multifocal lymphangioendotheliomatosis with thrombocytopenia: a newly recognized clinicopathological entity. Arch Dermatol 2004;140:599–606.
46. Prasad V, Fishman SJ, Mulliken JB, et al. Cutaneovisceral angiomatosis with thrombocytopenia. Pediatr Dev Pathol 2005;8:407–19.

47. Maronn M, Catrine K, North PE, et al. Expanding the phenotype of multifocal lymphangioendotheliomatosis with thrombocytopenia. Pediatr Blood Cancer 2009;52(4):531–4.
48. Shirley MD, Tang H, Gallione CJ, et al. Sturge-Weber syndrome and port-wine stains caused by somatic mutation in GNAQ. N Engl J Med 2013;368:1971–9.
49. Sudarsanam A, Ardern-Holmes SL. Sturge-Weber syndrome: from the past to the present. Eur J Paediatr Neurol 2014;18:257–66.
50. Wright DR, Frieden IJ, Orlow SJ, et al. The misnomer "macrocephaly-cutis marmorata telangiectatica congenital syndrome": report of 12 new cases and support for revising the name to macrocephaly-capillary malformations. Arch Dermatol 2009;145:287–93.
51. Lee MS, Liang MG, Mulliken JB. Diffuse capillary malformation with overgrowth: a clinical subtype of vascular anomalies with hypertrophy. J Am Acad Dermatol 2013;69(4):589–94.
52. Couto JA, Vivero MP, Kozakewich HP, et al. A somatic MAP3K3 mutation is associated with verrucous venous malformation. Am J Hum Genet 2015;96:480–6.
53. Rozas-Munoz E, Frieden IJ, Roe E, et al. Vascular stains: proposal for a clinical classification to improve diagnosis and management. Pediatr Dermatol 2016; 33(6):570–84.
54. Greene AK, Taber SF. Sturge-Weber syndrome: soft tissue and skeletal overgrowth. J Craniofac Surg 2009;20:1629–30.
55. Tallman B, Tan OT, Morelli JG, et al. Location of port-wine stains and the likelihood of ophthalmic and/or central nervous system complications. Pediatrics 1991;87:323–7.
56. Hennedige AA, Quaba AA, Al-Nakib K. Sturge-Weber syndrome and dermatomal facial port-wine stains: incidence, association with glaucoma, and pulsed tunable dye laser treatment effectiveness. Plast Reconstr Surg 2008;121: 1173–80.
57. Piram M, Lorette G, Sirinelli D, et al. Sturge-Weber syndrome in patients with facial port-wine stain. Pediatr Dermatol 2012;29:32–7.
58. Waelchli R, Aylett SE, Robinson K, et al. New vascular classification of port-wine stains: improving prediction of Sturge-Weber syndrome risk. Br J Dermatol 2014;171:861–7.
59. Comi AM. Advances in Sturge-Weber syndrome. Curr Opin Neurol 2006;19: 124–8.
60. Sujansky E, Conradi S. Sturge-Weber syndrome: age of onset of seizures and glaucoma and the prognosis for affected children. J Child Neurol 1995;10: 49–58.
61. Sujansky E. Outcome of Sturge-Weber syndrome in 52 adults. Am J Med Genet 1995;57:35–45.
62. Kossoff EH, Comi AM. Comorbidity of epilepsy and headache in patients with Sturge-Weber syndrome. J Child Neurol 2005;20:678–82.
63. North PE, Sanchez-Carpintero I, Mizeracki A, et al. The distinctive histology of lip enlargement in port-wine stains: a clinicopathological study. Lab Invest 2003; 83(1):96A.
64. Sanchez-Carpintero I, Mihm MC, Waner M, et al. Epithelial and mesenchymal hamartomatous changes in mature port-wine stains: morphological evidence for a multiple germ layer field defect. J Am Acad Dermatol 2004;50(4):606–12.
65. Finley JL, Clark RA, Colvin RB, et al. Immunofluorescent staining with antibodies to factor VIII, fibronectin, and collagenous basement membrane protein in normal human skin and port wine stains. Arch Dermatol 1982;118:971–5.

66. Barsky SH, Rosen S, Geer DE, et al. The nature and evolution of port wine stains: a computer-assisted study. J Invest Dermatol 1980;74:154–7.
67. Smoller BR, Rosen S. Port-wine stains. A disease of altered neural modulation of blood vessels? Arch Dermatol 1986;122:177–9.
68. Rydh M, Malm M, Jernbeck J, et al. Ectatic blood vessels in port-wine stains lack innervation: possible role in pathogenesis. Plast Reconstr Surg 1991;87: 419–22.
69. Couto JA, Huang L, Vivero MP, et al. Abstract 72: endothelial cells from capillary malformations are enriched for somatic GNAQ mutations and aberrantly express PDGFRβ. Plast Reconstr Surg 2015;135:56.
70. Weinstein LS, Shenker A, Gejman PV, et al. Activating mutations of the stimulatory G protein in the McCune-Albright syndrome. N Engl J Med 1991;325: 1688–95.
71. Van Raamsdonk CD, Bezrookove V, Green G, et al. Frequent somatic mutations of GNAQ in uveal melanoma and blue naevi. Nature 2009;457:599–602.
72. Zheng JW, Mai HM, Zhang L, et al. Guidelines for the treatment of head and neck venous malformations. Int J Clin Exp Med 2013;6(5):377–89.
73. Dubois J, Garel L. Imaging and therapeutic approach of hemangiomas and vascular malformations in the pediatric age group. Pediatr Radiol 1999;29: 879–93.
74. Calvert JT, Riney TJ, Kontos CD, et al. Allelic and locus heterogeneity in inherited venous malformations. Hum Mol Genet 1999;8:1279–89.
75. Vikkula M, Boon LM, Carraway KL 3rd, et al. Vascular dysmorphogenesis caused by an activating mutation in the receptor tyrosine kinase TIE2. Cell 1996;87:1181–90.
76. Wouters V, Limaye N, Uebelhoer M, et al. Hereditary cutaneomucosal venous malformations are caused by TIE2 mutations with widely variable hyperphosphorylating effects. Eur J Hum Genet 2010;18:414–20.
77. Limaye N, Wouters V, Uebelhoer M, et al. Somatic mutations in angiopoietin receptor gene TEK cause solitary and multiple sporadic venous malformations. Nat Genet 2009;41:118–24.
78. Soblet J, Limaye N, Uebelhoer M, et al. Variable somatic TIE2 mutations in half of sporadic venous malformations. Mol Syndromol 2013;4:179–83.
79. Uebelhoer M, Nätynki M, Kangas J, et al. Venous malformation–causative TIE2 mutations mediate an AKT-dependent decrease in PDGFB. Hum Mol Genet 2013;22:3438–48.
80. Hu HT, Huang YH, Chang YA, et al. Tie2-R849W mutant in venous malformations chronically activates a functional STAT1 to modulate gene expression. J Invest Dermatol 2008;128:2325–33.
81. Bean WB. Anomylous vascular spiders and related lesions of the skin. Springfield (IL): Charles C Thomas; 1958.
82. Nguyen H-L, Boon LM, Vikkula M. Genetics of vascular malformations. Semin Pediatr Surg 2014;23:221–6.
83. Mounayer C, Wassef M, Enjolras O, et al. Facial 'glomangiomas': large facial venous malformations with glomus cells. J Am Acad Dermatol 2001;45:239–45.
84. Gould EW, Manivel JC, Albores-Saavedra J, et al. Locally infiltrative glomus tumors and glomangiosarcomas. A clinical, ultrastructural, and immunohistochemical study. Cancer 1990;65:310–8.
85. Yang JS, Ko JW, Suh KS, et al. Congenital multiple plaque-like glomangiomyoma. Am J Dermatopathol 1999;21:454–7.

86. Rycroft RJ, Menter MA, Sharvill DE, et al. Hereditary multiple glomus tumours. Report of four families and a review of literature. Trans St Johns Hosp Dermatol Soc 1975;61:70–81.
87. Wood WS, Dimmick JE. Multiple infiltrating glomus tumors in children. Cancer 1977;40:1680–5.
88. Boon LM, Mulliken JB, Enjolras O, et al. Glomulovenous malformation (glomangioma) and venous malformation: distinct clinicopathologic and genetic entities. Arch Dermatol 2004;140:971–6.
89. Irrthum A, Brouillard P, Enjolras O, et al. Linkage disequilibrium narrows locus for venous malformation with glomus cells (VMGLOM) to a single 1.48 Mbp YAC. Eur J Hum Genet 2001;9:34–8.
90. Brouillard P, Olsen BR, Vikkula M. High-resolution physical and transcript map of the locus for venous malformations with glomus cells (VMGLOM) on chromosome 1p21-p22. Genomics 2000;67:96–101.
91. Brouillard P, Boon LM, Vikkula M. Mutations in a novel factor, glomulin, are responsible for glomuvenous malformations ("glomangiomas"). Am J Hum Genet 2002;70:866–74.
92. Brouillard P, Boon LM, Revencu N, et al, GVM Study Group. Genotypes and phenotypes of 162 families with a glomulin mutation. Mol Syndromol 2013;4: 157–64.
93. Amyere M, Aerts V, Brouillard P, et al. Somatic uniparental isodisomy explains multifocality of glomuvenous malformations. Am J Hum Genet 2013;92:188–96.
94. Grisendi S, Chambraud B, Gout I, et al. Ligand-regulated binding of FAP68 to the hepatocyte growth factor receptor. J Biol Chem 2001;276:46632–8.
95. Chambraud B, Radanyi C, Camonis JH, et al. FAP48, a new protein that forms specific complexes with both immunophilins FKBP59 and FKBP12: prevention by the immunosuppressant drugs FK506 and rapamycin. J Biol Chem 1996; 271:32923–9.
96. Tron AE, Arai T, Duda DM, et al. The glomuvenous malformation protein glomulin binds Rbx1 and regulates cullin RING ligase-mediated turnover of Fbw7. Mol Cell 2012;46:67–78.
97. McIntyre BA, Brouillard P, Aerts V, et al. Glomulin is predominantly expressed in vascular smooth muscle cells in the embryonic and adult mouse. Gene Expr Patterns 2004;4:351–8.
98. Enjolras O, Logeart I, Gelbert F, et al. Arteriovenous malformations: a study of 200 cases. Ann Dermatol Venereol 1999;127:17–22.
99. Bluefarb SM, Adams LA. Arteriovenous malformation with angiodermatitis. Stasis dermatitis simulating Kaposi's disease. Arch Dermatol 1967;96:176–81.
100. Richter G, North PE, Suen JY, et al. Arteriovenous malformations of the tongue: a spectrum of disease. Laryngoscope 2007;117(2):328–35.
101. Eerola I, Boon LM, Mulliken JB, et al. Capillary malformation–arteriovenous malformation, a new clinical and genetic disorder caused by RASA1 mutations. Am J Hum Genet 2003;73:1240–9.
102. Piccione M, Fragapane T, Antona V, et al. PTEN hamartoma tumor syndromes in childhood: description of two cases and a proposal for follow-up protocol. Am J Med Genet A 2013;161A(11):2902–8.
103. Guttmacher AE, Marchuk DA, White RI. Hereditary hemorrhagic telangiectasia. N Engl J Med 1995;333:918–24.
104. Abdalla SA, Letarte M. Hereditary haemorrhagic telangiectasia: current views on genetics and mechanisms of disease. J Med Genet 2006;43:97–110.

105. Revencu N, Boon LM, Mendola A, et al. RASA1 mutations and associated phenotypes in 68 families with capillary malformation-arteriovenous malformation. Hum Mutat 2013;34:1632–41.
106. Kim C, Ko CJ, Baker KE, et al. Histopathologic and ultrasound characteristics of cutaneous capillary malformations in a patient with capillary malformation-arteriovenous malformation syndrome. Pediatr Dermatol 2015;32:128–31.
107. Kozakewich HPW, Mulliken JB. Histopathology of vascular malformations. In: Mulliken JB, Burrows PE, Fishman SJ, editors. Mulliken & Young's vascular anomalies: hemangiomas and malformations. 2nd edition. Canada: Oxford University Press; 2013. p. 488, 500–1.
108. Hershkovitz D, Bercovich D, Sprecher E, et al. RASA1 mutations may cause hereditary capillary malformations without arteriovenous malformations. Br J Dermatol 2008;158:1035–40.
109. Thiex R, Mulliken JB, Revencu N, et al. A novel association between RASA1 mutations and spinal arteriovenous anomalies. AJNR Am J Neuroradiol 2010;31: 775–9.
110. Wooderchak-Donahue W, Stevenson DA, McDonald J, et al. RASA1 analysis: clinical and molecular findings in a series of consecutive cases. Eur J Med Genet 2012;55:91–5.
111. Henkemeyer M, Rossi DJ, Holmyard DP, et al. Vascular system defects and neuronal apoptosis in mice lacking ras GTPase-activating protein. Nature 1995;377:695–701.
112. Friedman E, Gejman PV, Martin GA, et al. Nonsense mutations in the C-terminal SH2 region of the GTPase activating protein (GAP) gene in human tumours. Nat Genet 1993;5:242–7.
113. Burrows PE, Gonzalez-Garay ML, Rasmussen JC, et al. Lymphatic abnormalities are associated with RASA1 gene mutations in mouse and man. Proc Natl Acad Sci U S A 2013;110:8621–6.
114. Lubeck BA, Lapinski PE, Bauler TJ, et al. Blood vascular abnormalities in Rasa1(R780Q) knockin mice: implications for the pathogenesis of capillary malformation-arteriovenous malformation. Am J Pathol 2014;184:3163–9.
115. Lapinski PE, Kwon S, Lubeck BA, et al. RASA1 maintains the lymphatic vasculature in a quiescent functional state in mice. J Clin Invest 2012;122:733–47.
116. Kawasaki J, Aegerter S, Fevurly RD, et al. RASA1 functions in EPHB4 signaling pathway to suppress endothelial mTORC1 activity. J Clin Invest 2014;124: 2774–84.
117. Kurek KC, Howard E, Tenant L, et al. PTEN hamartoma of soft tissue: a distinctive lesion in PTEN syndromes. Am J Surg Pathol 2012;36(5):671–87.
118. Sansal I, Sellers WR. The biology and clinical relevance of the PTEN tumor suppressor pathway. J Clin Oncol 2004;22:2954–63.
119. McAllister KA, Grogg KM, Johnson DW, et al. Endoglin, a TGF-beta binding protein of endothelial cells, is the gene for hereditary haemorrhagic telangiectasia type 1. Nat Genet 1994;8:345–51.
120. Johnson DW, Berg JN, Baldwin MA, et al. Mutations in the activin receptor-like kinase 1 gene in hereditary haemorrhagic telangiectasia type 2. Nat Genet 1996;13:189–95.
121. Gallione CJ, Repetto GM, Legius E, et al. A combined syndrome of juvenile polyposis and hereditary haemorrhagic telangiectasia associated with mutations in MADH4 32. (SMAD4). Lancet 2004;363(9412):852–9.
122. Tillet E, Bailly S. Emerging roles of BMP9 and BMP10 in hereditary hemorrhagic telangiectasia. Front Genet 2015;8(5):456.

123. Wooderchak-Donahue WL, McDonald J, O'Fallon B, et al. BMP9 mutations cause a vascular-anomaly syndrome with phenotypic overlap with hereditary hemorrhagic telangiectasia. Am J Hum Genet 2013;5(93):530–7.
124. Brewis C, Pracy JP, Albert DM. Treatment of lymphangiomas of the head and neck in children by intralesional injection of OK-432 (Picibanil). Clin Otolaryngol 2000;25:130–5.
125. Molitch HI, Unger EC, White EL, et al. Percutaneous sclerotherapy of lymphangiomas. Radiology 1995;194:343–7.
126. Esterly NB. Cutaneous hemangiomas, vascular stains and malformations, and associated syndromes [review]. Curr Probl Pediatr 1996;26(1):3–39.
127. Chitayat D, Kalousek DK, Bamforth JS, et al. Lymphatic abnormalities in fetuses with posterior cervical cystic hydroma. Am J Med Genet 1989;33:352–6, 207.
128. Luks VL, Kamitaki N, Vivero MP, et al. Malformative/overgrowth disorders are caused by somatic mutations in PIK3CA. J Pediatr 2015;166(4):1048–54.
129. Kurek KC, Luks VL, Ayturk UM, et al. Somatic activating mutations in PIK3CA cause CLOVES syndrome. Am J Hum Genet 2012;90:1108–15.
130. Lee JH, Huynh M, Silhavy JL, et al. De novo somatic mutations in components of the PI3K-AKT3-mTOR pathway cause hemimegalencephaly. Nat Genet 2012; 44:941–5.
131. Maclellan RA, Luks VL, Vivero MP, et al. PIK3CA activating mutations in facial infiltrating lipomatosis. Plast Reconstr Surg 2014;133:12e–9e.
132. Samuels Y, Wang Z, Bardelli A, et al. High frequency of mutations of the PIK3CA gene in human cancers. Science 2004;304:554.
133. Kinross KM, Montgomery KG, Kleinschmidt M, et al. An activating Pik3ca mutation coupled with Pten loss is sufficient to initiate ovarian tumorigenesis in mice. J Clin Invest 2012;122:553–7.

# Etiology and Genetics of Congenital Vascular Lesions

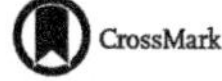

Angela Queisser, PhD[a], Laurence M. Boon, MD, PhD[a,b], Miikka Vikkula, MD, PhD[a,*]

**KEYWORDS**

- Malformation • Vascular • Gene • Mutation • Signaling pathway • Inhibitor
- Rapamycin

**KEY POINTS**

- Therapeutic options to treat vascular tumors and malformations are limited. Detection of genetic mutations, inherited or somatic, has opened up the field for understanding the underlying molecular mechanisms.
- RAS/MAPK/ERK signaling is increased because of mutations in *GNAQ* and *GNA11* in congenital hemangiomas and capillary malformation (CM), in *GNAQ*, *KRAS* and *BRAF* in pyogenic granuloma (PG), in *RASA1* in CM-AVM1, in *EPHB4* in CM-AVM2, in *KRIT1* in HCCVM, and in *MAP3K3* in verrucous venous malformations.
- PI3K/AKT/mTOR pathway is increased in hereditary hemorrhagic telangiectasia (HHT) with mutations in *BMP9/10*, *ALK1*, and *endoglin*, in sporadic venous malformations (VM and MVM), and blue rubber bleb nevus syndrome (BRBN), inherited cutaneomucosal venous malformations (VMCM), all with mutations in *TIE2*, and in sporadic VM and lymphatic malformations (LM) with mutations in *PIK3CA*.
- Increased hepatocyte growth factor/c-Met and TGF-ß signaling may occur in glomuvenous malformations (GVM) with mutations in *glomulin*.
- VEGFR1 expression is decreased and VEGF-A/VEGFR2 signaling is increased in infantile hemangioma (IH) with mutations in *TEM8* and *VEGFR2*.

## INTRODUCTION

Lesions of the vascular system are the most common congenital and neonatal abnormalities.[1] Vascular malformations of the head and neck region constitute approximately 60% of the lesions and occur approximately in 1 out of 22 children.[2]

---

Disclosure: The authors have nothing they wish to disclose.
[a] Human Molecular Genetics, de Duve Institute, University of Louvain, Avenue Hippocrate 74 (+5), Brussels B-1200, Belgium; [b] Division of Plastic Surgery, Center for Vascular Anomalies, Cliniques Universitaires St Luc, Avenue Hippocrate 10, B-1200 Brussels, Belgium
* Corresponding author. Human Molecular Genetics, de Duve Institute, University of Louvain, Avenue Hippocrate 74 (+5), bte B1.74.06, Brussels B-1200, Belgium.
*E-mail address:* miikka.vikkula@uclouvain.be

Otolaryngol Clin N Am 51 (2018) 41–53
https://doi.org/10.1016/j.otc.2017.09.006

Mulliken and Glowacki[3] laid out the foundation for a clear classification based on physical findings, clinical behavior, and cellular kinetics. Vascular anomalies are separated into two major categories: vascular tumors (mainly hemangiomas [congenital and infantile] and other vascular tumors) and vascular malformations (named according to the affected type of vessel: capillary, venous, lymphatic, arteriovenous, and mixed malformations).[3] Most types are known to be caused by inherited and/or somatic mutations. It is hoped that further studies on cellular effects of the mutations will lead to a better understanding of the underlying pathophysiology enabling development of novel treatments.

## VASCULAR TUMORS

### *Etiology and Genetics of Hemangiomas*

#### *Congenital hemangioma*

Congenital hemangiomas are rare lesions, and fully formed at birth.[2,4] There are three types: (1) rapidly involuting (RICH), (2) partially involuting, and (3) noninvoluting congenital hemangioma (NICH).[5] They do not express the glucose transporter-1 protein (GLUT1).[2]

Mutually exclusive, mosaic missense mutations in *GNAQ* and *GNA11* at position glutamine 209 (Gln209) have been identified.[6,7] *GNAQ* encodes the guanine nucleotide binding protein G(q) alpha, a subunit within a complex that hydrolyzes GTP to GDP.[6] The same somatic mutations have been reported in more than 80% of uveal melanomas.[8] In them, Gln209 missense mutations activate GTP-dependent signaling leading to constitutive activation of MAPK and/or YAP signaling.[6] These pathways may also be involved in RICH and NICH (**Fig. 1**).

#### *Pyogenic granuloma*

Pyogenic granuloma (PG) is a common benign vascular neoplasm and its occurrence within a capillary malformation (CM; see later) is a well-recognized event.[1,9] In such secondary PGs, a somatic GNAQ p.Arg183Gln mutation is present, reflecting an origin from cells of the underlying CM.[9] Moreover, 8 out of 10 secondary PGs have a BRAF p.Val600Glu somatic mutation and 1 out of 10 an NRAS p.Gln61Arg mutation. In contrast, in isolated PG, BRAF p.Val600Glu (in 3 of 25 cases) or p.Gly464Glu mutations or KRAS p.Gly13Arg (in 1 of 25) mutations were detected.[9] Therefore, it is speculated that the BRAF p.Val600Glu mutation is a driver event in isolated PGs, and a second-hit on a GNAQ p.Arg183Gln mutated CM-background in secondary PG.[9] Furthermore, mutations in *HRAS*, also identified in patients with colon cancer, play a role in PG (p.Q61R, p.E49K, Q61R, and p.G13S).[10] In summary, upregulated RAS/MAPK signaling seems to be the key mechanism (see **Fig. 1**, **Box 1**).

#### *Infantile hemangioma*

Infantile hemangioma (IH) ensues from endothelial cell (EC) hyperplasia. The cause of the aberrant EC proliferation remains unknown.[11] There are two theories: involvement of embolic placental angioblasts based on sharing of placental markers, such as GLUT1, Lewis Y antigen, and merosin; and Fcγ receptor II, with hemangiomas.[12] The embryonic endothelial precursor theory is based on detection of $CD133^+$/$CD34^+$ circulating progenitor and stem cells in hemangiomas and blood circulation of patients with hemangioma.[13] Moreover, injection of such “hemangioma stem cells” into nude mice led to development of hemangioma-like lesions.[14]

Vascular endothelial growth factor (VEGF)-A signaling seems to be a key in IH because changes in VEGF-A signaling pathway in hemangioma ECs leads to the formation of IH.[15] Sequencing 24 genes involved in EC proliferation, migration, adhesion, or

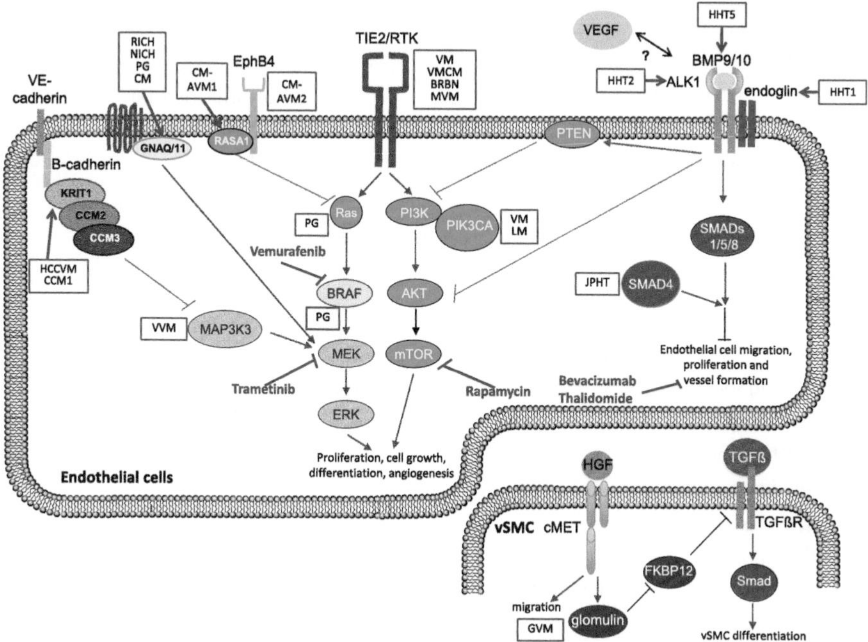


**Fig. 1.** Mutations and signaling pathways involved in vascular diseases and vascular tumors and hypothetical treatment options. Mutations in *GNAQ/GNA11*, *RASA1*, *EPHB4*, *MAP3K3*, and *KRIT1* lead to constitutive activation of RAS/MEK/ERK signaling. Mutations in *TIE2* and mutations in *ALK1*, *BMP9*, and *endoglin* lead to permanent activation of PI3K/AKT/mTOR pathway. In GVM, loss of glomulin may lead to the inhibition of TGF-ß signaling and thus to abnormal differentiated vSMCs. AVM, arteriovenous malformations; BMP, bone morphogenetic protein; BRBN, blue rubber bleb nevus syndrome; CCM, cerebral cavernous malformation; CM, capillary malformation; GVM, glomuvenous malformations; HCCVM, hyperkeratotic cutaneous capillary venous malformation; HGF,hepatocyte growth factor; HHT, hereditary hemorrhagic telangiectasia; JPHT, juvenile polyposis/HHT syndrome; LM, lymphatic malformation; MVM, multifocal venous malformation; TGF, transforming growth factor; VEGF, vascular endothelial growth factor; VM, venous malformation; VMCM, cutaneomucosal venous malformations; vSMC, vascular smooth muscle cells; VVM, verrucous venous malformations.

regulation of VEGF-A expression identified germ-line "risk-factor" variants in *integrin-like molecule tumor endothelial marker-8* (*TEM8*) and in *VEGFR2*.[15] The variant identified in *TEM8* may act in a dominant-negative fashion, whereas the variant in *VEGFR2* acts as a loss-of-function change.[15] Mutated TEM8 and VEGFR2 sequester ß-integrin in a complex, which negatively regulates ß-integrin activity and NFAT transcriptional function, leading to lowered VEGFR1 expression.[15,16] Subsequently, sequestration of VEGF is not possible and it binds to VEGFR2, activating downstream signaling, which results in increased proliferation of hemangioma ECs (**Box 1**, **Fig. 2**).[15,16]

## VASCULAR MALFORMATIONS

### *Etiology and Genetics of Capillary Malformations*

#### *Capillary malformations*

CMs (also known as "port-wine stains"), and the Sturge-Weber Syndrome, are associated with somatic Arg183 GNAQ mutations. This differs from the Gln209 mutations

**Box 1**
**Hemangioma**

*Congenital hemangioma*

- Three types: RICH, partially involuting congenital hemangioma, and NICH
- Already present at birth
- GLUT1 negative
- Activating somatic missense mutation in *GNAQ* or *GNA11* (at least RICH and NICH)
- Increased MAPK signaling?

*Isolated and secondary PG*

- Secondary PG arises on capillary malformations
- Activating somatic missense mutation in *GNAQ* and *KRAS*; driver and second-hit mutations in *BRAF*
- Increased MAPK signaling

*Infantile hemangioma*

- Endothelial cell hyperplasia
- Origin under discussion
  - Involvement of embolic placental angioblasts? (markers: GLUT1, Lewis Y antigen, merosin, Fcγ receptor II)
  - Endothelial progenitor cells? ($CD133^{+}/CD34^{+}$ circulating progenitor and stem cells)
- Variants in *TEM8* and *VEGFR2*
- Altered VEGF-A/VEGFR1 and VEGFR2 signaling?

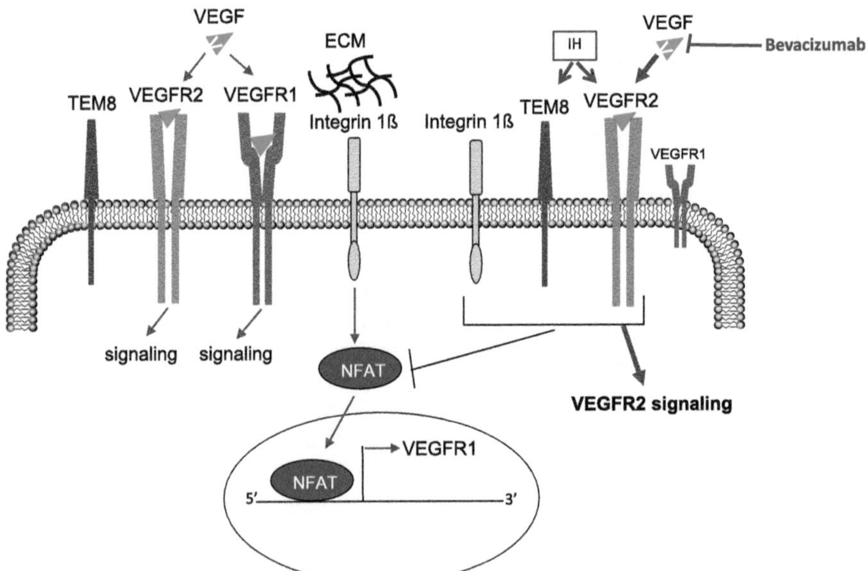


**Fig. 2.** Mutations and signaling pathways involved in infantile hemangioma and hypothetical treatment options. Mutations in *VEGFR2* and *TEM8* lead to sequestration of integrin 1ß and thus to inhibition of NFAT transcription and reduction of VEGFR1. VEGF exclusively binds to VEGFR2 triggering its signaling. IH, infantile hemangioma.

found in congenital hemangiomas.[6,17] As seen in melanomas, GNAQ p.Gln209Leu and GNAQ p.Arg183Gln induce activation of ERK after transfection of HEK293T cells, but this is more moderate for p.Arg183Gln than for p.Gln209Leu.[17]

Atypical CMs are associated with arteriovenous malformations (AVMs) in the same patient. This entity is called CM-AVM. The fast-flow lesions include arteriovenous fistula, AVM, or Parkes Weber syndrome.[18,19] CM-AVM is autosomal-dominantly inherited and caused by *RASA1* mutations.[20] One-third of patients have fast-flow lesions.[21] Thus, most (70%) have characteristic CMs. In about one-half of patients with CM-AVM a *RASA1* mutation is identified. This subentity is called CM-AVM1.[19]

*RASA1* mutations cause loss-of-function; more than 40 truncating mutations have been reported in more than 100 CM-AVM families.[16,19,20] According to phenotypic heterogeneity and reduced penetrance (98%), it is assumed that a somatic second mutation on the second allele of the same gene is involved.[16] These somatic mutations would be nonhereditary and lead to complete loss of the protein encoded by *RASA1*. This explains how inherited vascular malformations can be localized, multifocal, and increase in number with the age of a patient (paradominant inheritance).[22]

*RASA1* encodes the RAS p21 protein activator 1 (p120RasGAP), which inactivates RAS by enhancing its weak intrinsic GTPase activity (see **Fig. 1**).[16] p120RasGAP is recruited to the cell membrane on receptor tyrosine kinase activation, either alone or by Annexin A6.[16] p120RasGAP is essential for the organization of the EC networks, cellular growth, differentiation, and proliferation.[22,23] Moreover, it is involved in EC movement via interaction with p190RhoGAP or FAK.[16] p120RasGAP also protects cells from apoptosis through binding to AKT.[24] Thus, in patients with CM-AVM1, prolonged RAS/MAPK activation can lead to changes in several cellular behaviors.

A second CM-AVM subentity has been identified: CM-AVM2.[25] It is distinct from CM-AVM1. CM-AVM2 is caused by loss-of-function mutations in *EPHB4*[25] and patients with CM-AVM2 have typical small telangiectasias around the lips and on upper thorax, and less frequently intracerebral fast-flow lesions.

EPHB4 is a transmembrane receptor preferentially expressed in venous ECs during vascular development.[26] The ligand EphrinB2, also a transmembrane protein, is expressed on arterial ECs.[26] EPHB4 acts predominantly via the RAS/MAPK/ERK1/2 pathway and is responsible for suppression while interacting with p120RasGAP (see **Fig. 1**).[27] The latter is a direct effector of EPHB4. Consequently, loss-of-function of EPHB4 (CM-AVM2) or p120RasGAP (CM-AVM1) has similar effects, activation of RAS and the MAPK/ERK1/2 pathway.[25]

***Hereditary hemorrhagic telangiectasia***

Five loci are linked to hereditary hemorrhagic telangiectasia (HHT) and 90% of patients with HHT have a mutation in one of the three identified genes.[1,28,29] HHT1 is caused by loss-of-function mutations in *endoglin* (*ENG*)[30] and HHT2 in *activin receptor-like kinase 1* (*ALK1*).[31] Loss-of-function mutations in *MADH4*, encoding the downstream effector SMAD4, cause juvenile polyposis/HHT syndrome.[32] Linkage studies have identified additional loci on chromosome *5q31.3 to 32* (HHT3) and on *7p14* (HHT4).[33,34] In HHT5, substitutions were identified in the growth/differentiation factor-2 or bone morphogenetic protein (BMP)-9 (GDF2 or BMP9), the ligand for ALK1.[29,35]

All of these mutated genes encode proteins involved in BMP signaling pathway.[35] ALK1 and endoglin make a receptor complex expressed on EC membranes.[36] Endoglin, as a coreceptor, increases BMP9/BMP10/ALK1 signaling leading to phosphorylation of the receptor and activation of R-SMAD1/5/8 and co-SMAD, SMAD4. They act as transcription factors that can suppress EC migration and proliferation, and maintain a quiescent endothelial state (see **Fig. 1**).[36] Moreover, VEGF and AKT signaling are enhanced after *Alk1* deletion and BMP9/10 ligand blockade in human umbilical vein endothelial cells. This is caused by loss of BMP9/10 regulated inhibition of PTEN activity, which leads to uninhibited PI3K/AKT signaling (**Box 2**; see **Fig. 1**).[35]

## *Etiology and Genetics of Venous Anomalies*

### *Sporadic venous malformations, multifocal venous malformations, inherited cutaneomucosal venous malformations, and blue rubber bleb nevus syndrome*

Venous malformations (VMs), inherited cutaneomucosal venous malformations (VMCMs), and blue rubber bleb nevus syndrome (BRBN) are caused by mutations in the endothelial receptor tyrosine kinase TIE2 encoding *TEK* gene.[16,37] Mutations are located in the intracellular tyrosine kinase, kinase insert, or carboxyl-terminal tail, and result in amino acid substitutions or create C-terminal premature stop codons. They induce TIE2 receptor phosphorylation in the absence of a ligand.[16,37,38]

The somatic activating mutations in VMs, which usually occur as a unique lesion in the patient, are either single mutations or double mutations on the same allele.[37,38] The L914F is the most frequent, and exclusively identified in sporadic VMs. A few sporadic patients have multiple lesions (multifocal VM [MVM]). These patients tend to be mosaic for the first mutation, on top of which they generate a second-hit in lesional areas. The typical combination is Y897C-R915C.[39] The most common inherited VMCM-causing mutation is R849W, which causes weak TIE2 phosphorylation. It needs a somatic second-hit for lesions to develop, such as the mosaic mutations in patients with sporadic MVM.[37]

There are three known TIE2 ligands: (1) angiopoietin 1 (ANGPT1), (2) angiopoietin 2 (ANGPT2), and (3) angiopoietin 4 (ANGPT4).[40,41] ANGPT1 is able to activate TIE2 leading to phosphorylation of the receptor, whereas ANGPT2 is a context-dependent modulator of TIE2 activity.[16] In ECs, ligand binding leads to multimerization of TIE2 and its cross-phosphorylation resulting in activation of the canonical PI3K/AKT pathway, but also the MAPK pathway (see **Fig. 1**, **Box 3**).[16]

**Box 2**
**Capillary lesions**

*CM and CM-AVM*

- CM: somatic activating mutations in *GNAQ*
- Increased MAPK/ERK signaling?
- Inherited entities: CM-AVM1 and 2
- CM-AVM1: loss-of-function mutations in *RASA1*
- CM-AVM2: loss-of-function mutations in *EPHB4*
- Increased Ras/MAPK/ERK1/2 signaling? Downregulation of apoptosis?

*HHT*

- Mutations in endoglin (HHT1), activin receptor-like kinase 1 (HHT2), or SMAD4 (juvenile polyposis/HHT syndrome)
- Variants also in BMP9 (HHT5)
- Additional linked loci: chr. 5q31.3-32 (HHT3), on 7p14 (HHT4)
- Downregulated BMP9/10/ALK1 signaling and activation of PI3K/AKT/mTOR signaling through reduced PTEN; SMAD4?

**Box 3**
**Venous lesions**

*Sporadic VM and MVM, dominantly inherited VMCM, and BRBN*

- Activating mutations in endothelial receptor tyrosine kinase *TIE2* (TEK)
- *R849W* the most frequent germline mutation in VMCM
- In VMCM, different somatic second-hits in distant lesions of the patient
- *L914F* the most frequent somatic mutation in VM
- Y897C-R915C typical double-mutation in multifocal VM
- T1105N-T1106P typical double-mutation in BRBN
- Somatic activating mutations in *PIK3CA* in 20% of VM
- Increased PI3K/AKT/mTORC1 signaling

*HCCVM*

- Inherited loss-of-function mutations in *KRIT1/CCM1*
- Disruption of the KRIT1/CCM2/CCM3 complex leading to an increased MAP3K-signaling?

*Verrucous venous malformations*

- Somatic activating mutations in *MAP3K3*
- Increased MAP3K3/ERK signaling?

*GVM*

- Germline loss-of-function mutations in *glomulin*
- Glomulin is expressed in ECs and vSMCs
- 13 somatic second-hit mutations reported. Most common: acquired uniparental isodisomy of chromosome 1p.
- Increased hepatocyte growth factor/c-Met signaling with PI3K downstream target p70S6K, role in ubiquitination of proteins, TGF-ß signaling?

In VMs, the PI3K/AKT/mTOR signaling seems to be the major downstream signaling mechanism (see **Fig. 1**).[42] This is emphasized by identification of mutations in *PIK3CA* encoding the phosphatidylinositol-4,5-bisphosphate 3-kinase catalytic subunit alpha (p110alpha), an important part of the PI3K complex, in half of the VMs that lack a TIE2 mutation (see **Fig. 1**).[38,42–44] Overexpression of mutant forms of PIK3CA also activates AKT and disrupts characteristic EC monolayer morphology, and leads to loss of extracellular matrix fibronectin and downregulation of ANGPT2 and PDGF-B expression.[44]

BRBN lesions also contain point mutations in *TEK* leading to ligand-independent activation of the receptor.[39] Most of the patients have somatic *TEK* double-mutations (T1105N-T1106P, Y897F-R915L).[39] They also induce PI3K/AKT signaling. In BRBN, the same double-mutations are identified in distant lesions, although no trace of the mutations is detected in blood. Therefore, temporarily restricted circulating cells may be involved in inducing formation of new lesions.

### *Hyperkeratotic cutaneous capillary venous malformation and nodular venous malformation*

Hyperkeratotic cutaneous capillary venous malformation (HCCVM) is the most frequent cutaneous lesion associated with inherited cerebral cavernous malformation (CCM).[45] Cutaneous lesions are seen in 9% of patients with CCM.[46] Some have cutaneous CMs, others nodular type VMs. As in CCM1, patients with HCCVM with CCMs have an inherited loss-of-function mutation in *KRIT1*.[45,46] KRIT1 interacts with CCM2 and CCM3 to form a complex that regulates MAP3K3 function.[47] Loss of CCM complex function activates MAP3K3 signaling and its target genes *KLF2*, *KLF4*, *RHO*, and *ADAMTS* (see **Fig. 1**, **Box 3**).[47]

#### *Verrucous venous malformations*

Verrucous venous malformations are clinically reminiscent of HCCVMs. They are associated with somatic activating mutations in *MAP3K3*, underscoring a biologic dysfunction similar to that of HCCVMs.[48] MAP3K3 is a member of the MAP3K family of serine/threonine kinases, and also seems to be a downstream target of angiopoietin-1/TIE2 signaling.[48] Yet, it is implicated in the ERK-signaling pathway (see **Fig. 1**, **Box 3**).[48]

#### *Glomuvenous malformations*

Glomuvenous malformations (GVM) are distinguished from sporadic VMs and VMCMs. However, small lesions are indistinguishable clinically.[16] Loss-of-function mutations in *glomulin* (GLMN/FAP68) lead to abnormally differentiated vascular smooth muscle cells (vSMCs), called "glomus cells," located around distended venous channels.[49] More than 40 different mutations of *glomulin* are described.[50] GVM is the inherited vascular anomaly for which the highest number of somatic second-hits has been reported. Most of them are somatic chromosomal changes (acquired uniparental isodisomies) that are difficult to identify in heterogeneous tissues.[49,51]

Glomulin seems to be expressed in ECs and vSMCs. It interacts with the unphosphorylated hepatocyte growth factor receptor c-Met, but is released after ligand (hepatocyte growth factor) binding, which leads to phosphorylation of glomulin. This triggers activation of PI3K downstream targets including p70S6K.[16] Furthermore, glomulin interacts with Cul7 and forms an Skp1-Cul1-Fbox-like complex, which acts in protein degradation through ubiquitination.[52] Some data suggest that glomulin changes vSMCs phenotypes by interacting with transforming growth factor (TGF)-ß signaling. Glomulin binds FK506 binding protein 12 (FKBP12) (see **Fig. 1**), which inhibits TGF-ß signaling through TGF-ß type I receptor (TßRI) (**Box 3**).[23]

### *Etiology and Genetics of Lymphatic Malformations*

Lymphatic malformations (LMs) are caused by somatic activating mutations in *PIK3CA*.[53,54] Because the same mutations can give rise to LMs and VMs, the cellular origin should vary: lymphatic ECs versus venous ECs. Mutations in *PIK3CA* can enhance its binding to cell membrane and/or activate its kinase. This leads to activation of the AKT/mTOR cascade regulating cell growth, proliferation, and migration (**Box 4**; see **Fig. 1**).[53,54]

**Box 4**
**Lymphatic lesions**

*Lymphatic malformation*

- Activating somatic mutations in *PIK3CA*
- Increased AKT/mTOR signaling

## SUMMARY

Until now, therapeutic options to treat vascular tumors and malformations have been limited to classic approaches to destroy or remove abnormal vessels by laser, sclerotherapy, embolization, and/or surgery.[1] Detection of a genetic cause, inherited or somatic, has opened up the field for understanding the underlying molecular mechanisms. Most genetic defects alter directly intracellular signaling activities and subsequently various downstream actions. Even if all the downstream effects are not yet known, the identification of overt signaling opens these diseases to novel ideas to develop treatments.

Lesions that are caused by constitutively active PI3K/AKT/mTOR pathway (eg, VMCM, MVM, VM, BRBN, and LM) may benefit from mTOR inhibitors, such as rapamycin (see **Fig. 1**). A VM in vivo model was already generated by injecting TIE2-L914F mutated human umbilical vein endothelial cells into nude mice.[43] Treatment with rapamycin prevented VM growth. Additionally, in vitro, rapamycin significantly reduced mutant TIE2-induced AKT signaling.[43] Importantly, in a prospective clinical pilot study, six patients treated with rapamycin had reduced pain, bleeding, lesional size, and intravascular coagulopathy.[43,55] This has prompted large clinical studies to be set up, such as VASE (https://www.clinicaltrialsregister.eu/; EudraCT Number: 2015-001703-32).

Lesions where the RAS/BRAF/MAPK/ERK pathway plays a major role (eg, CM, CM-AVM1 and 2, PG, NICH, RICH, and verrucous venous malformation) another inhibitor may be needed. It would be conceivable to test a BRAF- (vemurafenib) or MEK-inhibitor (trametinib), which are used to treat metastatic *BRAF*-mutated melanoma[56] (see **Fig. 1**). Because many kinase inhibitors have variable affinities to several intracellular proteins, and multiple cross-talks occur between signaling pathways, numerous studies are needed to characterize the most efficient modalities.

In HHT, receptor mutations lead to decreased BMP signaling and this may lead in turn to an increase in angiogenic response. Thus, these patients could benefit from antiangiogenic agents, such as bevacizumab.[36] Yet, the diminished ALK activity also leads to increased PTEN phosphorylation and inactivation.[35] There is subsequent PI3K/AKT activation.[35] Rapamycin and other PI3K/AKT inhibitors may thus prove to be efficacious. General angiogenesis inhibitors, such as thalidomide or bevacizumab, the anti-VEGF antibody, may also be useful.[57–59] They can inhibit VEGF action whatever the underlying cause for expression may be. For example, they reduce nosebleeds in patients with HHT.[57–59] The pathophysiology of GVMs is less clear. If earlier data hold true, the TGF-ß pathway might serve as a target, in addition to modulation of mTOR (**Box 5**).[16]

**Box 5**
**Therapeutic hypotheses for the treatment of vascular diseases**

*Targeting the PI3K/AKT/mTOR pathway*

- mTOR inhibitors, such as rapamycin in VM, VMCM, MVM, BRBN, and LM; also HHT?

*Targeting the RAS/BRAF/MAPK/ERK pathway*

- Possible inhibitors could be the BRAF inhibitor vemurafenib or the MEK inhibitor trametinib in CM, CM-AVM1 and 2, PG, NICH, RICH, and verrucous venous malformations

*Targeting angiogenesis*

- Antiangiogenic agents, such as bevacizumab in HHT, IH

*Targeting TGF-ß pathway*

- GVM?

In conclusion, several mutations in key proteins of EC intracellular signaling have been identified to play a major role in the pathogenesis of vascular anomalies. In vitro and in vivo experiments are necessary to reveal the exact molecular mechanisms. To study repurposing of oncology drugs, in vivo models of vascular anomalies are urgently needed. Thereby preclinical testing can be performed, a prerequisite for development of novel and efficacious treatments for patients harboring vascular anomalies.

## REFERENCES


1. Mulliken JB, Fishman DJ. Mulliken and Young's vascular anomalies: hemangiomas and malformations. 2nd edition. New York: Oxford University Press; 2013.
2. Mahady K, Thust S, Berkeley R, et al. Vascular anomalies of the head and neck in children. Quant Imaging Med Surg 2015;5(6):886–97.
3. Mulliken JB, Glowacki J. Hemangiomas and vascular malformations in infants and children: a classification based on endothelial characteristics. Plast Reconstr Surg 1982;69(3):412–22.
4. Boon LM, Enjolras O, Mulliken JB. Congenital hemangioma: evidence of accelerated involution. J Pediatr 1996;128(3):329–35.
5. Nasseri E, Piram M, McCuaig CC, et al. Partially involuting congenital hemangiomas: a report of 8 cases and review of the literature. J Am Acad Dermatol 2014;70(1):75–9.
6. Ayturk UM, Couto JA, Hann S, et al. Somatic activating mutations in GNAQ and GNA11 are associated with congenital hemangioma. Am J Hum Genet 2016; 98(6):1271.
7. Funk T, Lim Y, Kulungowski AM, et al. Symptomatic congenital hemangioma and congenital hemangiomatosis associated with a somatic activating mutation in GNA11. JAMA Dermatol 2016;152(9):1015–20.
8. Van Raamsdonk CD, Bezrookove V, Green G, et al. Frequent somatic mutations of GNAQ in uveal melanoma and blue naevi. Nature 2009;457(7229):599–602.
9. Groesser L, Peterhof E, Evert M, et al. BRAF and RAS mutations in sporadic and secondary pyogenic granuloma. J Invest Dermatol 2016;136(2):481–6.
10. Lim YH, Douglas SR, Ko CJ, et al. Somatic activating RAS mutations cause vascular tumors including pyogenic granuloma. J Invest Dermatol 2015;135(6): 1698–700.
11. Buckmiller LM, Richter GT, Suen JY. Diagnosis and management of hemangiomas and vascular malformations of the head and neck. Oral Dis 2010;16(5): 405–18.
12. North PE, Waner M, Brodsky MC. Are infantile hemangiomas of placental origin? Ophthalmology 2002;109(4):633–4.
13. Yu Y, Flint AF, Mulliken JB, et al. Endothelial progenitor cells in infantile hemangioma. Blood 2004;103(4):1373–5.
14. Khan ZA, Boscolo E, Picard A, et al. Multipotential stem cells recapitulate human infantile hemangioma in immunodeficient mice. J Clin Invest 2008;118(7):2592–9.
15. Jinnin M, Medici D, Park L, et al. Suppressed NFAT-dependent VEGFR1 expression and constitutive VEGFR2 signaling in infantile hemangioma. Nat Med 2008; 14(11):1236–46.
16. Uebelhoer M, Boon LM, Vikkula M. Vascular anomalies: from genetics toward models for therapeutic trials. Cold Spring Harb Perspect Med 2012;2(8) [pii: a009688].

17. Shirley MD, Tang H, Gallione CJ, et al. Sturge-Weber syndrome and port-wine stains caused by somatic mutation in GNAQ. N Engl J Med 2013;368(21):1971–9.
18. Boon LM, Mulliken JB, Vikkula M. RASA1: variable phenotype with capillary and arteriovenous malformations. Curr Opin Genet Dev 2005;15(3):265–9.
19. Revencu N, Boon LM, Mulliken JB, et al. Parkes Weber syndrome, vein of Galen aneurysmal malformation, and other fast-flow vascular anomalies are caused by RASA1 mutations. Hum Mutat 2008;29(7):959–65.
20. Eerola I, Boon LM, Mulliken JB, et al. Capillary malformation-arteriovenous malformation, a new clinical and genetic disorder caused by RASA1 mutations. Am J Hum Genet 2003;73(6):1240–9.
21. Revencu N, Boon LM, Mendola A, et al. RASA1 mutations and associated phenotypes in 68 families with capillary malformation-arteriovenous malformation. Hum Mutat 2013;34(12):1632–41.
22. Boon LM, Ballieux F, Vikkula M. Pathogenesis of vascular anomalies. Clin Plast Surg 2011;38(1):7–19.
23. Brouillard P, Vikkula M. Genetic causes of vascular malformations. Hum Mol Genet 2007;16 Spec No. 2:R140–9.
24. Yue Y, Lypowy J, Hedhli N, et al. Ras GTPase-activating protein binds to Akt and is required for its activation. J Biol Chem 2004;279(13):12883–9.
25. Amyere M, Revencu N, Helaers R, et al. Germline loss-of-function mutations in EPHB4 cause a second form of capillary malformation–arteriovenous malformation (CM-AVM2) deregulating RAS-MAPK signaling. Circulation 2017;136(11): 1037–48.
26. Wang HU, Chen ZF, Anderson DJ. Molecular distinction and angiogenic interaction between embryonic arteries and veins revealed by ephrin-B2 and its receptor Eph-B4. Cell 1998;93(5):741–53.
27. Xiao Z, Carrasco R, Kinneer K, et al. EphB4 promotes or suppresses Ras/MEK/ERK pathway in a context-dependent manner: implications for EphB4 as a cancer target. Cancer Biol Ther 2012;13(8):630–7.
28. Bayrak-Toydemir P, McDonald J, Markewitz B, et al. Genotype-phenotype correlation in hereditary hemorrhagic telangiectasia: mutations and manifestations. Am J Med Genet A 2006;140(5):463–70.
29. Wooderchak-Donahue WL, McDonald J, O'Fallon B, et al. BMP9 mutations cause a vascular-anomaly syndrome with phenotypic overlap with hereditary hemorrhagic telangiectasia. Am J Hum Genet 2013;93(3):530–7.
30. McAllister KA, Grogg KM, Johnson DW, et al. Endoglin, a TGF-beta binding protein of endothelial cells, is the gene for hereditary haemorrhagic telangiectasia type 1. Nat Genet 1994;8(4):345–51.
31. Johnson DW, Berg JN, Baldwin MA, et al. Mutations in the activin receptor-like kinase 1 gene in hereditary haemorrhagic telangiectasia type 2. Nat Genet 1996; 13(2):189–95.
32. Gallione CJ, Repetto GM, Legius E, et al. A combined syndrome of juvenile polyposis and hereditary haemorrhagic telangiectasia associated with mutations in MADH4 (SMAD4). Lancet 2004;363(9412):852–9.
33. Bayrak-Toydemir P, McDonald J, Akarsu N, et al. A fourth locus for hereditary hemorrhagic telangiectasia maps to chromosome 7. Am J Med Genet A 2006; 140(20):2155–62.
34. Cole SG, Begbie ME, Wallace GM, et al. A new locus for hereditary haemorrhagic telangiectasia (HHT3) maps to chromosome 5. J Med Genet 2005;42(7):577–82.

35. Ola R, Dubrac A, Han J, et al. PI3 kinase inhibition improves vascular malformations in mouse models of hereditary haemorrhagic telangiectasia. Nat Commun 2016;7:13650.
36. Tillet E, Bailly S. Emerging roles of BMP9 and BMP10 in hereditary hemorrhagic telangiectasia. Front Genet 2014;5:456.
37. Limaye N, Wouters V, Uebelhoer M, et al. Somatic mutations in angiopoietin receptor gene TEK cause solitary and multiple sporadic venous malformations. Nat Genet 2009;41(1):118–24.
38. Natynki M, Kangas J, Miinalainen I, et al. Common and specific effects of TIE2 mutations causing venous malformations. Hum Mol Genet 2015;24(22):6374–89.
39. Soblet J, Kangas J, Natynki M, et al. Blue rubber bleb nevus (BRBN) syndrome is caused by somatic TEK (TIE2) mutations. J Invest Dermatol 2017;137(1):207–16.
40. Maisonpierre PC, Suri C, Jones PF, et al. Angiopoietin-2, a natural antagonist for Tie2 that disrupts in vivo angiogenesis. Science 1997;277(5322):55–60.
41. Valenzuela DM, Griffiths JA, Rojas J, et al. Angiopoietins 3 and 4: diverging gene counterparts in mice and humans. Proc Natl Acad Sci U S A 1999;96(5):1904–9.
42. Uebelhoer M, Natynki M, Kangas J, et al. Venous malformation-causative TIE2 mutations mediate an AKT-dependent decrease in PDGFB. Hum Mol Genet 2013;22(17):3438–48.
43. Boscolo E, Limaye N, Huang L, et al. Rapamycin improves TIE2-mutated venous malformation in murine model and human subjects. J Clin Invest 2015;125(9): 3491–504.
44. Limaye N, Kangas J, Mendola A, et al. Somatic activating PIK3CA mutations cause venous malformation. Am J Hum Genet 2015;97(6):914–21.
45. Eerola I, Plate KH, Spiegel R, et al. KRIT1 is mutated in hyperkeratotic cutaneous capillary-venous malformation associated with cerebral capillary malformation. Hum Mol Genet 2000;9(9):1351–5.
46. Sirvente J, Enjolras O, Wassef M, et al. Frequency and phenotypes of cutaneous vascular malformations in a consecutive series of 417 patients with familial cerebral cavernous malformations. J Eur Acad Dermatol Venereol 2009;23(9): 1066–72.
47. Zhou Z, Tang AT, Wong WY, et al. Cerebral cavernous malformations arise from endothelial gain of MEKK3-KLF2/4 signalling. Nature 2016;532(7597):122–6.
48. Couto JA, Vivero MP, Kozakewich HP, et al. A somatic MAP3K3 mutation is associated with verrucous venous malformation. Am J Hum Genet 2015;96(3):480–6.
49. Brouillard P, Boon LM, Mulliken JB, et al. Mutations in a novel factor, glomulin, are responsible for glomuvenous malformations ("glomangiomas"). Am J Hum Genet 2002;70(4):866–74.
50. Brouillard P, Boon LM, Revencu N, et al. Genotypes and phenotypes of 162 families with a glomulin mutation. Mol Syndromol 2013;4(4):157–64.
51. Amyere M, Aerts V, Brouillard P, et al. Somatic uniparental isodisomy explains multifocality of glomuvenous malformations. Am J Hum Genet 2013;92(2): 188–96.
52. Arai T, Kasper JS, Skaar JR, et al. Targeted disruption of p185/Cul7 gene results in abnormal vascular morphogenesis. Proc Natl Acad Sci U S A 2003;100(17): 9855–60.
53. Boscolo E, Coma S, Luks VL, et al. AKT hyper-phosphorylation associated with PI3K mutations in lymphatic endothelial cells from a patient with lymphatic malformation. Angiogenesis 2015;18(2):151–62.

54. Osborn AJ, Dickie P, Neilson DE, et al. Activating PIK3CA alleles and lymphangiogenic phenotype of lymphatic endothelial cells isolated from lymphatic malformations. Hum Mol Genet 2015;24(4):926–38.
55. Adams DM, Trenor CC 3rd, Hammill AM, et al. Efficacy and safety of sirolimus in the treatment of complicated vascular anomalies. Pediatrics 2016;137(2):e20153257.
56. Welsh SJ, Corrie PG. Management of BRAF and MEK inhibitor toxicities in patients with metastatic melanoma. Ther Adv Med Oncol 2015;7(2):122–36.
57. Ardelean DS, Letarte M. Anti-angiogenic therapeutic strategies in hereditary hemorrhagic telangiectasia. Front Genet 2015;6:35.
58. Peng HL, Yi YF, Zhou SK, et al. Thalidomide effects in patients with hereditary hemorrhagic telangiectasia during therapeutic treatment and in Fli-EGFP transgenic zebrafish model. Chin Med J (Engl) 2015;128(22):3050–4.
59. Thompson AB, Ross DA, Berard P, et al. Very low dose bevacizumab for the treatment of epistaxis in patients with hereditary hemorrhagic telangiectasia. Allergy Rhinol (Providence) 2014;5(2):91–5.

# Imaging of Vascular Lesions of the Head and Neck

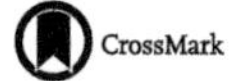

Jared M. Steinklein, MD*, Deborah R. Shatzkes, MD*

**KEYWORDS**

• Hemangioma • Lymphatic • Venous • Arteriovenous • Malformation • Pediatric • Head and neck • Radiology

**KEY POINTS**

- Diagnostic imaging plays an important role in the diagnosis of vascular lesions in the head and neck.
- Imaging provides precise lesional mapping of malformations, with MRI being the preferred imaging modality.
- Imaging may offer a differential diagnosis when a lesion differs from classic patterns, which are discussed in this article.

## INTRODUCTION

Diagnostic imaging has an important role in both the diagnosis and management of vascular lesions of the head and neck. Imaging confirms the diagnosis, maps the lesion, identifies associated anomalies, and provides surveillance of disease and/or response to therapy.[1] The true nature and extent of a clinically evident vascular lesion may not be fully appreciated until the lesion is imaged.[2] In addition, imaging provides a means for guided therapy for some vascular anomalies. With advances in imaging technology, including multiplanar and cross-sectional technique, imaging provides intricate detail as to lesional mapping and relationship to adjacent vital structures. Furthermore, discovery of additional anomalies may lead to the diagnosis of a clinical syndrome. This article provides an overview of imaging techniques and discusses and displays imaging findings of vascular tumors, such as hemangiomas, vascular malformations, and other anomalies.

In the armamentarium of a radiologist are varied imaging modalities, each having their advantages and disadvantages. Ultrasound is readily available and noninvasive,

Disclosure Statement: The authors have nothing to disclose.
Department of Radiology, Lenox Hill Hospital, 100 East 77th Street, Radiology 3rd Floor, New York, NY 10075, USA
* Corresponding authors.
*E-mail addresses:* jsteinklein@northwell.edu (J.M.S.); dshatzkes@northwell.edu (D.R.S.)

Otolaryngol Clin N Am 51 (2018) 55–76
https://doi.org/10.1016/j.otc.2017.09.007
oto.theclinics.com

can be performed without anesthesia, and best evaluates superficial lesions while limited in evaluating deeper soft tissue and bony anatomy. Computed tomography (CT) is the traditional cross-sectional technique for evaluating both the bony and the deeper anatomy, but its use of ionizing radiation makes it less preferable in the pediatric population, particularly when multiple imaging examinations are required for follow-up. In the last few decades, MRI has become an indispensable imaging tool with its superior contrast resolution for soft tissues and lack of ionizing radiation. Disadvantages of MRI include lengthy acquisition time and the need for the patient to stay still. In the pediatric population, this may require anesthesia or moderate sedation to ensure diagnostic image quality. With the evolution of noninvasive imaging techniques, catheter angiography is generally reserved for treatment; a discussion of transcatheter treatment applications and techniques is beyond the scope of this article.

Because MRI provides the most discriminatory detail of soft tissue, it is the mainstay in the imaging evaluation of vascular anomalies. This article focuses therefore on the MRI findings of specific lesions and presents a simplified algorithm for the radiologist and clinician to best narrow the differential diagnosis.

## TECHNICAL CONSIDERATIONS

Using a high-frequency transducer, ultrasonography provides excellent spatial resolution of superficial structures. Deeper lesions are seen but at a lower spatial resolution, and sometimes incompletely if obscured by bony anatomy.[3,4] Vascular anatomy is often imaged with ultrasound because of its real-time ability to demonstrate flowing objects and Doppler technique to quantify flow. As a first-line diagnostic tool, ultrasound confirms the presence of a vascular mass and can assess for venous or arterial-type flow.[4,5]

CT uses ionizing radiation akin to conventional radiography and is generally less preferred than MRI. Current multidetector systems allow the postprocessing of image data into multiplanar reconstructed image sets.[6] Although soft tissue resolution of CT is inferior to MRI, CT is well suited to assess bony anatomy and the presence of calcification, for example, a phlebolith of a venous malformation (VM). Another benefit of CT is its quick acquisition time, with most scans performed in less than 1 minute. This benefit is useful in an emergency care situation or when sedation for MRI is not available.

Cellular injury from ionizing radiation is a cumulative phenomenon. Although a single CT examination may impose a minimal amount of radiation, repeated examinations do incur cumulative dose. Total cumulative dose is causally related with increased risk of pediatric cancers.[7] In recent years, CT manufacturers have developed algorithms to process and reconstruct imaging data of lower dose scans while maintaining image quality.[8] The Image Gently campaign and the Society of Pediatric Radiology provide guidelines and resources to minimize ionizing radiation dose for imaging procedures, available at their Web site www.imagegently.org.

For the most part, vascular lesions, as the name implies, have some connection to local vascular supply and will enhance following intravenous contrast administration. Contrast-enhanced imaging is the standard of care for both CT and MRI. For CT, iodinated contrast agents are generally safe for use in children. Contrast reactions may be mild and include hives or rash, or, rarely, may be more severe, resulting in anaphylaxis. Contrast-induced nephropathy may occur in patients with underlying renal insufficiency.

MRI has emerged as the primary modality for the evaluation of most vascular anomalies.[5] Using a superconducting magnet and selective image parameters, MRI quantifies differences in local proton density within tissue. This translates to superior soft tissue resolution, making it the preferred imaging tool when evaluating any soft tissue mass.[9,10] In addition to identifying a vascular lesion and providing information regarding its specific histologic composition, MRI is effective in identifying more aggressive imaging features with local invasion that may suggest a malignant alternative diagnosis.[10,11]

Whereas CT maps physical density and radiograph attenuation of tissue, MRI better depicts the local proton environment and gives more relevant information about soft tissue composition.[5] For instance, T2-weighted imaging highlights the signal of hypocellular and water-rich environments, such as within a macrocystic lymphatic malformation (LM), with lesser intense signal encountered in cellular neoplasms, such as hemangioma.[9] Rapidly flowing blood will be void of signal, with arteries commonly referred to as "flow voids" on routine spin-echo sequences. More detailed discussion of MRI characteristics of the most common vascular lesions is provided in later discussion.

MRI has evolved since its inception and development over the end of the last century but still has its limitations. First, MRI requires time to complete and requires the patient to be completely still for optimal image quality. Despite recent advances in technology, an MRI examination currently requires at least 30 minutes of scan acquisition for routine imaging of the head and neck. For an infant or child, remaining still for 30 minutes or more is challenging, if not impossible. To ensure diagnostic quality of the examination, the patient may require sedation and/or anesthesia, each entailing its own risks, although considered generally safe in the absence of a major preexisting condition.[12] A child younger than 2 months of age can be scanned without anesthesia with a "feed-and-wrap" technique. An older child may be better able to cooperate and remain still with or without moderate sedation instead of general anesthesia. Regardless of age or medical condition, anesthesiology staff must be available during the entirety of the procedure. The resources and cost required to complete these examinations must not be underestimated.[12,13]

Basic MRI protocols should include precontrast and postcontrast T1-weighted imaging. Postcontrast imaging is performed with fat saturation, as lesion conspicuity and bony involvement are better depicted with suppression of normally T1-hyperintense fat in the soft tissues and bone marrow.[9,10] On the other hand, fatty tissue in the head and neck provides excellent intrinsic contrast, and fat suppression should never be applied to noncontrast T1-weighted images. T2-weighted imaging may be performed both with and without fat saturation, which can be achieved either with chemical fat-saturation techniques or by use of an inversion recovery sequence such as short TI inversion recovery (STIR). These sequences are acquired in at least 2 planes, preferably in the axial and coronal plane. Imaging field of view should be tailored to cover the lesion with optimal signal-to-noise ratio and provide visualization of adjacent vital structures, namely the orbit and intracranial compartment.[14] Time-resolved MR angiography may be used to evaluate high-flow malformations, depicting both early arterial components and subsequent venous drainage.[15]

A summary of imaging modalities and their strengths and weaknesses is provided in **Table 1**.

## IMAGING OF HEMANGIOMAS (INFANTILE AND CONGENITAL)

Although the vast majority of hemangiomas are diagnosed clinically, imaging may prove helpful if physical examination findings are not specific or a deep soft tissue component is suspected. Imaging can provide information about tumor behavior

**Table 1**
**Summary of imaging modalities**

| Modality | Advantages/Applications | Disadvantages |
|---|---|---|
| Ultrasound | • Excellent spatial resolution of superficial lesions<br>• Readily available<br>• No ionizing radiation<br>• Noninvasively quantifies flow | • Limited evaluation of deeper lesions and relation to bony anatomy<br>• Limited soft tissue contrast resolution |
| CT | • Cross-sectional evaluation of deep lesions<br>• Optimal depiction of calcifications (eg, phleboliths) and impact on facial skeleton | • Use of ionizing radiation, especially if repeated examinations are required<br>• Limited soft tissue contrast resolution |
| MRI | • Best soft tissue contrast resolution<br>• No ionizing radiation exposure<br>• MR angiography techniques provide noninvasive vascular information | • Long acquisition time may require use of sedation or anesthesia<br>• Most expensive and least available |
| Angiography | • Provides optimal spatial and temporal resolution of lesion vascularity<br>• Allows for catheter directed or percutaenous therapy | • Invasive<br>• Use of ionizing radiation |

and may suggest the possibility of a more aggressive, perhaps malignant, alternative diagnosis.[9,11] The role of the radiologist here is to understand common appearances of all common vascular anomalies and to identify features that are worrisome for malignancy. After initial diagnostic imaging, tissue sampling may be recommended for definitive diagnosis.

Hemangiomas are most commonly imaged during their proliferative phase, where they typically appear as well-defined and lobulated masses on all imaging modalities.[2,10,11] Ultrasound typically reveals a lobulated and hyperechoic mass (**Fig. 1**A), with diffuse vascularity on color flow analysis (**Fig. 1**B), and Doppler interrogation reveals low-resistance arterial flow. Paltiel and colleagues[4] demonstrated that the presence of a discrete soft tissue mass on ultrasound was a reliable discriminator between hemangiomas and other high-flow lesions such as AVMs.

Proliferating infantile hemangiomas are of similar density to muscle on noncontrast CT imaging and will avidly enhance after contrast administration (**Fig. 2**). Small adjacent feeding and draining vessels may also be visible.[16,17] On MRI, proliferative phase

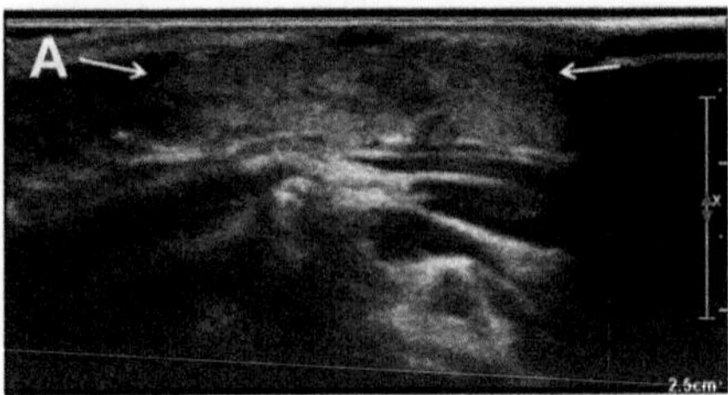


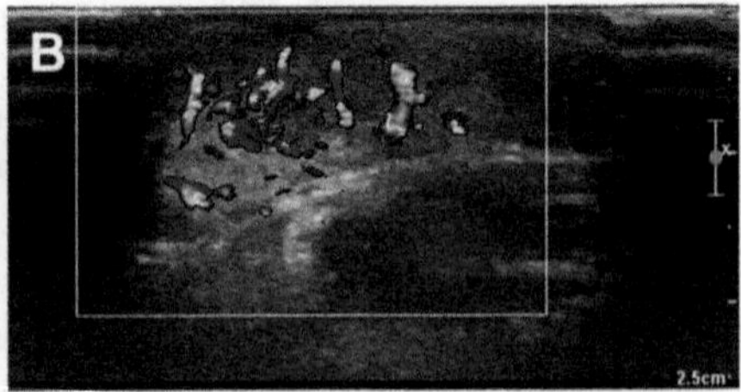


**Fig. 1.** Infantile hemangioma, ultrasound. (*A*) Ultrasound image of the right cheek shows an oblong mildly hyperechoic mass with well-defined borders (*arrows*). (*B*) Color spectral ultrasound image shows diffuse vascularity of the proliferating hemangioma.

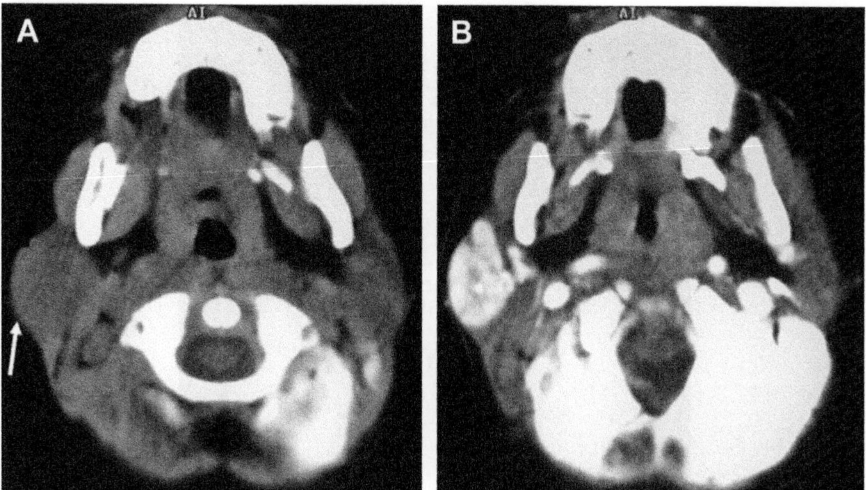


**Fig. 2.** Infantile hemangioma, CT. (*A*) Noncontrast CT of a right parotid hemangioma (*arrow*) shows similar density of the mass to muscle and other soft tissues. (*B*) Postcontrast CT shows avid and diffuse enhancement of the mass with well-circumscribed margins. Note the parotid gland is a common site for hemangioma.

hemangiomas appear as lobulated masses of isointense signal to muscle on T1-weighted imaging and moderately intense signal on T2-weighted imaging (**Fig. 3**A, B). Postcontrast T1-weighted imaging will show homogenous and avid enhancement of the mass (**Fig. 3**C), Small linear foci of signal void may be identified both within and surrounding the mass; these represent flow voids that reflect the hypervascularity of proliferating phase hemangiomas (**Fig. 4**).[10]

When distinguishing between hemangiomas and vascular malformations on MRI, T2 signal characteristics are particularly useful. Hemangiomas possess moderately hyperintense signal relative to skeletal muscle on T2-weighted imaging, but considerably lower signal than that of cerebrospinal or vitreous fluid (**Fig. 5**). Hemangiomas also typically demonstrate lower T2 signal than the relatively hypocellular venous or

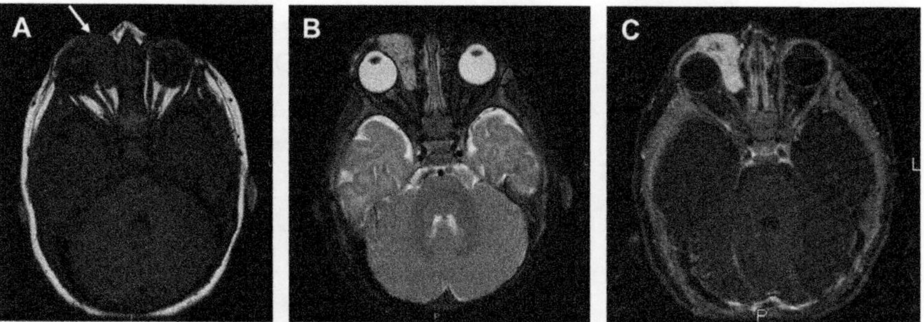


**Fig. 3.** Infantile hemangioma, MRI. (*A*) Precontrast T1-weighted image of a right periorbital hemangioma (*arrow*) with postseptal extraconal extension and deviation of the globe. (*B*) STIR image shows moderate T2 signal intensity, less than that of vitreous humor in the adjacent globe. Small central flow voids are seen. (*C*) Postcontrast T1-weighted image shows diffuse and avid enhancement.

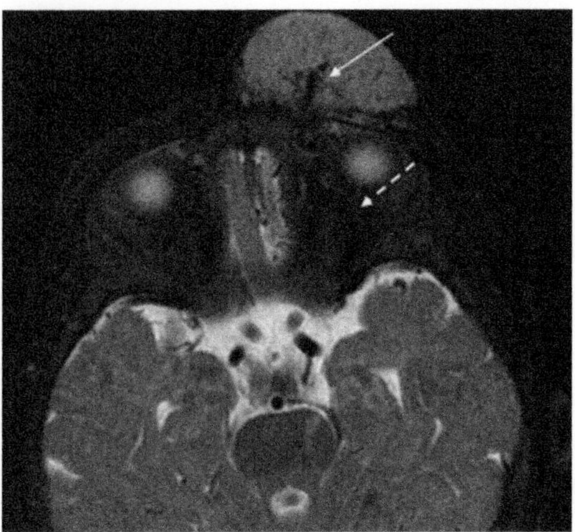

**Fig. 4.** Infantile hemangioma, flow voids. Axial STIR MRI of a left supraorbital hemangioma with prominent tubular flow voids both within the lesion (*solid arrow*) and in the superior orbit (*dashed arrow*).

LMs discussed later in this article. Generally speaking, a lesion is more likely to be hypercellular if it possesses intermediate to low signal on T2-weighted imaging.[9,11]

During the involutional phase, there is decreased bulk of tumor and less enhancing component when compared with initial imaging. MRI may depict fatty or fibrofatty changes within the lesion, visible as increased signal on T1-weighted imaging (**Fig. 6**). Further involution and fibrofatty replacement of the lesion is identified at the

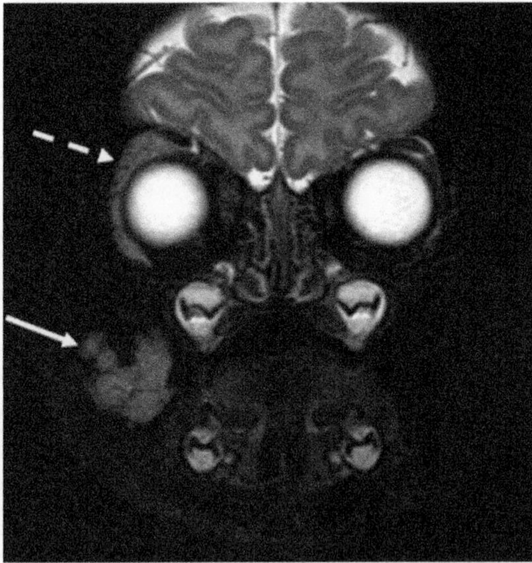

**Fig. 5.** Infantile hemangioma. Coronal STIR MRI of multifocal hemangioma in the right buccal space (*solid arrow*) and right orbit at the lacrimal fossa (*dashed arrow*). Note the moderate signal intensity, less than that of vitreous humor in the adjacent globe. Multiplicity of lesions occurs in up to 20% of cases.

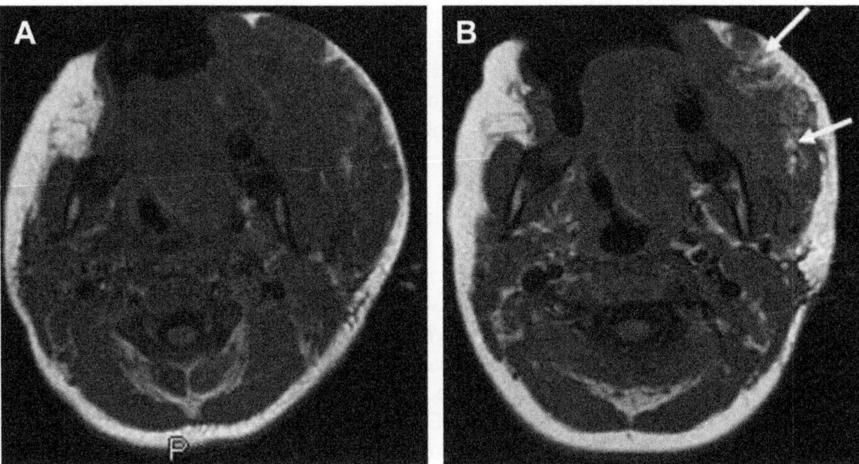


**Fig. 6.** Involuting infantile hemangioma, phase II. (*A*) Axial T1-weighted MRI of a left facial hemangioma at diagnosis. (*B*) Follow-up axial T1-weighted MRI in phase II shows decreased bulk of the mass with areas of interspersed hyperintense signal representing fatty change (*arrows*).

involuted phase. At this stage, imaging findings may be confined to local distortion of tissue without visible mass[1] (**Fig. 7**A). Longstanding hyperemia may result in overgrowth of the adjacent bony skeleton, which may contribute to persistent facial asymmetry following lesional involution (**Fig. 7**B). Complementary to MRI, CT imaging with volume-rendered 3D reconstructions of the skeleton and navigational data may then be used to assist in cosmetic surgical planning.

Additional utilities of cross-sectional imaging, specifically MRI, are to establish the depth and extent of a lesion and to identify any associated regional anomalies. Specifically, lesions of the face may involve the orbit or may be associated with intracranial

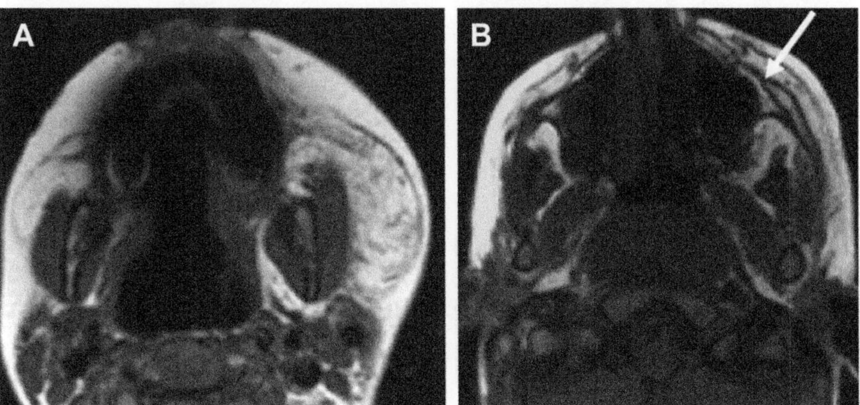


**Fig. 7.** Involuted infantile hemangioma, phase III. (*A*) Axial T1-weighted MRI through the face shows a predominantly hyperintense left buccal space mass. Signal represents adipose hypertrophy of an involuted hemangioma. (*B*) Axial T1-weighted MRI at superior margin of the lesion shows bony overgrowth at the left zygomaticomaxillary suture.

abnormalities. Involvement of the central nervous system by an infantile hemangioma is rare, occurring in only 1% of cases.[1,3] MRI and MR angiography of the brain are useful in evaluating the anomalies associated with PHACES syndrome, namely cerebellar hypoplasia and arterial stenosis or dysgenesis (**Fig. 8**).[14,16] The intracranial anomalies are typically ipsilateral to the facial hemangioma, and there is often ipsilateral enlargement of Meckel cave (see **Fig. 8**B). Periorbital and intraorbital hemangiomas are very common (see **Fig. 3**), and treatment may be necessary in the setting of visual axis disturbance that may ultimately result in amblyopia. When reviewing imaging studies in a patient with a periorbital hemangioma, it is particularly important to note the presence of any postseptal or intraconal component of the lesion (see **Fig. 3**; **Fig. 9**). Hemangiomas may involve the aerodigestive tract (**Fig. 10**), and potential airway narrowing may be an indication for therapeutic intervention.

Congenital hemangiomas (CHs) are present at birth, as the name implies, and are much less common than the infantile type. Histologically, these are distinguished by their lack of GLUT-1 protein expression.[1] Distinction between infantile hemangiomas and CHs is primarily based on their clinical behavior: A rapidly involuting congenital hemangioma typically involutes by 14 months of age, whereas a noninvoluting congenital hemangioma (NICH) may continue to exhibit somatic growth late into childhood.[18,19] Gorincour and colleagues[18] have described imaging features that may help distinguish between infantile and CHs. A greater proportion of CHs possessed a more heterogeneous imaging appearance, and lesional borders tended to be less well defined. Interestingly, a portion of CHs showed calcifications, whereas none of the common hemangiomas had visible calcification. Venous thrombosis was also more common in CHs.[3,8,18,19] An example of NICH with follow-up imaging is shown in **Fig. 11**.

The kaposiform hemangioendothelioma is an endothelial-derived spindle cell neoplasm that is nonmetastasizing but locally aggressive and is classified as a "borderline" vascular tumor. This lesion presents as a rapidly growing postnatal mass and may be mistaken at first for an infantile hemangioma. On imaging, these lesions are considerably less well defined than infantile hemangiomas and often

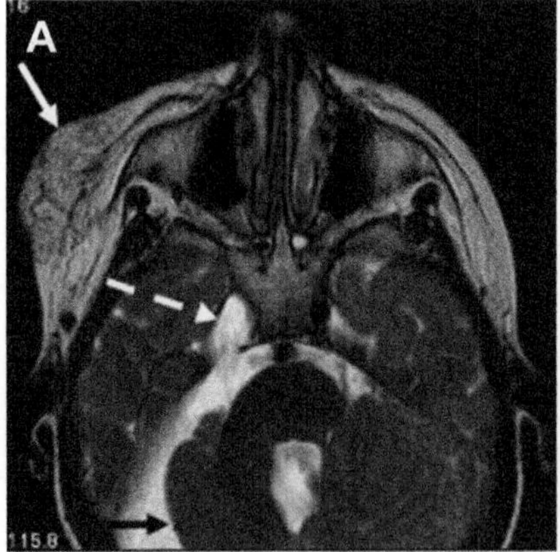


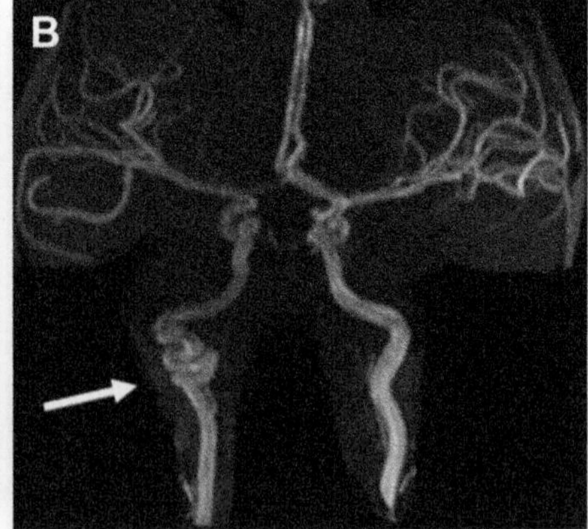


**Fig. 8.** PHACES. (*A*) Axial T2-weighted MRI of the brain in a patient with known right facial segmental infantile hemangioma (*white arrow*) shows ipsilateral enlargement of right Meckel's cave (dashed *arrow*), and hypoplasia of the right cerebellar hemisphere (*black arrow*). (*B*) MR angiogram volume-rendered anteroposterior view in the same patient shows tortuosity of a dysplastic right internal carotid artery (*arrow*).

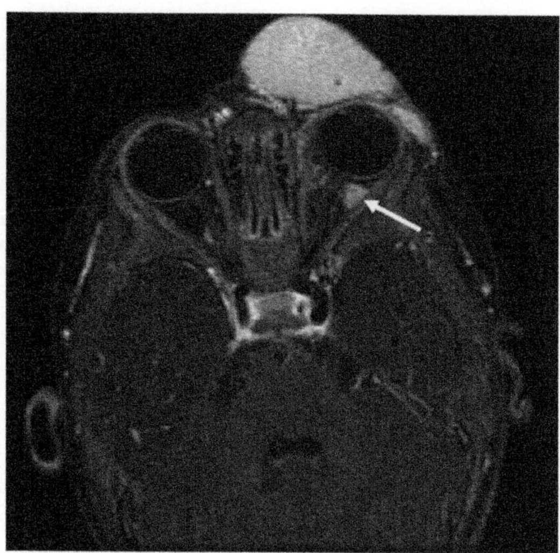

**Fig. 9.** Intraorbital infantile hemangioma. Postcontrast axial T1-weighted fat-suppressed image of a left orbital infantile hemangioma with intraconal component adjacent to the optic nerve (*arrow*).

demonstrate invasive borders[3] (**Fig. 12**), and, rarely, bony invasion. Platelet sequestration and a consumption coagulopathy ensue in more than 50% of cases, constituting Kasabach-Merritt syndrome.[20,21]

In general, the presence of a rapidly growing soft tissue lesion in a child may be worrisome to the parent and, on occasion, the primary health care provider, and imaging may be called upon to distinguish between a hemangioma and a malignant

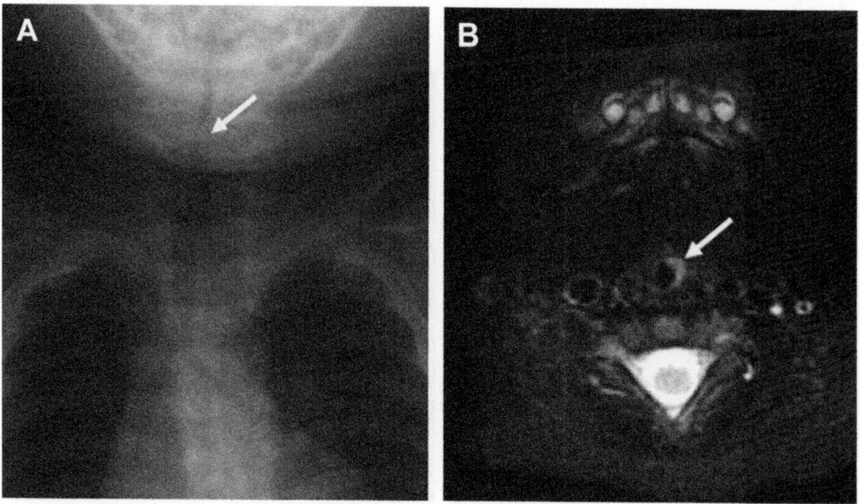


**Fig. 10.** Subglottic infantile hemangioma. (*A*) Frontal radiograph of the neck shows a rounded lesion along the left lower larynx with narrowing of the airway. (*B*) Axial STIR MRI shows a left subglottic submucosal mass contributing to airway narrowing, with moderately intense signal.

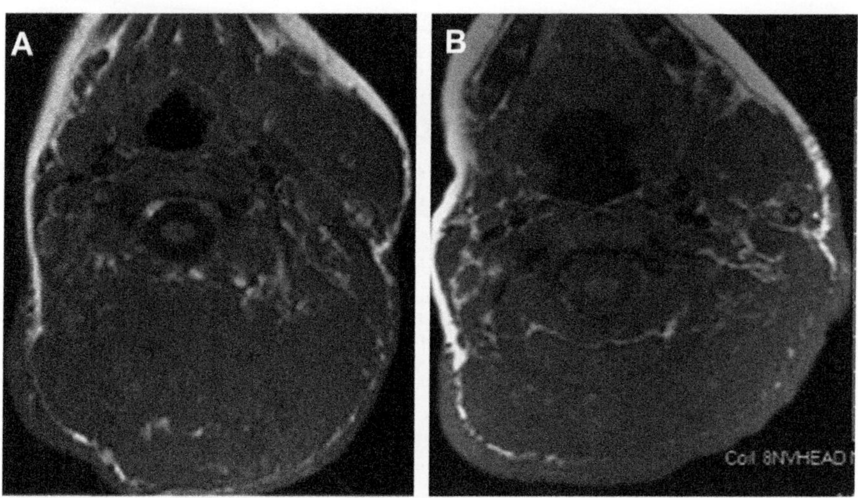


**Fig. 11.** NICH. (*A*) Axial T1-weighted MRI shows an extensive and multispatial left facial and posterior neck mass. (*B*) Axial T1-weighted MRI in the same patient 5 years later shows persistence of the mass in keeping with a NICH.

tumor, such as rhabdomyosarcoma. Confirmation of a well-defined lesion with the classic imaging features of hemangioma is reassuring. Teo and colleagues[11] described morphologic features that are significantly more common in hemangioma: lobulation, septation, and central signal voids. However, they found no reliable MRI feature that could distinguish between hemangioma and malignancy. As a general rule, a less well-circumscribed or infiltrative lesion suggests a malignant process such as rhabdomyosarcoma or metastatic neuroblastoma, especially when there is associated bone destruction (**Fig. 13**).[11]

Imaging features of infantile hemangiomas are summarized in **Table 2**.

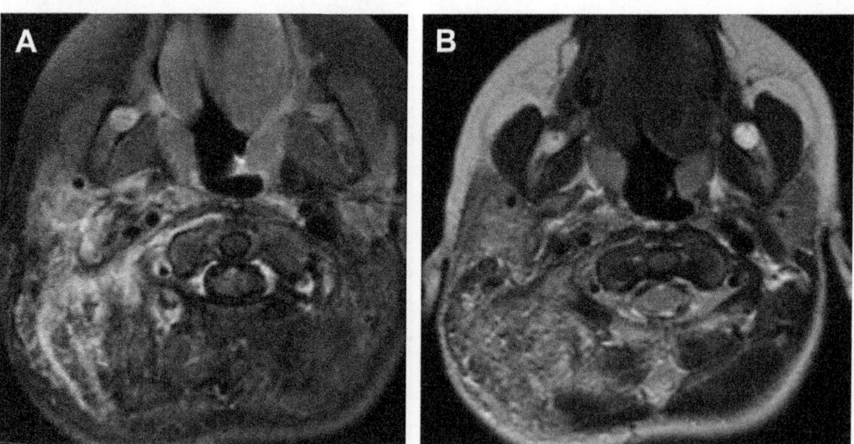


**Fig. 12.** Kaposiform hemangioendothelioma. (*A*) Axial T1-weighted contrast-enhanced fat-saturated MRI shows an ill-defined and more invasive enhancing lesion with infiltration of myofascial and deep facial planes. (*B*) Corresponding T2-weighted MRI shows ill-defined margins and infiltrative appearance.

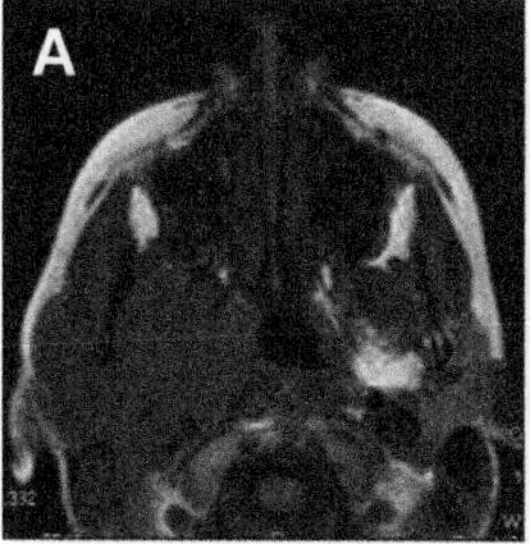

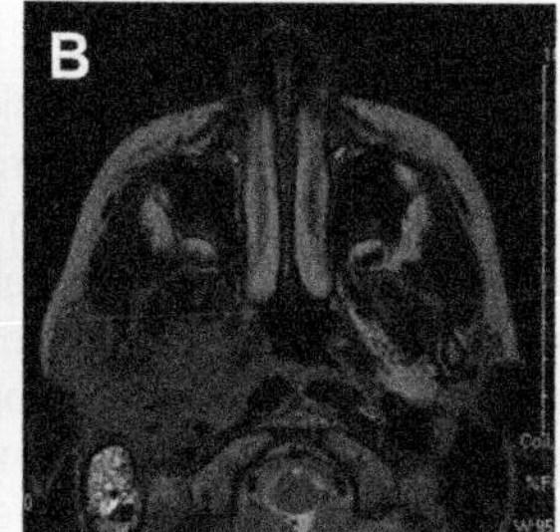

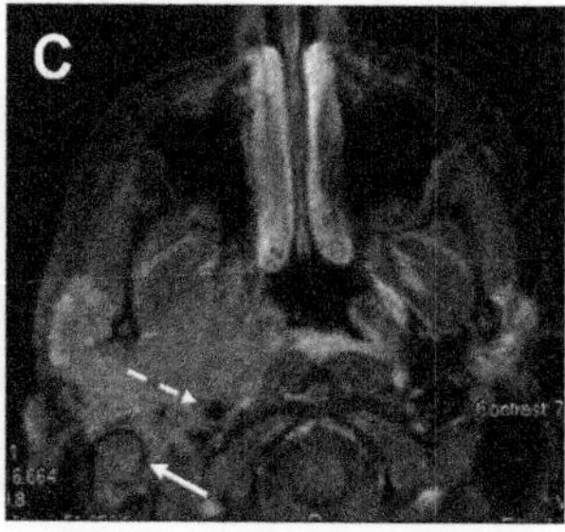


**Fig. 13.** Rhabdomyosarcoma. (*A*) Axial T1-weighted image shows an ill-defined mass in the right infratemporal fossa, masticator, and parapharyngeal space. (*B*) Corresponding T2-weighted MRI shows intermediate signal indicating hypercellularity of the mass. (*C*) Post-contrast axial T1-weighted fat-suppressed image shows enhancement of the mass, ill-defined margins, and invasive borders. There is encasement of the right internal carotid artery (*dashed arrow*), and enhancement may involve the mastoid cortex (*solid arrow*). Note that bony erosion or destruction may be more readily seen on CT.

**Table 2**
**Summary of imaging features of major vascular anomalies**

| Hemangioma Imaging Features | AVM Imaging Features | VM Imaging Features | LM Imaging Features |
|---|---|---|---|
| • Multilobular mass with distinct margins<br>• *Proliferative phase*: hypervascular with large internal and feeding/draining vessels on ultrasound/CT/MRI<br>• *Proliferative phase*: MRI shows avid enhancement and only moderate T2 hyperintensity reflecting hypercellularity<br>• *Involuting phase*: progressive diminution in enhancement with increasing fatty component<br>• *Involuted phase*: residual fibrofatty tissue and skeletal overgrowth may result in persistent facial asymmetry | • Ultrasound<br>○ Ill-defined vascular flow on color sonography<br>○ Doppler: high-velocity low-resistance arterial flow, pulsatile flow in venous drainage<br>• CT<br>○ Enlarged feeding and draining vessels<br>○ Osseous overgrowth and/or lysis<br>• MRI<br>○ No distinct mass<br>○ Tissue is permeated by vascular flow voids<br>○ Enlarged feeding and draining vessels<br>○ Mild enhancement and T2 hyperintensity reflect tissue edema | • Ultrasound<br>○ Tubular vascular channels with low-flow Doppler waveforms<br>○ Flow may augment with compression or Valsalva<br>• CT<br>○ Dynamically enhancing focal or transspatial mass<br>○ Presence of phleboliths is pathognomonic<br>• MRI<br>○ Dynamically enhancing focal or transspatial mass<br>○ Marked hyperintensity on T2-weighted imaging<br>○ No arterial flow voids | • Macrocystic LM<br>○ Image like cysts on US/CT/MRI with well-defined fluid-filled masses<br>○ MRI: fluid (low T1, high T2) signal without central enhancement. May have enhancement of thin capsule and/or internal septations<br>○ MRI: frequent internal hemorrhage results in fluid-fluid levels<br>• Microcystic LM<br>○ Multiple small "microcysts" with intervening solid septations, often with ill-defined, infiltrative margins<br>○ MRI: smaller relative fluid volume may result in lower T2 signal |

## IMAGING OF VASCULAR MALFORMATIONS

Vascular malformations, also known as vasoformative lesions, are a varied group of lesions that represent defects of vascular morphogenesis rather than neoplasms.[16] If small and deep, clinical presentation may be delayed into infancy or even childhood. Vascular malformations are named by their vessel of origin and further categorized into high-flow and slow-flow lesions.[5] High-flow lesions include arteriovenous malformations (AVM) or arteriovenous fistulae. The more common slow-flow malformations include VM, LM, or rarely combined lesions such as venolymphatic malformations (VLM). Imaging confirms the diagnosis, establishes involvement of deeper anatomy, and aims to exclude an alternative or more worrisome lesion. Imaging can also facilitate therapeutic intervention with angiographic and percutaneous treatment, for both diagnostic and therapeutic purposes.[1,16]

Ultrasound plays a role in the initial evaluation particularly for superficial lesions and is often the first line of imaging because of its availability and noninvasive technique. Color spectral imaging confirms the presence or absence of internal vascularity, and Doppler interrogation can distinguish between high- and low-flow lesions.

Cross-sectional imaging evaluation of vascular malformations mostly entails the use of MRI given its superior resolution of soft tissues. There is added utility of time-resolved MR angiography, allowing for depiction of arterial flow and venous drainage of an AVM or AV fistula, and pooling of contrast within a VM.[3] CT can be complementary to MRI, especially in the setting of a VM, where the presence of phleboliths is pathognomonic. CT also plays a role if there is any osseous involvement of a malformation.

An AVM is a high-flow lesion defined as an abnormal tangle or nidus of vessels with aberrant connection between arteries and veins. These may be clinically apparent as a reddish/purplish deformity with a palpable thrill. Chronic hyperemia to the regional anatomy may result in bony and muscular hypertrophy in some cases.[1] As there is no true intervening parenchyma, the malformation permeates the soft tissues, and imaging often fails to depict a discrete or circumscribed mass.[10]

Ultrasound may demonstrate an ill-defined lesion if the nidus is of sufficient volume. Doppler interrogation is helpful to establish flow characteristics. As an AVM bypasses a normal capillary bed, high velocity flow is met with low resistance.[4] Pulsatile and arterial type flow may be identified in its draining veins. The most specific imaging feature for AVM on MRI is the presence of flow voids, reflecting arterial flow within the lesion (**Fig. 14**).[10] AVMs appear as ill-defined regions of signal

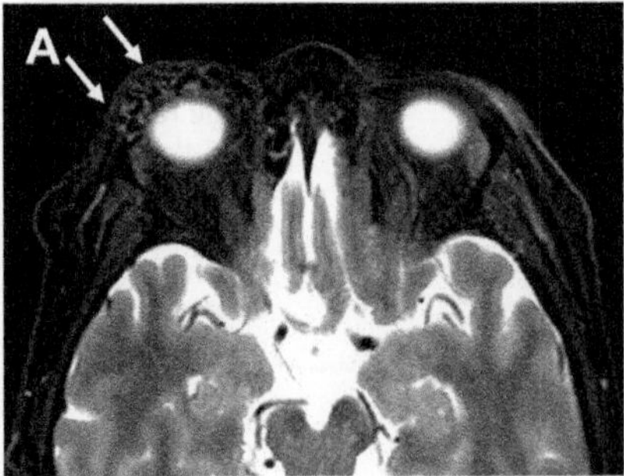


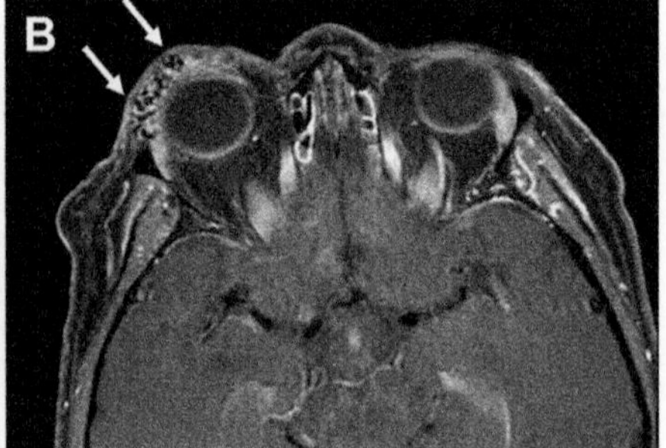


**Fig. 14.** AVM. (*A*) Axial STIR MRI of a right periorbital AVM shows a grouping of flow voids (*arrows*) without discrete mass. (*B*) Corresponding axial T1-weighted contrast-enhanced fat-suppressed MRI shows mild enhancement of in between flow voids (*arrows*) but, again, no discrete enhancing mass lesion. Enhancement mostly represents local hyperemia and edema.

abnormality with mild or no contrast enhancement and without discrete mass lesion (**Fig. 15**). Furthermore, early arterial flow as well as shunting into venous drainage can be established on time-resolved MR angiography.[3,15] CT is used primarily to evaluate the impact of an AVM on regional osseous structures, whether it be overgrowth secondary to chronic hyperperfusion or lysis reflecting intraosseous components of the lesion (**Fig. 16**). Conventional angiography is the gold standard for diagnosis and characterization of an AVM because this examination provides the best spatial resolution and temporal resolution to study vascular anatomy.[5] Therapeutic interventional procedures such as arterial or venous embolization can be performed using angiographic guidance or delivery.[6,16] The imaging features of AVMs are summarized in **Table 2**.

Slow-flow vascular malformations are relatively more common. The prototypical superficial lesion is the capillary malformation. Capillary malformations are readily apparent on clinical examination, and imaging plays little role in their diagnosis. The primary utility of imaging in the setting of facial capillary malformation, often referred to as "port wine stain," is to search for associated intracranial findings that may indicate the presence of underlying Sturge-Weber syndrome. These include ipsilateral cerebral pial angiomatosis that appears as characteristic tram-track cortical and subcortical calcifications on CT (**Fig. 17**), and as pial enhancement on MRI (**Fig. 18**). Chronic vascular steal phenomenon results in volume loss of the affected cerebral hemisphere (see **Figs. 17** and **18**).

VMs are composed of interconnected and sinusoidal venous channels that form as a result of a defect in vascular morphogenesis between the fourth and 10th weeks of gestation.[16] Classically, VMs involve multiple spaces of regional anatomy, especially in the neck, because they are not encapsulated lesions. Imaging therefore plays a vital role in precisely mapping the extent of a lesion. Figuratively speaking, a clinically evident bluish mass may be the tip of the iceberg, with voluminous malformation occupying deeper structures (**Fig. 19**). VM is common in the

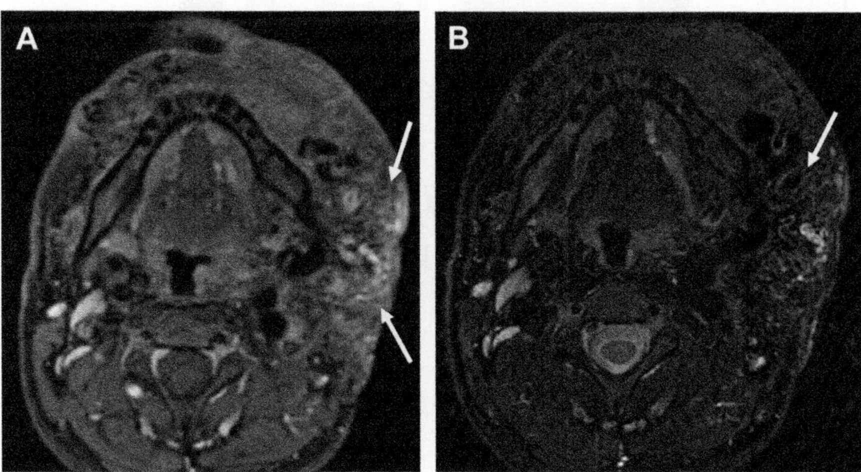


**Fig. 15.** AVM. (*A*) Axial T1-weighted contrast-enhanced fat-suppressed MRI shows a large and extensive facial AVM with mild and diffuse enhancement (*arrows*) between flow voids. (*B*) Corresponding axial STIR MRI shows multiple and extensive flow voids, one of which is marked with an arrow.

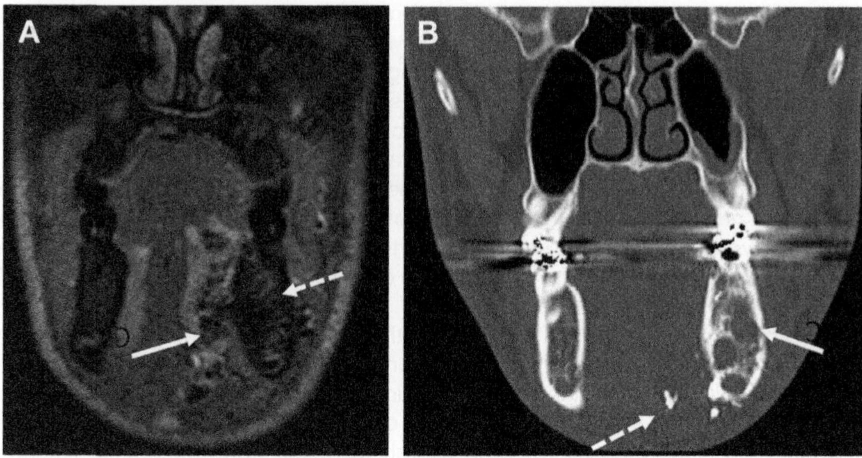


**Fig. 16.** AVM. (*A*) Coronal STIR MRI of a left floor of mouth AVM with internal flow voids (*solid arrow*) with enlargement of the adjacent mandible, which also contains flow voids within the medullary space (*dashed arrow*). (*B*) Corresponding coronal CT image of the same lesion shows expansion of the left hemimandible with several areas of bony lysis (*solid arrow*). There are amorphous dense foci in the left floor of mouth AVM that represent therapeutic embolization material (*dashed arrow*).

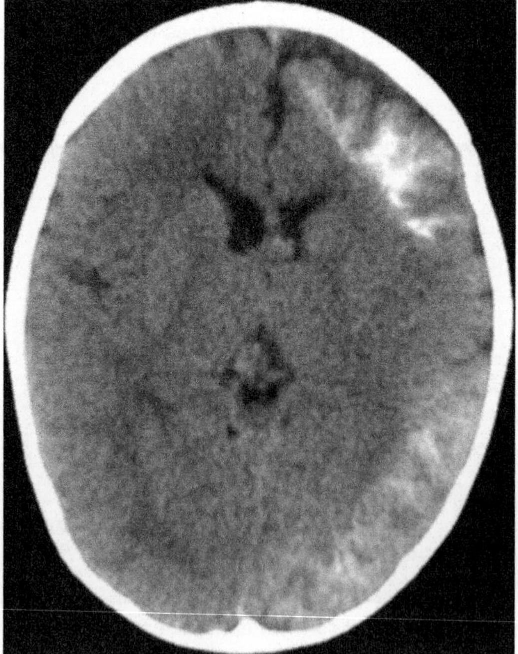

**Fig. 17.** Sturge-Weber. Axial CT image shows left cerebral hemisphere volume loss with diffuse cortical and subcortical calcification.

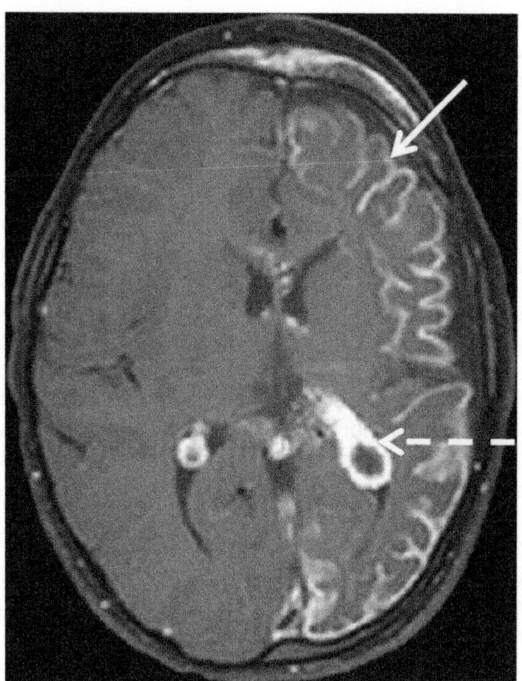

**Fig. 18.** Sturge-Weber. Axial T1-weighted postcontrast MRI shows diffuse pial enhancement representing angiomatosis (*solid arrow*) as well as a left choroid plexus angioma (*dashed arrow*). Note the diffuse volume loss of the left cerebral hemisphere.

parotid, buccal, and masticator spaces with deeper pharyngeal or palatal extension. Thrombi within a lesion may calcify over time and form phleoboliths, a specific and pathognomonic imaging feature of VM. Imaging features of a VM are summarized in **Table 2**.

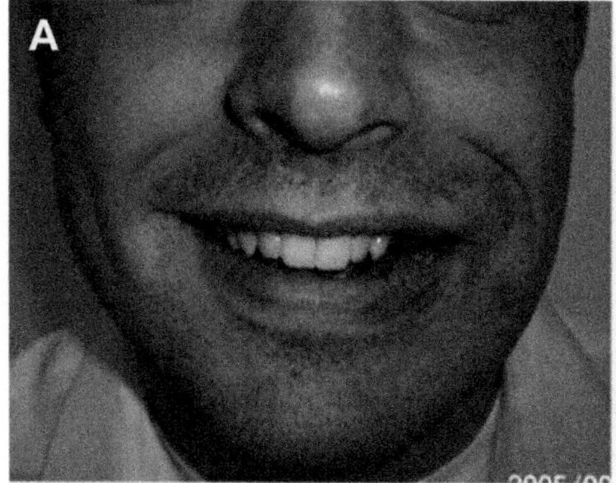


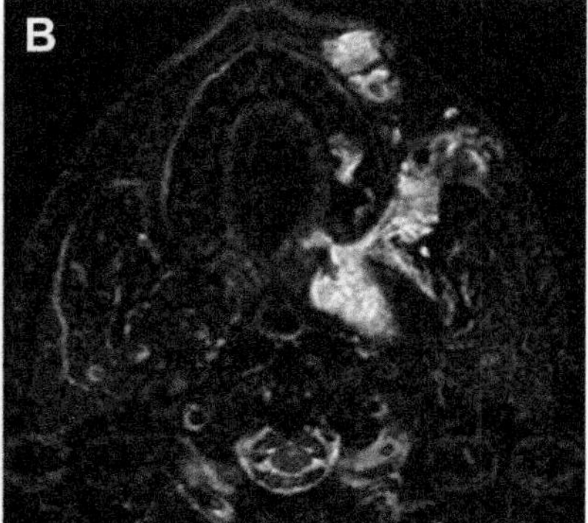


**Fig. 19.** VM. (*A*) Photograph of a patient with clinically evident bluish lip mass. (*B*) Axial STIR MRI shows the left lip VM with multispatial involvement, not clinically apparent, involving the buccal space, muscles of mastication, and deep parapharyngeal space and oral cavity at the palate.

On ultrasound, a VM is seen as a lobulated hypoechoic mass with tubular or sinusoidal regions of vascular flow. Doppler interrogation may depict venous waveforms with augmentation occurring during local compression or a Valsalva maneuver, for example, when an infant cries. Phleboliths may be seen as shadowing echogenic foci on ultrasound (**Fig. 20**) and are even better depicted as radiodense rounded calcified foci on CT (**Fig. 21**).[5]

Because VMs are composed of tubules or channels of slowly flowing blood, there is high water content within the lesion and therefore very hyperintense signal on T2-weighted MRI (**Fig. 22**A). This imaging feature may be helpful in distinguishing a VM from a hemangioma, which will typically demonstrate more intermediate T2 signal. Phleboliths appear as rounded foci of signal void within the lesion that are visible on T2-weighted imaging and sometimes on T1-weighted imaging (**Fig. 22**B). Gadolinium will accumulate slowly within these vascular channels, with early patchy enhancement that will demonstrably "fill in" on delayed images (**Fig. 22**C, D). Neither conventional nor MR angiography plays an important role in the assessment of slow-flow malformations such as VM. Interventional radiologists do have a role in treatment of VMs, as sclerotherapy performed via direct lesional puncture is an important component of therapy.[16]

LMs are composed of endothelium-lined channels akin to their venous counterparts, but represent a defect in lymphatic morphogenesis. Failure of lymphatic channel assimilation results in a malformation with pools of sequestered lymph. LMs can be classified as macrocystic, microcystic, or mixed based on the size of the lymphatic channels, with corresponding differences in their imaging appearance. Small and/or deep LMs may remain undetected until adulthood, when rapid enlargement in the setting of infection or intralesional hemorrhage may first bring the lesion to clinical attention. Of note, the vast majority of LMs occur in the head and neck, reported at an incidence of 70% to 80%.[16]

As with their venous counterparts, LMs are often multispatial, and thus, MRI is most useful in depicting precise mapping of the malformation. CT is best used to evaluate bony abnormalities; for example, an enlarging malformation may remodel or scallop the adjacent bone, and LMs in the "beard" distribution frequently result in facial skeletal abnormalities.[22]

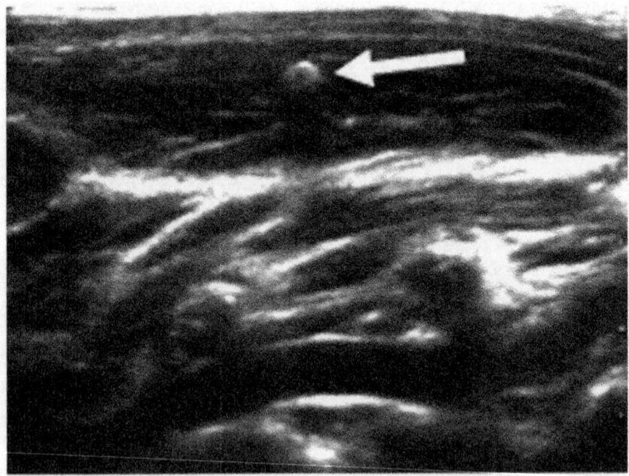

**Fig. 20.** VM, ultrasound. Grayscale ultrasound image shows a lobular hypoechnoic mass with a small rounded echogenic focus (*arrow*). Note the acoustic shadowing deep to the focus. Appearance is diagnostic of a small calcified phlebolith.

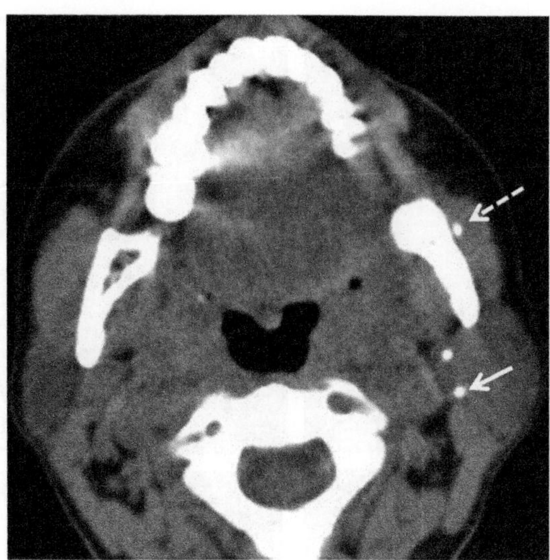

**Fig. 21.** VM, CT. Axial noncontrast CT image in a patient with a left facial VM shows small calcified phleboliths in both the left masseter muscle (*dashed arrow*) and the parotid gland (*solid arrow*).

Imaging features of LMs, summarized in **Table 2**, vary depending on whether there is macrocystic or microcystic composition. Macrocystic LMs on ultrasound will appear as hypoechoic and avascular masses with occasional thin septations (**Fig. 23**). On MRI, these lesions image like cysts, with very low T1 and high T2 signal (**Fig. 24**A). Contrast enhancement of a macrocystic LM is typically minimal in the absence of infection or inflammation (**Fig. 24**B). When there is hemorrhage into a retrobulbar orbital LM, acute and often dramatic proptosis may result. The presence of hemorrhagic fluid-fluid levels within these macrocystic spaces is virtually diagnostic of an LM[10] (**Fig. 25**).

Macrocystic LMs are soft and compressible lesions that tend to insinuate around structures rather than displacing them. In fact, an intraorbital LM may be indented by the optic nerve sheath and extraocular muscles, a useful finding that may help distinguish them from more ominous lesions (**Fig. 26**). Orbital LM and VLMs have additional association with intracranial vascular anomalies, and contrast-enhanced MRI of the brain is suggested for complete workup.[23]

Microcystic LMs are composed of much smaller cystic spaces and a larger proportion of solid septations. On ultrasound, a microcystic LM may appear more echogenic than its macrocystic counterpart due to increased number of interfaces between microcyst walls.[4] On MRI, this results in less intense signal on T2-weighted imaging. Microcystic LMs appear ill defined and infiltrative with occasional mild enhancement. A common presentation is the so-called beard distribution, where a multispatial LM crosses midline at the level of the oral cavity (**Fig. 27**). Rarely, a lesion will demonstrate both enhancing and nonenhancing dysplastic vascular components and will be classified as a VLM.

LMs occasionally occur in a syndromic fashion, and imaging may identify asymptomatic associated lesions. Multifocal or diffuse lymphangiomatosis is associated with frequent skeletal involvement that may be asymptomatic in the absence of pathologic fracture (**Fig. 28**). It is crucial to establish the presence of osseous involvement

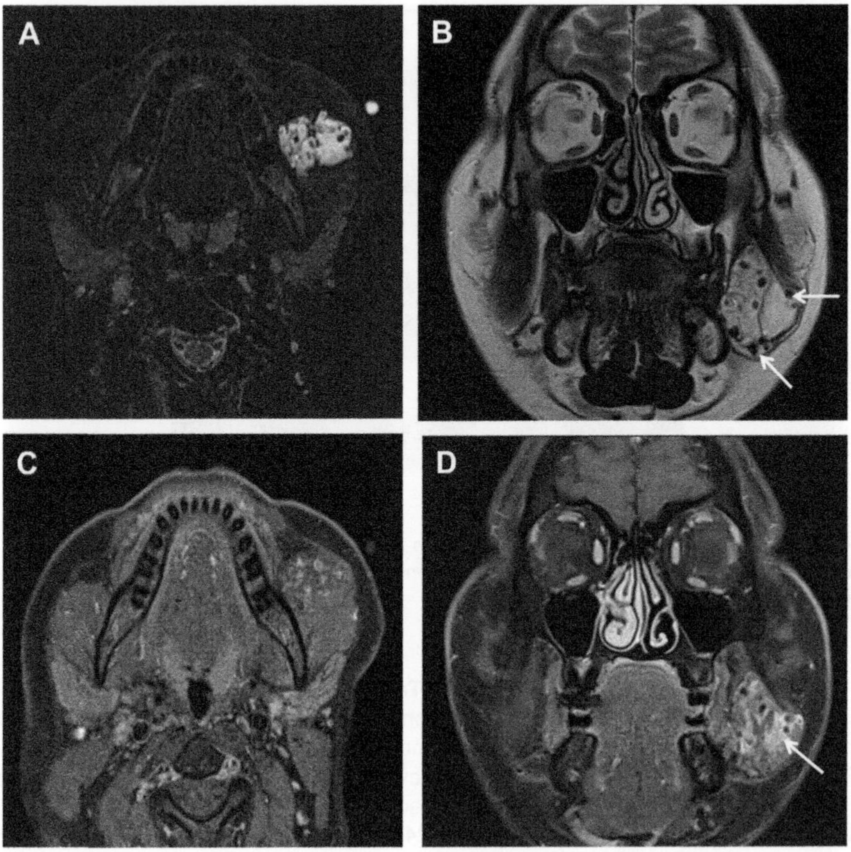

**Fig. 22.** VM, MRI. (*A*) Axial STIR MRI shows a lobulated and very hyperintense mass along the anterior margin of the left masseter muscle. (*B*) Coronal T2-weighted MRI shows several round foci of signal void representing phleboliths. (*C*) Axial T1-weighted postcontrast and fat-suppressed MRI shows incomplete central enhancement. (*D*) Coronal T1-weighted postcontrast and fat-suppressed MRI acquired 6 minutes after the axial acquisition shows further central enhancement, characteristic of a slow-flow VM.

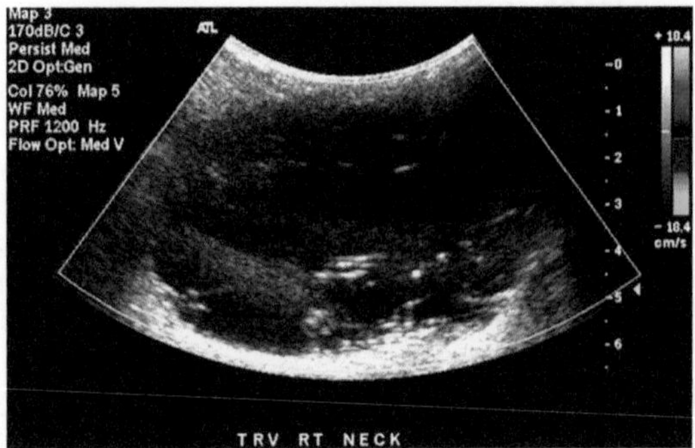


**Fig. 23.** LM, ultrasound. Ultrasound image shows a lobulated hypoechoic mass with internal echogenic septa. Color flow shows no visible color signal to imply vascular flow.

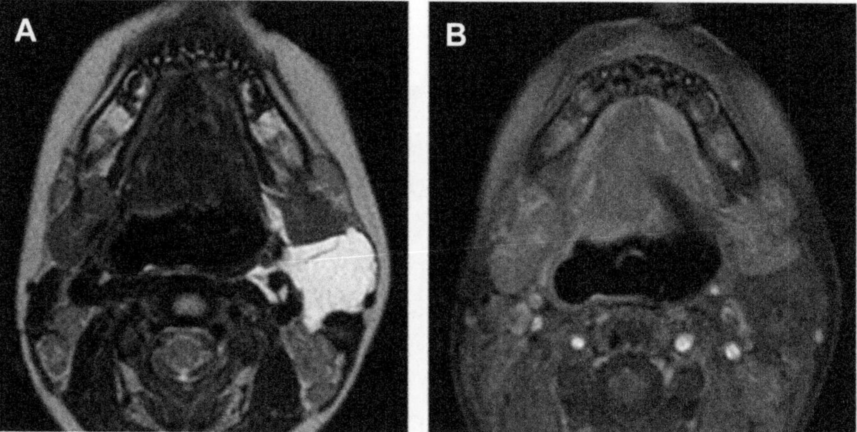


**Fig. 24.** LM, MRI. (*A*) Axial T2-weighted MRI of the neck shows a markedly hyperintense lesion in the left parotid space, which insinuates along fascial planes medially. Homogenous appearance favors a macrocystic form of LM. (*B*) Axial T1-weighted contrast-enhanced fat-suppressed MRI shows no evidence of internal or peripheral enhancement.

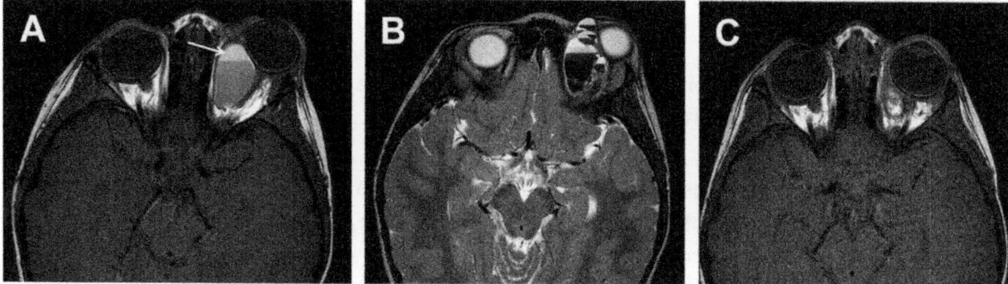


**Fig. 25.** LM, orbital. (*A*) Axial T1-weighted MRI shows a left orbital mass with internal fluid level with fluid of hyperintense signal on T1-weighted imaging (*arrow*). Appearance is consistent with hemorrhage in a LM. Note the mass effect upon the left globe and proptosis. (*B*) Axial T2-weighted MRI at a level just superior to that of A is an appearance of multiple cystic spaces with fluid-fluid levels (*solid arrows*). Note recent blood products appear hypointense on T2-weighted imaging (*dashed arrow*). (*C*) Axial T1-weighted MRI obtained after percutaneous sclerotherapy of the left orbital LM shows marked reduction in volume of the lesion and near resolution of proptosis.

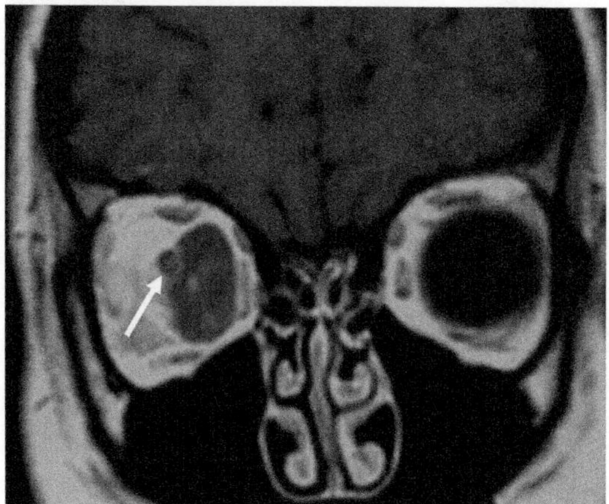

**Fig. 26.** LM, orbital. Coronal T1-weighted MRI shows a right orbital intraconal mass, which is contoured by the optic nerve (*arrow*), a sign of a noninvasive and compressible lesion, a feature that argues against a more worrisome lesion or neoplasm.

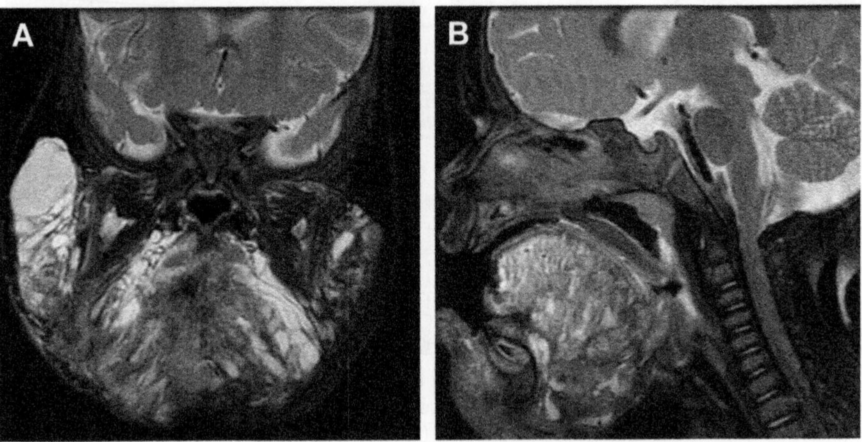

**Fig. 27.** LM, microcystic. (*A*) Coronal STIR MRI of a microcystic LM demonstrates innumerable rounded components of T2-hyperintense malformation with transspatial involvement in the face. Lesions that involve the oral cavity tend to cross midline in a so-called beard distribution. (*B*) Sagittal STIR MRI of the same patient again shows the transspatial extent of the malformation in the oral cavity and floor of mouth. MR appearance is that of a more ill-defined lesion compared with a macrocystic LM.

because lesions may enlarge with somatic growth of the child and with hormonal stimulation. Another entity of note is Gorham-Stout disease, also described as "vanishing bone disease." In this rare entity, intraosseous proliferation of lymphatic vessels results in progressive and often dramatic skeletal osteolysis.

### *Imaging Differential Diagnosis*

A simplified MRI-based diagnostic algorithm can be used to differentiate between the most common vascular lesions. **Table 3** summarizes this simplified approach using discriminatory MRI features.

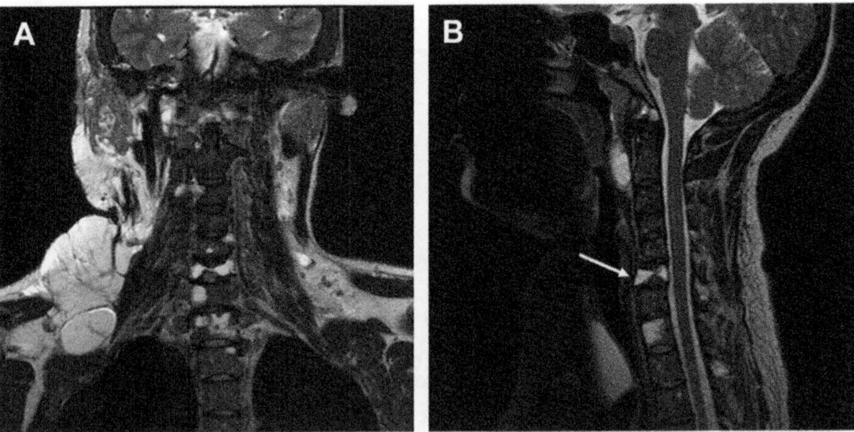

**Fig. 28.** Lymphangiomatosis. (*A*) Coronal T2-weighted MRI shows a right neck LM with osseous involvement seen in the C5 through T1 vertebral bodies. (*B*) Sagittal T2-weighted image of the same patient shows pathologic compression deformity of C6 (*arrow*). Note malformation in the retropharyngeal space and at the thoracic inlet as well.

**Table 3**
**Simplified algorithm of magnetic resonance appearance of major vascular anomalies**

| | (+) Enhancement | (−) Enhancement |
|---|---|---|
| Intermediate T2 signal | Hemangioma | AVM |
| High T2 signal | VM | LM |

The first discriminatory imaging finding is the presence or absence of contrast enhancement. Hemangiomas and VMs will enhance intensely. AVMs and LMs will enhance minimally, if at all.

The second discriminatory imaging finding is appearance on T2-weighted imaging. VMs and macrocystic LMs will exhibit very intense T2-weighted signal because of their cystic composition with pooling of slowly flowing blood or lymph, respectively. Hemangiomas as vascular neoplasms have a cellular composition and will show more intermediate T2 signal intensity. AVMs typically show similar mild T2 hyperintensity reflecting tissue edema.

## SUMMARY

Imaging plays an important role in evaluating vascular lesions not fully amenable to clinical examination and in the diagnostic work-up of lesions that are of uncertain cause. Although ultrasonography may provide important information about vascularity and morphology in lesions that are superficial, it has limited application in the assessment of deeper structures and their relation to bony anatomy. Because of its superior tissue contrast and lack of ionizing radiation, MRI has emerged as an important tool for both initial diagnosis of vascular lesions and assessment of treatment response. CT is generally reserved as a complementary examination for identification of calcified elements that may confirm a suspected diagnosis (eg, phleboliths in VM) or in assessing lesional impact on the facial skeleton.

## REFERENCES


1. Mulliken JB, Burrows PE, Fishman SJ. Mulliken & Young's vascular anomalies: hemangiomas and malformations. New York: Oxford University Press; 2013.
2. Burrows PE, Laor T, Paltiel H, et al. Diagnostic imaging in the evaluation of vascular birthmarks. Dermatol Clin 1998;16(3):455–88.
3. Dubois JCA, Alison M. Vascular anomalies: what a radiologist needs to know. Pediatr Radiol 2010;40(6):895–905.
4. Paltiel HJ, Burrows PE, Kozakewich HPW, et al. Soft-tissue vascular anomalies: utility of US for diagnosis. Radiology 2000;214(3):747–54.
5. Abernethy LJ. Classification and imaging of vascular malformations in children. Eur Radiol 2003;13(11):2483–97.
6. Bittles MA, Sidhu MK, Sze RW, et al. Multidetector CT angiography of pediatric vascular malformations and hemangiomas: utility of 3-D reformatting in differential diagnosis. Pediatr Radiol 2005;35(11):1100–6.
7. Bulas DI, Goske MJ, Applegate KE, et al. Image gently: why we should talk to parents about CT in children. AJR Am J Roentgenol 2009;192(5):1176–8.
8. Strauss KJ, Goske MJ, Kaste SC, et al. Image gently: ten steps you can take to optimize image quality and lower CT dose for pediatric patients. AJR Am J Roentgenol 2010;194(4):868–73.

9. Meyer JS, Hoffer FA, Barnes PD, et al. Biological classification of soft-tissue vascular anomalies: MR correlation. AJR Am J Roentgenol 1991;157(3):559–64.
10. Stein-Wexler R. MR imaging of soft tissue masses in children. Magn Reson Imaging Clin N Am 2009;17(3):489–507.
11. Teo E-LHJ, Strouse PJ, Hernandez RJ. MR imaging differentiation of soft-tissue hemangiomas from malignant soft-tissue masses. AJR Am J Roentgenol 2000; 174(6):1623–8.
12. Cauldwell C. Anesthesia risks associated with pediatric imaging. Pediatr Radiol 2011;41(8):949–50.
13. Schulte-Uentrop L, Goepfert MS. Anaesthesia or sedation for MRI in children. Curr Opin Anaesthesiol 2010;23(4):513–7.
14. Viswanathan V, Smith E, Mulliken J, et al. Infantile hemangiomas involving the neuraxis: clinical and imaging findings. AJNR Am J Neuroradiol 2009;30(5): 1005–13.
15. Krishnamurthy R, Muthupillai R, Chung T. Pediatric body MR angiography. Magn Reson Imaging Clin N Am 2009;17(1):133–44.
16. Dubois JE, Garel L. Imaging and therapeutic approach of hemangiomas and vascular malformations in the pediatric age group. Pediatr Radiol 1999;29(12): 879–93.
17. Judd CD, Chapman PR, Koch B, et al. Intracranial infantile hemangiomas associated with PHACE syndrome. AJNR Am J Neuroradiol 2007;28(1):25–9.
18. Gorincour G, Kokta V, Rypens F, et al. Imaging characteristics of two subtypes of congenital hemangiomas: rapidly involuting congenital hemangiomas and non-involuting congenital hemangiomas. Pediatr Radiol 2005;35(12):1178–85.
19. Enjolras O, Mulliken JB, Boon LM, et al. Noninvoluting congenital hemangioma: a rare cutaneous vascular anomaly. Plast Reconstr Surg 2001;107(7):1647–54.
20. Lalaji TA, Haller JO, Burgess RJ. A case of head and neck kaposiform hemangioendothelioma simulating a malignancy on imaging. Pediatr Radiol 2001; 31(12):876–8.
21. Khong P-L, Burrows PE, Kozakewich HP, et al. Fast-flow lingual vascular anomalies in the young patient: is imaging diagnostic? Pediatr Radiol 2003;33(2): 118–22.
22. O TM, Kwak R, Portnof JE, et al. Analysis of skeletal mandibular abnormalities associated with cervicofacial lymphatic malformations. Laryngoscope 2010; 121(1):91–101.
23. Bisdorff AJNR, Mulliken JB, Carrico J, et al. Intracranial vascular anomalies in patients with periorbital lymphatic and lymphaticovenous malformations. AJNR Am J Neuroradiol 2007;28(2):335–41.

# Infantile Hemangiomas in the Head and Neck Region

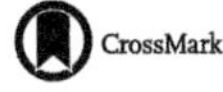

Denise M. Adams, MD[a,b,c,*], Kiersten W. Ricci, MD[a,b,c]

**KEYWORDS**

- Infantile hemangioma • Focal • Segmental/regional/diffuse hemangioma
- Hepatic hemangioma • Propranolol • Timolol

**KEY POINTS**

- Infantile hemangioma occurs in 4% to 5% of infants and is the most common benign vascular tumor of infancy.
- Infantile hemangiomas are also classified into 3 distinct morphologic patterns that include focal, segmental/regional/diffuse, or multifocal lesions.
- Most infantile hemangiomas can be diagnosed by clinical history and physical examination.

## NATURAL HISTORY

Infantile hemangioma (IH) occurs in 4% to 5% of infants and is the most common benign vascular tumor of infancy. They are not present at birth; but commonly there is a precursor lesion, such as an area of pallor, telangiectasia, or small purple area, that then brightens in color and increases in size becoming more apparent at 3 to 7 weeks of age.[1–3] The lesion then proliferates for an average of 3 to 5 months and then involutes over several years. With involution, the overlying skin is not normal and at times areas of abnormal texture, color, or residual fibroadipose tissue can be seen.

IHs are categorized as superficial, deep, or compound[1–3] (**Fig. 1**). Superficial hemangiomas appear at birth as red plaquelike lesions with minimal elevation. Deep hemangiomas are soft masslike lesions that can have a blue hue and are warm on palpation. They appear later (2–3 months), especially in areas with excess fatty tissue,

Disclosure: The authors have nothing to disclose.

[a] Division of Hematology, Vascular Anomalies Center, Boston Children's Hospital, 300 Longwood Avenue, Boston, MA 02115, USA; [b] Oncology, Boston Children's Hospital, 300 Longwood Avenue, Boston, MA 02115, USA; [c] Division of Hematology, Hemangioma and Vascular Malformation Center, Cancer and Blood Diseases Institute, Cincinnati Children's Hospital Medical Center, Cincinnati, OH, USA

* Corresponding author. Vascular Anomalies Center, Boston Children's Hospital, 300 Longwood Avenue, Fegan 3rd Floor, Boston, MA 02115.

*E-mail address:* denise.adams@childrens.harvard.edu

Otolaryngol Clin N Am 51 (2018) 77–87
https://doi.org/10.1016/j.otc.2017.09.009
0030-6665/18/

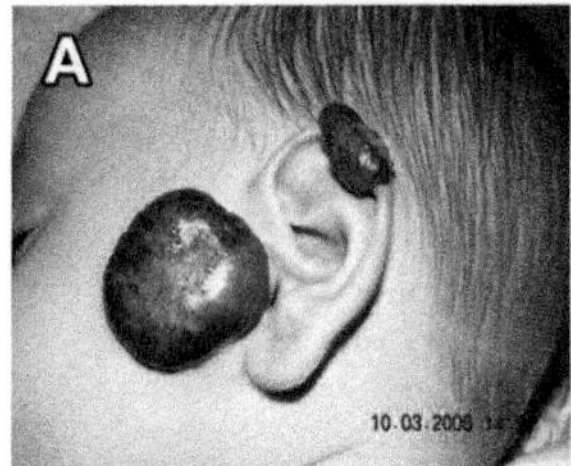

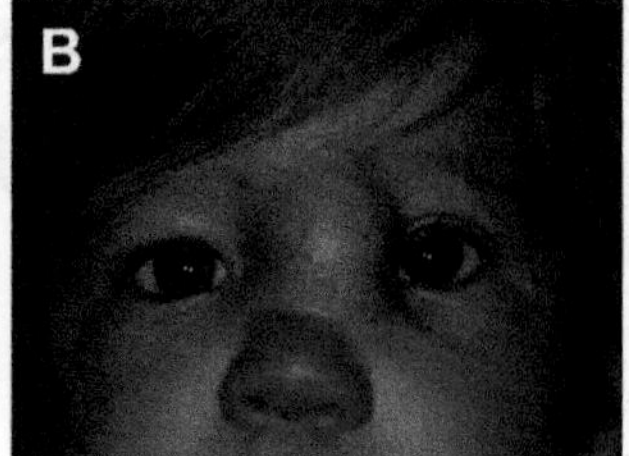

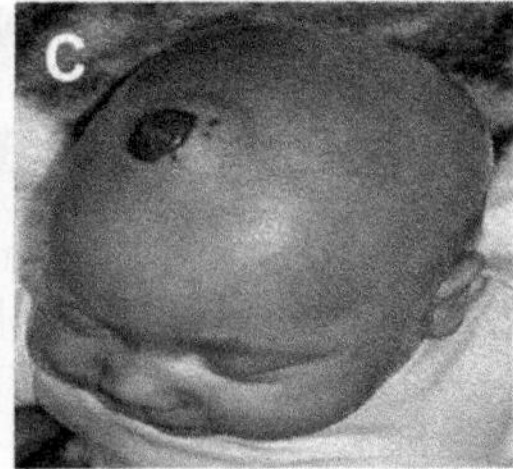


**Fig. 1.** IH; (*A*) superficial, local pedunculated infantile hemangioma; (*B*) deep, focal hemangioma; (*C*) compound hemangioma with deep and superficial components.

such as the neck and axilla. At times, these are confused with other soft tissue tumors; ultrasound will reveal a high-flow lesion with a typical wave characteristic of an infantile hemangioma. Mixed hemangiomas have both superficial and deep components that allow easier identification.

IHs are also classified into 3 distinct morphologic patterns that include solitary, segmental/regional/diffuse, or multifocal lesions.[1–3] These patterns are significant as they can be a clue to the possibility of other underlying syndromes. Solitary lesions are the most common, are usually uncomplicated, and commonly do not require intervention unless on an area that has a high risk for complications. IHs that cover a diffuse area have a higher risk of complications, such as ulceration, and also can be associated with syndromes, such as PHACE (posterior fossae abnormalities, hemangiomas, arterial/aortic anomalies, cardiac anomalies, eye abnormalities) (**Table 1**) and LUMBAR (lower-body hemangioma and other cutaneous defects, urogenital anomalies, ulceration, myelopathy, bony deformities, anorectal malformations, arterial anomalies, and renal anomalies) or be in a bearded distribution and have an increased risk of

**Table 1**
**PHACE syndrome**

| PHACE | Anomalies | Risk |
|---|---|---|
| *P*osterior fossa anomalies | Cerebellar anomalies (Dandy-Walker malformation) | Developmental delay<br>Pituitary dysfunctions |
| *H*emangioma | Large facial hemangioma >5 cm, large bearded distribution, shoulder, neck, back | Disfigurement, airway lesion, ulceration |
| *A*rterial | Cerebrovascular anomalies of major vessels: dysplasia, stenosis/occlusion, hypoplasia/aplasia, aberrant origin, saccular aneurysm<br>Persistent embryonic arteries | Progressive arterial occlusion<br>Stroke<br>Other neurologic issues |
| *C*ardiac | Aortic arch anomalies including coarctation of the aorta, aortic dysplasia, aberrant subclavian artery, right-sided aortic arch, ventricular septal defect, atrial septal defect | Congenital heart disease requiring surgical repair |
| *E*ye | Microphthalmos, retinal vascular abnormalities, persistent fetal retinal vessels, exophthalmos, coloboma, and optic nerve atrophy | Visual loss |

airway lesions. Finally, multiple IHs are defined as greater than 5 lesions that can occur over the body. They are usually small in size (millimeters) and can be associated with internal lesions most commonly in the liver.

Most IHs can be diagnosed by clinical history and physical examination. A biopsy is rarely needed and performed only if there are atypical features and/or an atypical history and/or presentation. For most hemangiomas, imaging is also not necessary. For deep hemangiomas, ultrasound imaging is beneficial for diagnosis, as it reveals a high-flow lesion with a typical Doppler wave characteristic.[4] MRI is rarely needed unless there is a question about diagnosis, internal lesions, or associated syndromes.

## PATHOLOGY AND BIOLOGY

IHs are benign cutaneous tumors that primarily consist of capillaries and proliferating endothelial cells and histologically stain positive for glucose transporter 1 (GLUT-1) during all phases of their life cycle.[2] IHs are more common in female patients, white non-Hispanic patients, and premature infants.[1,5] They are associated with advanced maternal age and placental complications.[1–3]

Most IHs occur sporadically and are not inherited; however, they may be caused by a rare autosomal dominant abnormality of chromosome 5.[6] Interestingly, IH proliferation is based on vasculogenesis or the formation of new blood vessels from angioblasts.[7–16] During the proliferative phase, angiogenic factors, such as vascular endothelial growth factor (VEGF), fibroblast growth factor (FGF), CD34, CD31, CD133, LYVE-1, and insulinlike growth factor 2 (IGF-2) are expressed while in involution and IHs express increased apoptosis. During involution, there are also increased mast cells and levels of metalloproteinase as well as upregulation of interferon and decreased basic FGF. Research has shown that IH endothelial cells are clonal in nature; throughout their development, they express a particular phenotype showing positive staining for GLUT-1.[17] GLUT-1 is also expressed on placental endothelial cells but is absent in other vascular malformations and most other vascular tumors.

Because IHs are associated with conditions related to placental hypoxia and multiple targets of hypoxia[1–4] are demonstrated in proliferating hemangiomas, such as VEGF-A, GLUT-1, and IGF-2,[18,19] preliminary research had focused on the role of hypoxia in hemangioma pathogenesis. The hypotheses suggest that a proliferating hemangioma is an attempt to normalize hypoxic tissue that occurred in utero.

## COMPLICATIONS

Although IHs are considered benign and most do not require intervention, complications can be life threatening (visceral lesions) or cause significant disfigurement with possible long-term psychological issues. It is, thus, very important for physicians to be aware of these issues and monitor patients closely. Knowledge of the lesions at high potential risk for complications is critical for early intervention and ultimate improvement of patients' quality of life. High-risk anatomic sites and potential complications include periorbital location (visual compromise), mandibular or beard distribution (airway lesions), nasal tip (disfigurement), auricular (ulceration and disfigurement), lumbosacral (LUMBAR syndrome), large facial lesions (PHACE syndrome, ulceration, and disfigurement), and multifocal presentation (internal lesions).

## ULCERATION

Ulceration can cause significant pain and disfigurement.[20–22] Risk factors include certain anatomic locations (lip, anogenital area, ear, chest, upper back, lumbar/sacral region, and gluteal region) as well as large diffuse lesions over the face or extremities. Ulceration is the most frequent and urgent complication for IHs. Ulcerations occur in the proliferative phase, and early warning signs can be a black central pinpoint area or a white/gray discoloration. Rapid treatment is critical, as ulceration causes pain, dysfunction, and scarring. Treatment includes proper wound care, pain control, and decreasing hemangioma proliferation with medical therapy.

Appropriate wound care should be initiated with a plastic surgery and dermatology team and includes topical ointments to help reduce crusting and decrease friction as well as the use of topical antibiotics, especially for the anogenital area to reduce infection. Nonstick dressing is also beneficial. If crusting occurs, wet to dry dressings can be applied or other techniques to debride the wound. A pulse dye laser has been used to improve pain and augment healing. Most important to healing is decreasing the proliferation of the hemangioma by systemic treatments, which are discussed later in this article.

## AIRWAY INFANTILE HEMANGIOMA

Airway IHs are usually associated with segmental hemangiomas in a bearded distribution, which may include all or some of the following: the preauricular skin, mandible, lower lip, chin, or anterior neck, although they can be found without skin lesions.[23] It is important for an otolaryngologist to proactively assess lesions in this distribution before signs of stridor occur. The incidence of an airway IH increases with increased area of bearded involvement. Medical management is essential for airway hemangiomas. Most physicians will use higher dosages of propranolol (3 mg/kg/d), and medical therapy is usually needed for a longer period of time. The presentation and management of airway IH are covered in more detail in this chapter.

## PERIORBITAL INFANTILE HEMANGIOMA

Periorbital hemangiomas can cause visual compromise.[24] This compromise usually occurs with hemangiomas of the upper medial eyelid, but any hemangioma around the eye that is large enough can obstruct the visual axis. The clinician should be aware of subcutaneous periocular hemangiomas, as these lesions can extend into the orbit, causing exophthalmos or globe displacement with only limited cutaneous manifestations. Issues with these lesions are astigmatism from direct pressure of the growing hemangioma, ptosis, proptosis, and strabismus. One of the leading causes of preventable blindness in children is stimulus-deprivation amblyopia caused by hemangioma obstruction. All periorbital hemangiomas or those with any possibility of potential visual impairment should have an ophthalmologic evaluation and follow-up until the hemangioma has undergone involution.

## SYNDROMES ASSOCIATED WITH INFANTILE HEMANGIOMA

### *Please Check this Listing of "PHACE Items"*

PHACE syndrome is the association of large facial (most commonly IH) with other structural or developmental anomalies (**Fig. 2**). PHACE syndrome is more common in girls, full-term, normal-birth-weight, and singleton infants.[25,26] The syndrome is not rare among patients with IHs. A prospective study of 108 infants with large facial hemangiomas observed 31% of patients had PHACE syndrome.[27] The cause for this condition is still unknown. The diagnostic criteria for PHACE association have previously been published.[28] The most common extracutaneous manifestations of PHACE association are cerebrovascular anomalies followed by congenital heart disease, ocular abnormalities, and midline defects. Importantly, the cerebrovascular and

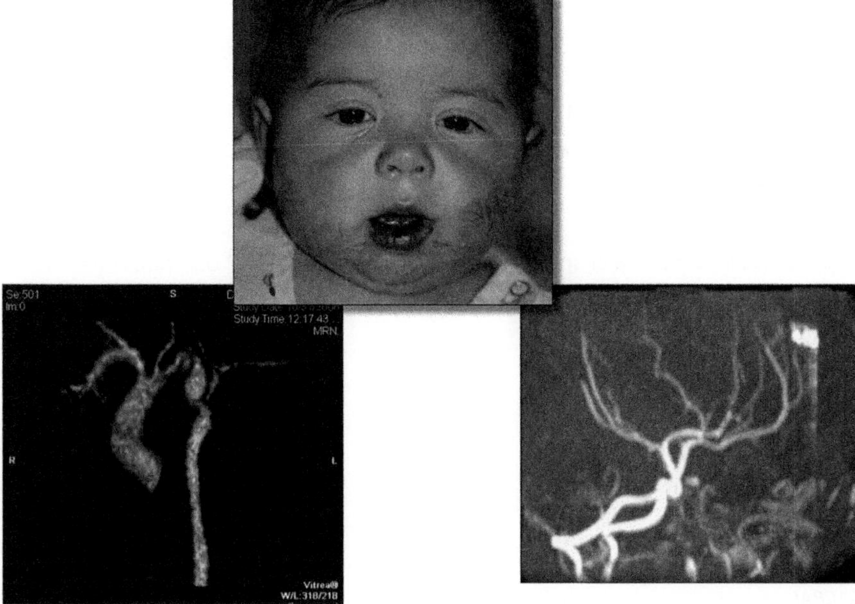


**Fig. 2.** PHACE syndrome. patient with PHACE: hemangioma in a bearded distribution (airway lesions), coarctation of the aorta, absent left carotid, and left vertebral artery.

cardiac/aortic arch anomalies often occur in the same patient, compounding the risk for ischemic events and stroke.[29–34] The diagnosis of PHACE requires clinical examination, cardiac evaluation with echocardiogram, ophthalmologic evaluation, and MRI/magnetic resonance angiogram (MRA) of the head, neck, and mediastinum. Patients need to be monitored for short- and long-term effects as noted earlier. Other issues include speech and language delay, swallowing dysfunction, hearing loss (conductive and sensorineural), and early onset migraines.[35–38] A report of 2 patients with retro-orbital IH and arteriopathy suggested a possible new presentation of PHACE syndrome.[39] For patients with proptosis, globe deviation, and strabismus, an MRI/MRA is recommended. Further workup for PHACE may be needed because of central nervous system (CNS) findings.

Patients with PHACE association and large facial IHs often require systemic therapy for their hemangiomas. In these cases, special consideration must be given to the possibility of underlying cerebrovascular disease and pretreatment workup, including MRI/MRA of the head and neck and cardiac evaluation, is generally recommended before the initiation of therapy. If cerebrovascular issues are found, consultation with neurology or a neurovascular team should be initiated before therapy with beta-blockers.

### *Lower-Body Hemangioma and Other Cutaneous Defects, Urogenital Anomalies, Ulceration, Myelopathy, Bony Deformities, Anorectal Malformations, Arterial Anomalies, Renal Anomalies/Perineal Hemangioma, External Genital Malformations, Lipomyelomeningocele, Vesicorenal Abnormalities, Imperforate Anus, Skin Tag/Spinal Dysraphism, Anogenital, Cutaneous, Renal and Urologic Anomalies, Associated with an Angioma of Lumbosacral Localization Syndrome*

IHs located over the lumbar or sacral spine may be associated with genitourinary, anorectal anomalies, or neurologic issues, such as tethered cord (**Box 1**).[40,41] The

**Box 1**
**Segmental lower body infantile hemangioma syndromes**

*LUMBAR*

- *L*ower-body hemangioma and other cutaneous defects
- *U*rogenital anomalies or ulceration
- *M*yelopathy
- *B*ony deformities
- *A*norectal malformations or arterial anomalies
- *R*enal anomalies

*PELVIS*

- *P*erineal hemangioma
- *E*xternal genital malformations
- *L*ipomyelomeningocele
- *V*esicorenal abnormalities
- *I*mperforate anus
- *S*kin tag

*SACRAL*

- *S*pinal dysraphism
- *A*nogenital
- *C*utaneous
- *R*enal and urologic anomalies
- *A*ssociated with an angioma of
- *L*umbosacral localization

following criteria have been used to describe segmental IH syndrome in the lumbar, pelvic, and sacral areas. This syndrome has been described in the literature using several acronyms. Segmental lesions over the gluteal cleft and lumbar spine need to be evaluated with either ultrasound or MRI, depending on the age of patients.

### *Multiple Infantile Hemangiomas*

Infants with more than 5 IHs need to be evaluated for visceral hemangiomas (**Fig. 3**). The most common site of involvement is the liver, in which multiple or diffuse lesions can be noted.[42] Often these lesions are asymptomatic; but in a minority of cases, symptoms, such as heart failure secondary to large vessel shunts, compartment syndrome, or profound hypothyroidism due to the expression of iodothyronine deiodinase, can occur.[43]Multiple or diffuse liver hemangiomas can occur in the absence of skin lesions. Other rare potential complications of visceral hemangiomas that depend on specific organ involvement include gastrointestinal hemorrhage, obstructive jaundice, and CNS sequelae, caused by mass effects.

### *Medical Management*

Most uncomplicated IHs do not require intervention (**Fig. 4**). Watchful observation and anticipatory guidance is the most common treatment. Complicated hemangiomas and those in high-risk anatomic sites, as described previously, require active intervention.

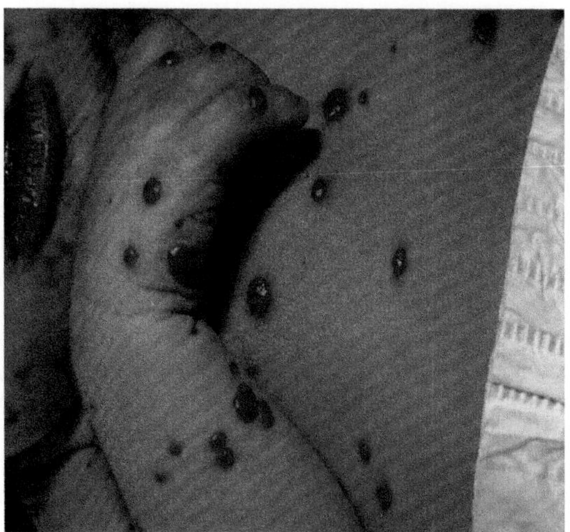

**Fig. 3.** Multiple cutaneous hemangiomas.

Propranolol, a nonselective adrenergic blocker, is the first-line treatment of complicated IHs and is generally initiated for those that are potentially life-threatening, disfiguring, ulcerated, and refractory to other treatments or causing functional impairment. Since the discovery of propranolol for treatment of IHs in 2008, 2 randomized control trials (RCTs) and numerous case reports and retrospective studies have been published supporting its safety and effectiveness, with an estimated treatment failure rate of only 1% to 2%.[44–48] Although both RCTs demonstrated equivalent efficacy of oral propranolol and corticosteroids, propranolol was better tolerated than steroids and substantially more efficacious than placebo. In 2014, the US Food and Drug Administration (FDA) approved an oral formulation of propranolol specifically for the treatment of IHs in children. Oral propranolol is typically initiated at doses of 1 mg/kg/d or less and escalated to 2 to 3 mg/kg/d divided in 2 or 3 doses. In infants, propranolol is generally well tolerated with minimal significant side effects. The most concerning potential side effects are hypoglycemia, bradycardia, and hypotension, which can generally be avoided by incremental dose escalation, close monitoring, and precautionary measures. Propranolol should be held before procedures requiring anesthesia and/or fasting. Other oral beta-blockers, such as atenolol and nadolol, also seem to be safe and efficacious, but much less evidence is available.[49–51]

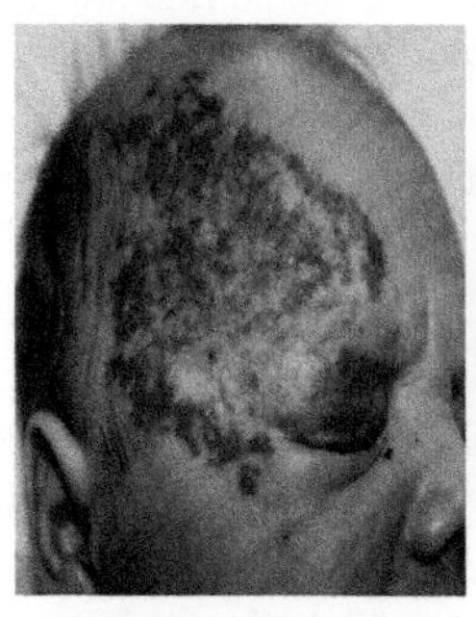


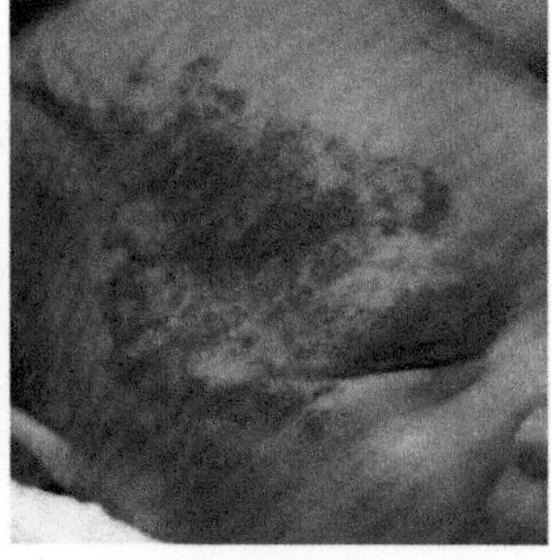


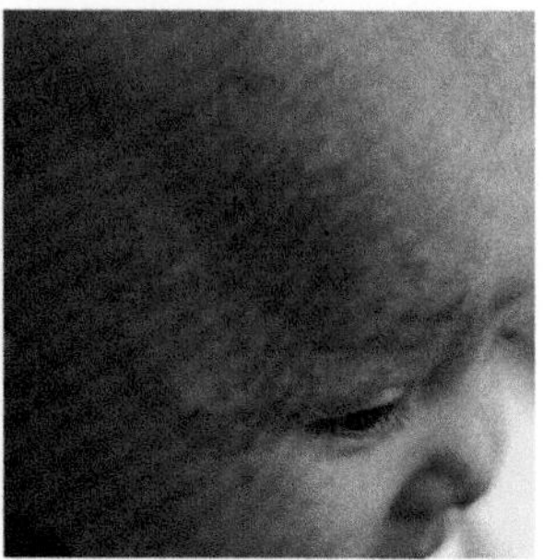


**Fig. 4.** Propranolol results.

Although not yet approved by the FDA for the treatment of IHs, topical timolol has become the favored treatment in less aggressive IHs because of the decreased potential for serious side effects. Timolol maleate is readily available as an ophthalmic preparation in a solution or gel form, which is easily and directly applied to IHs. Multiple studies have shown that timolol is effective at diminishing the color, size, and volume of IHs, particularly when used on young infants with superficial IHs in the rapid proliferative phase.[52–58] Both timolol solution and gel seem to be more effective than topical corticosteroids in reducing the size of IHs . As would be expected, the onset of effect with topical timolol is generally more gradual and modest than that typically seen with oral propranolol. Several studies have demonstrated that topical timolol is safe, with the most common side effect being local skin irritation. Although systemic absorption may occur, the degree is unknown and does not seem to be clinically relevant in most children. However, a recent study suggests that adverse events are more likely to occur in infants who are very young (<1 month adjusted age), weigh less than 2500 g, or have a history of prematurity, apnea, or bradycardia.[58] The risk of side effects also increases with timolol application in or near the eye and to mucosal and ulcerated areas.

Although no longer the first-line treatment, oral corticosteroids are still an effective method of treatment of IHs and may be used in conjunction with oral propranolol while achieving target dosing and initial responses. Corticosteroids are also considered when beta-blockers are contraindicated, causing intolerable side effects or ineffective. Other systemic and more toxic therapies, such as interferon and vincristine, are now rarely used because of unfavorable side effect profiles and need for a central venous catheter for administration. Sirolimus, an inhibitor of mammalian target of rapamycin, has shown to have an antiproliferative and antiangiogenic effect in in vitro studies of hemangioma endothelial cells, suggesting a potential role in the treatment of IHs.[59,60] One case report described the successful use of sirolimus in the treatment of a cutaneous hemangioma associated with PHACE syndrome that had otherwise failed conventional therapies.[61] As a treatment of complex vascular anomalies, oral sirolimus has been well tolerated and efficacious; but further studies are necessary to determine its role in the treatment of complicated IHs.

There have been great advances in the epidemiology, pathogenesis, and medical management of IHs. Prospective clinical trials have resulted in FDA-approved medication that has improved the outcome for these patients.

## REFERENCES

1. Munden A, Butschek R, Tom WL, et al. Prospective study of infantile haemangiomas: incidence, clinical characteristics and association with placental anomalies. Br J Dermatol 2014;170(4):907–13.
2. Darrow DH, Greene AK, Mancini AJ, et al. Diagnosis and management of infantile hemangioma. Pediatrics 2015;136(4):e1060–104.
3. Darrow DH, Greene AK, Mancini AJ, et al. Diagnosis and management of infantile hemangioma: executive summary. Pediatrics 2015;136(4):786–91.
4. Dubois J, Patriquin HB, Garel L, et al. Soft-tissue hemangiomas in infants and children: diagnosis using Doppler sonography. AJR Am J Roentgenol 1998;171(1):247–52.
5. Haggstrom AN, Drolet BA, Baselga E, et al. Prospective study of infantile hemangiomas: demographic, prenatal, and perinatal characteristics. J Pediatr 2007;150(3):291–4.

6. Blei F, Walter J, Orlow SJ, et al. Familial segregation of hemangiomas and vascular malformations as an autosomal dominant trait. Arch Dermatol 1998; 134(6):718–22.
7. North PE, Waner M, Mizeracki A, et al. A unique microvascular phenotype shared by juvenile hemangiomas and human placenta. Arch Dermatol 2001;137(5): 559–70.
8. Barnés CM, Huang S, Kaipainen A, et al. Evidence by molecular profiling for a placental origin of infantile hemangioma. Proc Natl Acad Sci U S A 2005; 102(52):19097–102.
9. Walter JW, North PE, Waner M, et al. Somatic mutation of vascular endothelial growth factor receptors in juvenile hemangioma. Genes Chromosomes Cancer 2002;33(3):295–303.
10. Khan ZA, Boscolo E, Picard A, et al. Multipotential stem cells recapitulate human infantile hemangioma in immunodeficient mice. J Clin Invest 2008;118(7):2592–9.
11. Ritter MR, Reinisch J, Friedlander SF, et al. Myeloid cells in infantile hemangioma. Am J Pathol 2006;168(2):621–8.
12. Bielenberg DR, Bucana CD, Sanchez R, et al. Progressive growth of infantile cutaneous hemangiomas is directly correlated with hyperplasia and angiogenesis of adjacent epidermis and inversely correlated with expression of the endogenous angiogenesis inhibitor, IFN-beta. Int J Oncol 1999;14(3):401–8.
13. Nguyen VA, Kutzner H, Fürhapter C, et al. Infantile hemangioma is a proliferation of LYVE-1-negative blood endothelial cells without lymphatic competence. Mod Pathol 2006;19(2):291–8.
14. Yu Y, Flint AF, Mulliken JB, et al. Endothelial progenitor cells in infantile hemangioma. Blood 2004;103(4):1373–5.
15. Ritter MR, Dorrell MI, Edmonds J, et al. Insulin-like growth factor 2 and potential regulators of hemangioma growth and involution identified by large-scale expression analysis. Proc Natl Acad Sci U S A 2002;99(11):7455–60.
16. Takahashi K, Mulliken JB, Kozakewich HP, et al. Cellular markers that distinguish the phases of hemangioma during infancy and childhood. J Clin Invest 1994; 93(6):2357–64.
17. Boye E, Yu Y, Paranya G, et al. Clonality and altered behavior of endothelial cells from hemangiomas. J Clin Invest 2001;107(6):745–52.
18. Colonna V, Resta L, Napoli A, et al. Placental hypoxia and neonatal haemangioma: clinical and histological observations. Br J Dermatol 2010;162(1):208–9.
19. de Jong S, Itinteang T, Withers AH, et al. Does hypoxia play a role in infantile hemangioma? Arch Dermatol Res 2016;308(4):219–27.
20. Chamlin SL, Haggstrom AN, Drolet BA, et al. Multicenter prospective study of ulcerated hemangiomas. J Pediatr 2007;151(6):684–9, 689.e1.
21. Maguiness SM, Hoffman WY, McCalmont TH, et al. Early white discoloration of infantile hemangioma: a sign of impending ulceration. Arch Dermatol 2010;146(11): 1235–9.
22. Di Maio L, Baldi A, Dimaio V, et al. Use of flashlamp-pumped pulsed dye laser in the treatment of superficial vascular malformations and ulcerated hemangiomas. In Vivo 2011;25(1):117–23.
23. Elluru RG, Friess MR, Richter GT, et al. Multicenter evaluation of the effectiveness of systemic propranolol in the treatment of airway hemangiomas. Otolaryngol Head Neck Surg 2015;153(3):452–60.
24. Xue L, Sun C, Xu DP, et al. Clinical outcomes of infants with periorbital hemangiomas treated with oral propranolol. J Oral Maxillofac Surg 2016;74(11):2193–9.

25. Metry DW, Garzon MC, Drolet BA, et al. PHACE syndrome: current knowledge, future directions. Pediatr Dermatol 2009;26(4):381–98.
26. Frieden IJ, Reese V, Cohen D. PHACE syndrome. The association of posterior fossa brain malformations, hemangiomas, arterial anomalies, coarctation of the aorta and cardiac defects, and eye abnormalities. Arch Dermatol 1996;132(3): 307–11.
27. Metry DW, Haggstrom AN, Drolet BA, et al. A prospective study of PHACE syndrome in infantile hemangiomas: demographic features, clinical findings, and complications. Am J Med Genet A 2006;140(9):975–86.
28. Metry D, Heyer G, Hess C, et al. Consensus statement on diagnostic criteria for PHACE syndrome. Pediatrics 2009;124(5):1447–56.
29. Drolet BA, Dohil M, Golomb MR, et al. Early stroke and cerebral vasculopathy in children with facial hemangiomas and PHACE association. Pediatrics 2006; 117(3):959–64.
30. Burrows PE, Robertson RL, Mulliken JB, et al. Cerebral vasculopathy and neurologic sequelae in infants with cervicofacial hemangioma: report of eight patients. Radiology 1998;207(3):601–7.
31. Heyer GL, Dowling MM, Licht DJ, et al. The cerebral vasculopathy of PHACES syndrome. Stroke 2008;39(2):308–16.
32. Haggstrom AN, Garzon MC, Baselga E, et al. Risk for PHACE syndrome in infants with large facial hemangiomas. Pediatrics 2010;126(2):e418–26.
33. Poindexter G, Metry DW, Barkovich AJ, et al. PHACE syndrome with intracerebral hemangiomas, heterotopia, and endocrine dysfunction. Pediatr Neurol 2007; 36(6):402–6.
34. Hess CP, Fullerton HJ, Metry DW, et al. Cervical and intracranial arterial anomalies in 70 patients with PHACE syndrome. AJNR Am J Neuroradiol 2010;31(10): 1980–6.
35. Yu J, Siegel DH, Drolet BA, et al. Prevalence and clinical characteristics of headaches in PHACE syndrome. J Child Neurol 2016;31(4):468–73.
36. Martin KL, Arvedson JC, Bayer ML, et al. Risk of dysphagia and speech and language delay in PHACE syndrome. Pediatr Dermatol 2015;32(1):64–9.
37. Chiu YE, Siegel DH, Drolet BA, et al. Tooth enamel hypoplasia in PHACE syndrome. Pediatr Dermatol 2014;31(4):455–8.
38. Duffy KJ, Runge-Samuelson C, Bayer ML, et al. Association of hearing loss with PHACE syndrome. Arch Dermatol 2010;146(12):1391–6.
39. Antonov NK, Spence-Shishido A, Marathe KS, et al. Orbital hemangioma with intracranial vascular anomalies and hemangiomas: a new presentation of PHACE syndrome? Pediatr Dermatol 2015;32(6):e267–72.
40. Iacobas I, Burrows PE, Frieden IJ, et al. LUMBAR: association between cutaneous infantile hemangiomas of the lower body and regional congenital anomalies. J Pediatr 2010;157(5):795–801.e1-7.
41. Girard C, Bigorre M, Guillot B, et al. PELVIS syndrome. Arch Dermatol 2006; 142(7):884–8.
42. Hsi Dickie B, Fishman SJ, Azizkhan RG. Hepatic vascular tumors. Semin Pediatr Surg 2014;23(4):168–72.
43. Huang SA, Tu HM, Harney JW, et al. Severe hypothyroidism caused by type 3 iodothyronine deiodinase in infantile hemangiomas. N Engl J Med 2000;343(3):185–9.
44. Léauté-Labrèze C, Hoeger P, Mazereeuw-Hautier J, et al. A randomized, controlled trial of oral propranolol in infantile hemangioma. N Engl J Med 2015; 372(8):735–46.

45. Hoeger PH, Harper JI, Baselga E, et al. Treatment of infantile haemangiomas: recommendations of a European expert group. Eur J Pediatr 2015;174:855–65.
46. Drolet BA, Frommelt PC, Chamlin SL, et al. Initiation and use of propranolol for infantile hemangioma: report of a consensus conference. Pediatrics 2013; 131(1):128–40.
47. Malik MA, Menon P, Rao KL, et al. Effect of propranolol vs prednisolone vs propranolol with prednisolone in the management of infantile hemangioma: a randomized controlled study. J Pediatr Surg 2013;48:2453–9.
48. Bauman NM, Shin JJ, Oh AK, et al. Propranolol vs prednisolone for symptomatic proliferating infantile hemangiomas: a randomized clinical trial. JAMA Otolaryngol Head Neck Surg 2014;140:323–30.
49. Ábarzúa-Araya A, Navarrete-Dechent CP, Heusser F, et al. Atenolol versus propranolol for the treatment of infantile hemangiomas: a randomized controlled study. J Am Acad Dermatol 2014;70(6):1045–9.
50. Ji Y, Wang Q, Chen S, et al. Oral atenolol therapy for proliferating infantile hemangioma: a prospective study. Medicine (Baltimore) 2016;95(24):e3908.
51. Pope E, Chakkittakandiyil A, Lara-Corrales I, et al. Expanding the therapeutic repertoire of infantile haemangiomas: cohort-blinded study of oral nadolol compared with propranolol. Br J Dermatol 2013;168(1):222–4.
52. Chakkittakandiyil A, Phillips R, Frieden IJ, et al. Timolol maleate 0.5% or 0.1% gel-forming solution for infantile hemangiomas: a retrospective, multicenter, cohort study. Pediatr Dermatol 2012;29(1):28–31.
53. Yu L, Li S, Su B, et al. Treatment of superficial infantile hemangiomas with timolol: evaluation of short-term efficacy and safety in infants. Exp Ther Med 2013;6(2): 388–90.
54. Chan H, McKay C, Adams S, et al. RCT of timolol maleate gel for superficial infantile hemangiomas in 5- to 24-week-olds. Pediatrics 2013;131(6):e1739–47.
55. Danarti R, Ariwibowo L, Radiono S, et al. Topical timolol maleate 0.5% for infantile hemangioma: its effectiveness compared to ultrapotent topical corticosteroids - A single-center experience of 278 cases. Dermatology 2016;232(5):566–71.
56. Püttgen K, Lucky A, Adams D, et al. Topical timolol maleate treatment of infantile hemangiomas. Pediatrics 2016;138(3):e20160355.
57. Weibel L, Barysch MJ, Scheer HS, et al. Topical timolol for infantile hemangiomas: evidence for efficacy and degree of systemic absorption. Pediatr Dermatol 2016; 33(2):184–90.
58. Frommelt P, Juern A, Siegel D, et al. Adverse events in young and preterm infants receiving topical timolol for infantile hemangioma. Pediatr Dermatol 2016;33(4): 405–14.
59. Greenberger S, Yuan S, Walsh LA, et al. Rapamycin suppresses self-renewal and vasculogenic potential of stem cells isolated from infantile hemangioma. J Invest Dermatol 2011;131(12):2467–76.
60. Medici D, Olsen BR. Rapamycin inhibits proliferation of hemangioma endothelial cells by reducing HIF-1-dependent expression of VEGF. PLoS One 2012;7(8): e42913.
61. Kaylani S, Theos AJ, Pressey JG. Treatment of infantile hemangiomas with sirolimus in a patient with PHACE syndrome. Pediatr Dermatol 2013;30(6):e194–7.

# Congenital Vascular Tumors

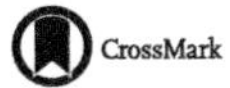

Jeremy A. Goss, MD[a], Arin K. Greene, MD, MMSc[b,*]

**KEYWORDS**

- Vascular tumors • Pyogenic granuloma • Congenital hemangioma
- Kaposiform hemangioendothelioma • Tufted angioma • Infantile myofibroma
- Epithelioid hemangioendothelioma • Enzinger intramuscular hemangioma
- Angiosarcoma • Cutaneovisceral angiomatosis with thrombocytopenia

**KEY POINTS**

- Vascular tumors and malformations comprise the field of vascular anomalies.
- Although the majority of tumors affect the skin, lesions involving the mucous membranes have been noted.
- Tufted angioma, or angioblastoma of Nakagawa, shares clinical and histopathologic features with kaposiform hemangioendothelioma, suggesting these vascular tumors exist together along a spectrum.
- Fewer than 1% of soft tissue sarcomas are classified as angiosarcoma and only 1% of angiosarcomas affect children.

## INTRODUCTION

Vascular tumors are benign neoplasms, which result from proliferating endothelial cells. These lesions present during infancy or childhood, may affect any location, and exhibit postnatal growth. Local complications include bleeding, tissue destruction, and pain whereas systemic sequelae include thrombocytopenia, congestive heart failure, and death. Vascular tumors should be differentiated from vascular malformations, which present at birth, have a quiescent endothelium, and grow in proportion to the child. Together, vascular tumors and malformations comprise the field of vascular anomalies.

Infantile hemangioma is the most common vascular tumor of childhood. For more information on this topic, see Denise M. Adams's article, "Infantile Hemangiomas in the Head and Neck Region", Marcelo Hochman's article, "The Role of Surgery in the Management

---

Disclosure: J.A. Goss and A.K. Greene have nothing they wish to disclose.

[a] Department of Plastic and Oral Surgery, Boston Children's Hospital, Harvard Medical School, 300 Longwood Avenue Boston, MA, 02115, USA; [b] Department of Plastic and Oral Surgery, Vascular Anomalies Center, Boston Children's Hospital, Harvard Medical School, 300 Longwood Avenue Boston, MA, 02115, USA

* Corresponding author.

*E-mail address:* arin.greene@childrens.harvard.edu

Otolaryngol Clin N Am 51 (2018) 89–97

https://doi.org/10.1016/j.otc.2017.09.008

of Infantile Hemangiomas: What is the Best Timing?" and Milton Waner's article, "The Surgical Management of Infantile Hemangiomas" in this issue. Other congenital tumors, in order of most common, include pyogenic granuloma (PG), congenital hemangioma (CH), kaposiform hemangioendothelioma (KHE), tufted angioma (TA), infantile myofibroma (IM), epithelioid hemangioendotheloma (EHE), Enzinger intramuscular hemangioma, angiosarcoma, cutaneovisceral angiomatosis with thrombocytopenia (CAT).

## PYOGENIC GRANULOMA

A small, solitary, red, bleeding or ulcerated lesion that presents in childhood (**Fig. 1**) is pathognomonic for PG, formerly *lobular capillary hemangioma*. These tumors are small compared with other vascular tumors, with 75% measuring less than 1 cm in diameter.[1] PGs are twice as common in boys and the mean age of onset is 7 years; only 12% develop during the first year of life. Although a majority of tumors affect the skin (88%), lesions involving the mucous membranes (12%) have been noted. Lesions affect the head and neck (62%), trunk (19%), and extremities (18%). Within the head and neck, specific sites include cheek (29%), oral cavity (14%), scalp (11%), forehead (10%), eyelid (9%), or lips (9%).[1] Complications include bleeding (64%) and ulceration (36%). Twenty-five percent of patients have a history of preexisting trauma or underlying cutaneous conditions, such as a capillary malformation or arteriovenous malformation. History and physical examination are sufficient for diagnosis; imaging is unnecessary.

With bleeding and crusting, PG may shrink, but regrowth is common. Treatment with curettage, shave excision, or laser therapy is ineffective because the lesion extends into the reticular dermis, which is often inaccessible by these approaches.[1,2] These modalities have recurrence rates as high as 50%.[1,2] Cure rate of approximately 100% is achieved after full-thickness skin excision.[1,2] Alternatively, the lesion can be shaved and the base cauterized with a Bovie through the thickness of the dermis.

## CONGENITAL HEMANGIOMA

CHs are solitary, red-violaceous lesions with coarse telangiectasias, central pallor, and peripheral pale halos. The incidence of CH is currently unknown. CH more commonly

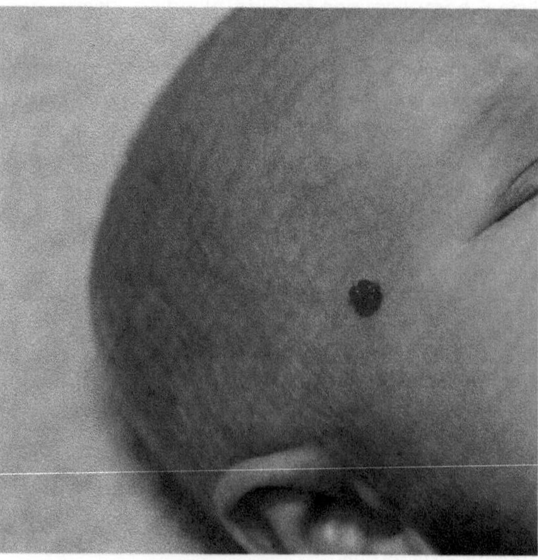

**Fig. 1.** Two-month-old boy with PG of the face.

affects an extremity and shows equal distribution among sexes. There are 2 forms of CH: rapidly involuting CH (RICH) and noninvoluting CH (NICH). RICH and NICH are distinguished by their clinical course; CHs that become smaller after birth are RICH.

RICH (**Fig. 2**) affects the limbs (52%) more often than the head and neck (42%) or trunk (6%).[3,4] It involutes shortly after birth, with 50% of lesions having completed regression by 7 months of age and the remaining tumors fully involuting by 14 months.[3,4] After involution, the skin usually is atrophic and deficient of subcutaneous adipose tissue. By contrast, NICH (**Fig. 3**) involves the head and neck (43%) more frequently than the limbs (38%) or trunk (19%).[5] These lesions do not undergo involution after birth but instead remain unchanged.[5] Imaging is rarely indicated, but in instances where the diagnosis is equivocal, ultrasound and MRI findings of CHs show fast-flow, shunting, and parenchymal masses with enhancement.[6]

The mainstay of management for CH is observation. RICH begins to involute shortly after birth and resolves by 1 year of age. Drug treatment has not been shown to accelerate involution. Atrophic tissue after involution may require reconstruction with grafting (dermal, fat, and acellular dermis) or resection. Rarely, a large lesion may cause high-output cardiac failure and require embolization or excision. NICHs are stable lesions that do not involute or respond to pharmacologic treatment. If a NICH causes disfigurement and psychosocial morbidity, it can be resected. Alternatively, the lesion's color may be improved with pulsed dye laser and/or sclerotherapy.

## KAPOSIFORM HEMANGIOENDOTHELIOMA

KHE is a benign vascular tumor that is locally aggressive but does not metastasize (**Fig. 4**). The incidence is 1 in 100,000. Sixty percent of lesions are observed in the neonatal period.[7] KHEs are solitary, red-purple lesions that have an equal male-female distribution. KHE affects the head/neck (40%), extremities (30%), or trunk (30%).[8] KHE proliferates in early childhood and partially regresses after 2 years of age. Adult-onset KHE also may occur.[9] In adults, the average age at diagnosis is 42.9 years, there is a strong male predominance (80%), and anatomic distribution is similar to that of affected children.[9] History and physical examination usually are sufficient for definitive diagnosis; however, MRI may help determine the extent of disease. MRI shows hyperintense, infiltrative lesions that enhance with contrast on T2-weighted images.[6]

More than half of all children with KHE develop Kasabach-Merritt phenomenon (KMP), a profound thrombocytopenia (<25,000/mm$^3$) compounded by low fibrinogen

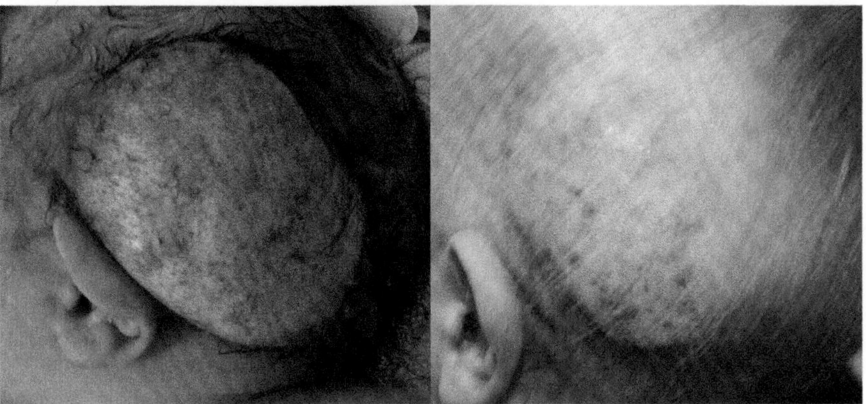

**Fig. 2.** Male newborn with a RICH of the scalp (*Left*). The tumor has regressed at 1 year of age (*Right*).

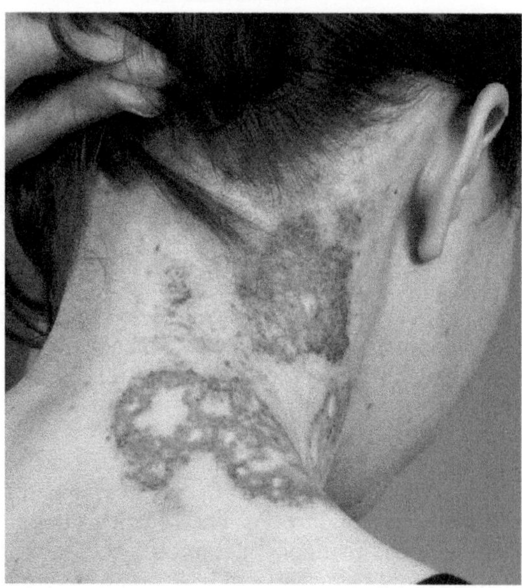

**Fig. 3.** NICH affecting the neck of a female adult.

and elevated fibrin-split products (D-dimers). Mortality from KMP ranges from 12% to 24%.[10] Tumors larger than 8 cm in diameter, those that present during infancy, and those that affect the viscera and/or muscle more commonly exhibit KMP.[7] Adult-onset KHE does not cause KMP, which may be attributed to smaller tumor size.[9]

By 2 years of age, children with KHE often experience partial involution of the lesion, but the tumor persists without intervention and may cause chronic pain and/or contracture. Resection usually is not possible because lesions are large and involve multiple tissues and vital structures. Patients with KMP require systemic treatment with chemotherapeutic agents to prevent life-threatening complications. The authors' current first-line treatment is sirolimus and second-line treatment is vincristine.[11] Patients without KMP are usually treated as well to minimize the risk of fibrosis, chronic pain, and contracture.

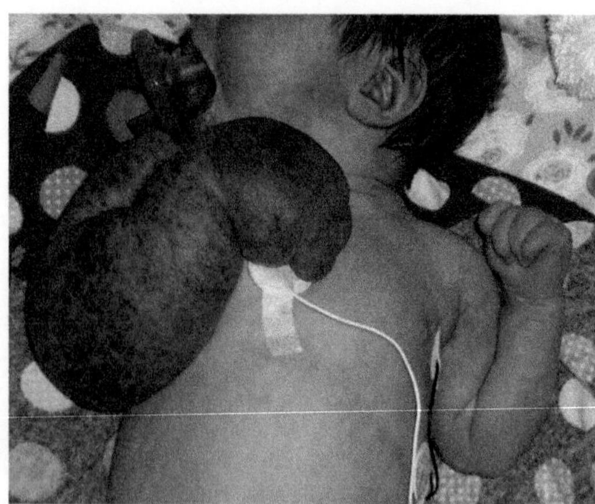

**Fig. 4.** Male newborn with KHE of the upper extremity.

Platelet levels should normalize with involution and systemic therapy. Platelet transfusion should be avoided if KMP is suspected, unless there is evidence of active bleeding or excision is indicated. Heparin may stimulate tumor growth, result in platelet sequestration within the lesion, and worsen bleeding.

## TUFTED ANGIOMA

TA, or angioblastoma of Nakagawa, shares clinical and histopathologic features with KHE, suggesting these vascular tumors exist together along a spectrum. Lesions may be locally invasive but never metastasize. TA has a variable appearance; it may present as a violaceous plaque (**Fig. 5**), solitary tumor, or diffuse cutaneous stain over the trunk or neck.[12] Regardless, onset is usually during infancy or early childhood and similar to KHE, KMP may occur. TA is distinguishable from KHE through histopathology. Rounded tufts of capillary nodules in the dermis or subcutis, colloquially referred to as "cannonballs," help differentiate between the two.[12] Symptomatic, localized tumors may be resected, but diffuse lesions or those that induce KMP require systemic pharmacotherapy with sirolimus or vincristine.

## INFANTILE MYOFIBROMA

IM, previously called infantile hemangiopericytoma, is the most common benign fibrous tumor of infancy. IM may be solitary (most common form), multifocal (infantile myofibromatosis), or generalized (viscera involved). There is slight male predominance. Sixty percent of lesions are present at birth.[13] Red-violaceous, ulcerating skin with rubbery, mobile subcutaneous nodules are typical and affect the head and neck (**Fig. 6**), trunk, or extremities. Handheld Doppler demonstrates fast flow. MRI indicating hypointensity-isointensity on T1-weighted images helps distinguish these lesions from lymphatic malformations, infantile fibrosarcoma, and teratoma.[14] Biopsy may be necessary for elucidating the diagnosis. Typical findings include eosinophilic myfibroblasts in nodules, whorls, and/or fascicles surrounded by poorly differentiated spindle cells containing hyperchromatic nuclei.

The solitary form shows regression in 30% to 60% of cases and can be managed with observation or with resection if symptomatic.[14] Likewise, the multifocal variant has a favorable prognosis, and management approach is similar to that of solitary lesions. Visceral involvement of the heart, lungs, gastrointestinal tract, and pancreas

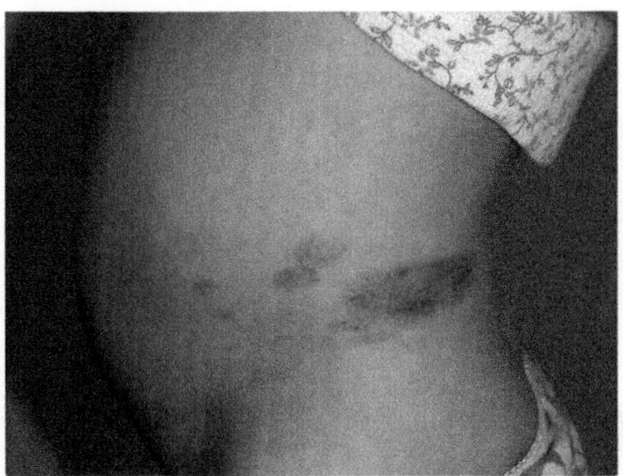

**Fig. 5.** TA in a 3-year-old girl.

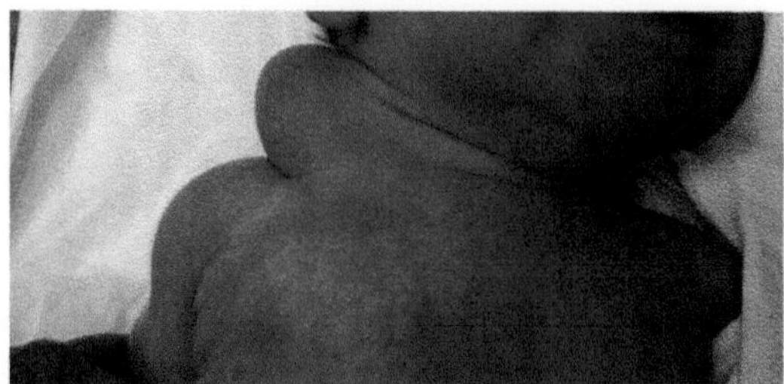

**Fig. 6.** Newborn with IM affecting the neck.

typify generalized IM, which is present in 25% to 40% of IM. Mortality for generalized type IM is 75% and treatment involves chemotherapy, radiation, and/or resection.[14]

## EPITHELIOID HEMANGIOENDOTHELIOMA

EHEs are multifocal tumors with a variable clinical course. EHE may remain stable, grow indolently, progress rapidly, undergo apoptosis, or metastasize (25%).[15] These lesions can involve the skin, bone, liver, or lung (**Fig. 7**). Histopathology reveals round or polygonal epithelioid endothelial cells with eosinophilic hyaline cytoplasm. These tumors often appear as infiltrative nests or cords of epithelioid cells.[16] Because of their potential for metastasis, serial imaging should be obtained. Lesions are managed with systemic chemotherapy, radiation, and/or resection; otherwise, stable lesions may be observed.[17] In cases that primarily affect the liver, transplantation may be indicated.

## ENZINGER INTRAMUSCULAR HEMANGIOMA

Enzinger intramuscular hemangioma, or intramuscular hemangioma (capillary-type), are solitary, benign, painless vascular tumors that primarily affect skeletal muscle (**Fig. 8**). The median age at diagnosis is 25 years, and as many as 25% of patients are in the pediatric age group.[13] Affected areas include the extremities (38%), trunk (32%), and head/neck (30%).[13] Skin overlying the affected muscle is grossly normal and biopsy is necessary for diagnosis. Unencapsulated lobules containing capillary-like vessels embedded within skeletal muscle, and possibly extending into the subcutaneous fat and dermis, are characteristic. Treatment options include embolization

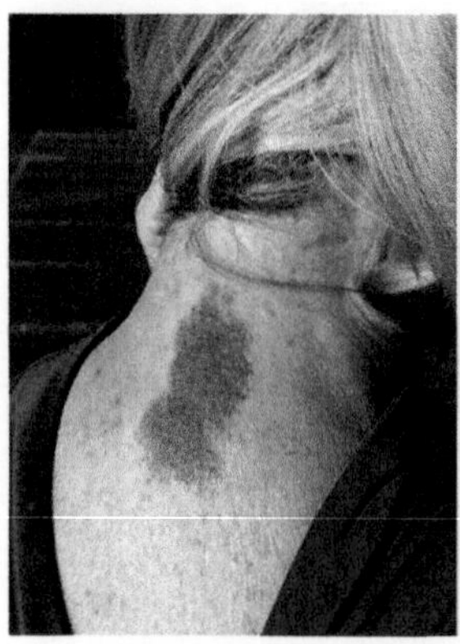

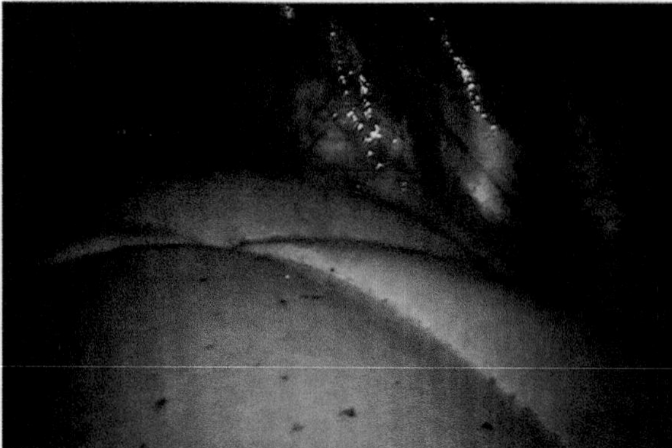

**Fig. 7.** Adult patient with EHEs of the skin (*Left*) and lung (*Right*).

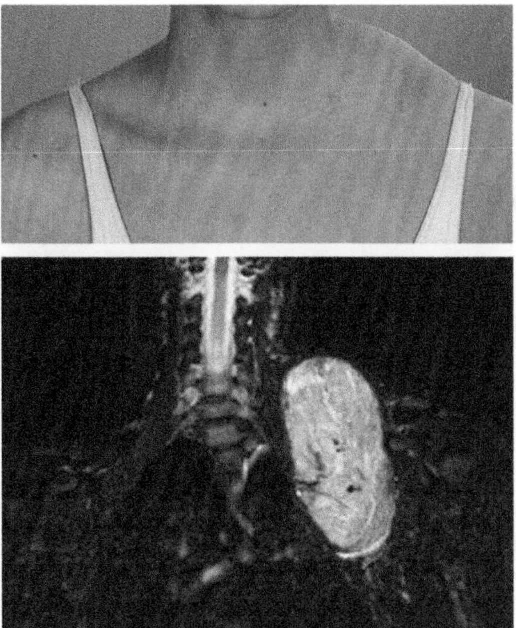

**Fig. 8.** Adolescent female with Enzinger hemangioma of the neck and shoulder (*Top*). Imaging showing intramuscular involvement (*Bottom*).

and/or resection when lesions become symptomatic; however, 20% of tumors recur after excision.[13]

## ANGIOSARCOMA

Fewer than 1% of soft tissue sarcomas are classified as angiosarcoma and only 1% of angiosarcomas affect children.[18–20] There is equal male and female distribution, and the median age of diagnosis is 11 years[18] (**Fig. 9**). Lesions most often affect the

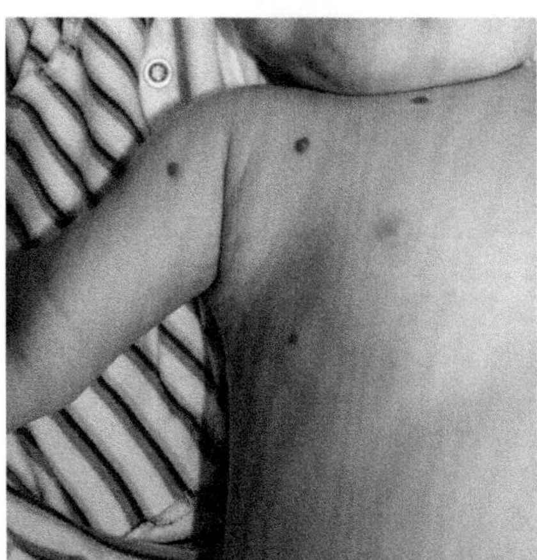

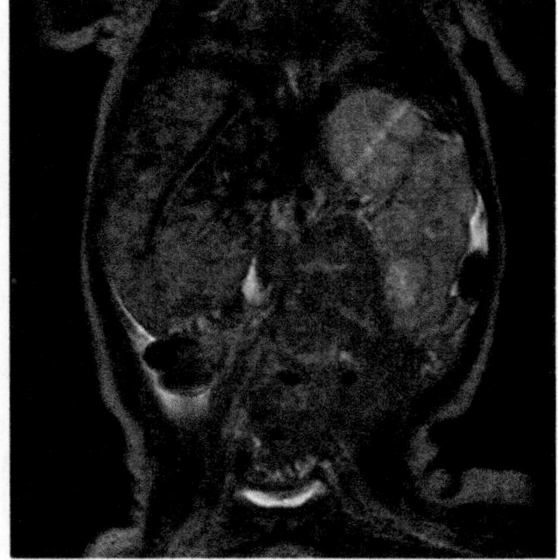

**Fig. 9.** Angiosarcoma in a male infant involving the skin (*Left*) with metastasis to the liver and spleen (*Right*).

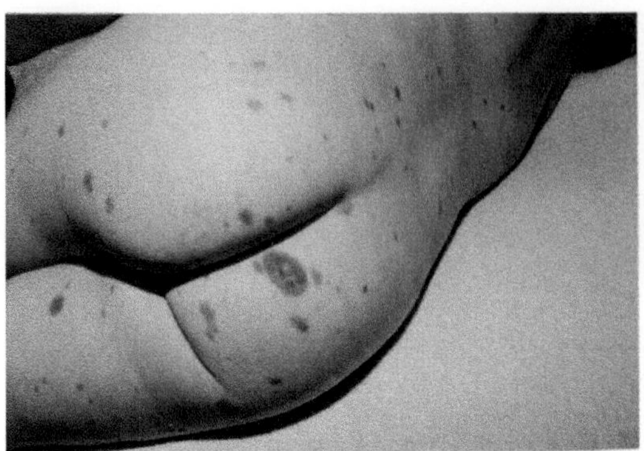
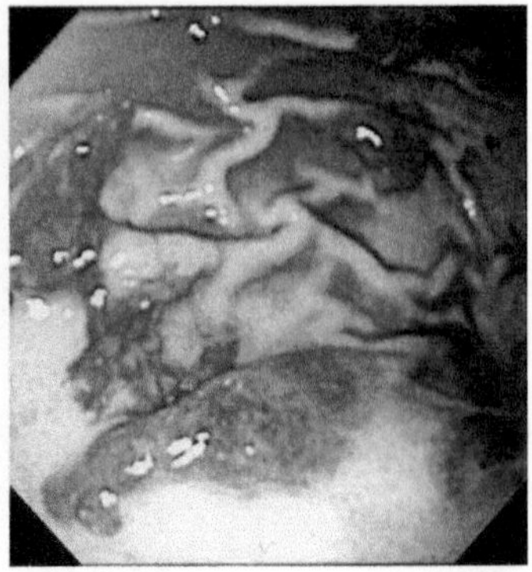

**Fig. 10.** A 3-year-old girl with CAT (*Left*). Endoscopy reveals diffuse lesions of the stomach with areas of hemorrhage (*Right*).

mediastinum (heart and pericardium) (46%), liver (13%), and breast (13%), whereas the spleen, mesentery, pelvis, and upper extremities may each be involved (7%).[18] These malignant tumors are capable of metastasis and often spread to regional lymph nodes, the lungs, or the liver. Mortality is high (67%).[18] Histology shows either convoluted vessels infiltrating normal tissue or solid nests of cells. Management includes chemotherapy, radiation, and/or resection.

## CUTANEOVISCERAL ANGIOMATOSIS WITH THROMBOCYTOPENIA

CAT, or multifocal lymphangioendotheliomatosis with thrombocytopenia, may affect the skin (extremities and trunk), gastrointestinal tract (mucosa), lung, bone, liver, spleen, and muscle[21] (**Fig. 10**). Infants have an increased risk of thrombocytopenia secondary to hematemesis and/or melena from numerous mucosal lesions involving the gastrointestinal tract, which are prone to bleeding.[21] Characteristic skin lesions are red-brown macules-plaques or blue plaques and papules. CAT can be distinguished from similarly presenting lesions, such as hemangiomatosis, lymphangiomatosis, and blue rubber bleb nevus syndrome by histology; thin-walled, blood-filled vascular channels with endothelial hyperplasia are typical findings.[21] Treatment with systemic corticosteroids, interferon, thalidomide, or vincristine is effective in reducing the size of the lesion and the potential for hemorrhage.

## REFERENCES


1. Patrice SJ, Wiss K, Mulliken JB. Pyogenic granuloma (lobular capillary hemangioma): a clinicopathologic study of 178 cases. Pediatr Dermatol 1991;8:267–76.
2. Lee J, Sinno H, Tahiri Y, et al. Treatment options for cutaneous pyogenic granulomas: a review. J Plast Reconstr Aesthet Surg 2011;64:1216–20.
3. Boon LM, Enjolras O, Mulliken JB. Congenital hemangioma: evidence of accelerated involution. J Pediatr 1996;128:329–35.
4. Berenguer B, Mulliken JB, Enjolras O, et al. Rapidly involuting congenital hemangioma: clinical and histopathologic features. Pediatr Dev Pathol 2003;6:495–510.
5. Enjolras O, Mulliken JB, Boon LM, et al. Noninvoluting congenital hemangioma: a rare cutaneous vascular anomaly. Plast Reconstr Surg 2001;107:1647–54.
6. Arnold R, Chaudry G. Diagnostic imaging of vascular anomalies. Clin Plast Surg 2011;38:21–9.

7. Croteau SE, Liang MG, Kozakewich HP, et al. Kaposiform hemangioendothelioma: atypical features and risks of Kasabach-Merritt phenomenon in 107 referrals. J Pediatr 2013;162:142–7.
8. Mulliken JB, Anupindi S, Ezekowitz RA, et al. Case records of the Massachusetts General Hospital. Weekly clinicopathological exercises. Case 13-2004. A newborn girl with a large cutaneous lesion, thrombocytopenia, and anemia. N Engl J Med 2004;350:1764–75.
9. Karnes JC, Lee BT, Phung T, et al. Adult-onset kaposiform hemangioendothelioma in a posttraumatic site. Ann Plast Surg 2009;62:456–8.
10. Sarkar M, Mulliken JB, Kozakewich HP, et al. Thrombocytopenic coagulopathy (Kasabach-Merritt phenomenon) is associated with Kaposiform hemangioendothelioma and not with common infantile hemangioma. Plast Reconstr Surg 1997;100:1377–86.
11. Adams DM. Special considerations in vascular anomalies: hematologic management. Clin Plast Surg 2011;38:153–60.
12. Jones EW, Orkin M. Tufted angioma (angioblastoma). A benign progressive angioma, not to be confused with Kaposi's sarcoma or low-grade angiosarcoma. J Am Acad Dermatol 1989;20:214–25.
13. Greene AK. Rare vascular tumors. In: Berger M, editor. Vascular anomalies: classification, diagnosis, and management. St Louis (MO): Quality Medical Publishing; 2013. p. 69–79.
14. Merrell SC, Rahbar R, Alomari AI, et al. Infantile myofibroma or lymphatic malformation: differential diagnosis of neonatal cystic cervicofacial lesions. J Craniofac Surg 2010;21:422–6.
15. Hristov AC, Wisell J. A "high-risk" epithelioid hemangioendothelioma presenting as a solitary, ulcerated, subcutaneous tumor. Am J Dermatopathol 2011;33:e88–90.
16. Weiss SW, Enzinger FM. Epithelioid hemangioendothelioma: a vascular tumor often mistaken for a carcinoma. Cancer 1982;50:970–81.
17. Lai FM, Allen PW, Yuen PM, et al. Locally metastasizing vascular tumor. Spindle cell, epithelioid, or unclassified hemangioendothelioma? Am J Clin Pathol 1991;96:660–3.
18. Deyrup AT, Miettinen M, North PE, et al. Angiosarcomas arising in the viscera and soft tissue of children and young adults: a clinicopathologic study of 15 cases. Am J Surg Pathol 2009;33:264–9.
19. Coffin CM, Dehner LP. Vascular tumors in children and adolescents: a clinicopathologic study of 228 tumors in 222 patients. Pathol Annu 1993;28 Pt 1:97–120.
20. Ferrari A, Casanova M, Bisogno G, et al. Malignant vascular tumors in children and adolescents: a report from the Italian and German Soft Tissue Sarcoma Cooperative Group. Med Pediatr Oncol 2002;39:109–14.
21. Prasad V, Fishman SJ, Mulliken JB, et al. Cutaneovisceral angiomatosis with thrombocytopenia. Pediatr Dev Pathol 2005;8:407–19.

# Psychosocial Impact of Vascular Anomalies on Children and Their Families

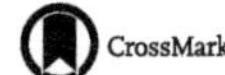

Alexandra G. Espinel, MD, Nancy M. Bauman, MD*

**KEYWORDS**

- Vascular anomalies • Psychosocial impact • Propranolol
- Facial neoplasm/psychology

**KEY POINTS**

- Measuring the psychosocial impact of vascular anomalies is made difficult by the wide range of presentation and severity of the lesions as well as the relatively rare incidence.
- There is no linear relationship between the degree of deformity and degree of distress.
- Patients with more severe lesions may have better coping mechanisms for the impact developed through multiple medical encounters.
- Early treatment can be protective against developing a negative self-image, regardless of the aesthetic effect.
- Providers must also be sensitive to the psychologic impact of vascular anomalies on the parents.

## INTRODUCTION

Based on their clinical and cytologic attributes, vascular anomalies are divided into tumors and malformations. Infantile hemangiomas (IHs) are the most common vascular tumor and frequently affect visible areas of the face, head, and neck Although hemangiomas involute with age, approximately 70% of children show residual lesions after involution.[1] Persistent telangiectasia, sagging skin, scarring, and pigment changes (**Fig. 1**) can cause obvious deformity of the face that may be particularly disfiguring depending on the size and location. Vascular malformations are further subcategorized as low-flow lymphatic, venous, capillary, or mixed lesions and as high-flow arteriovenous malformations. Vascular malformations typically grow as a child grows although they may acutely enlarge under certain conditions. These lesions may also cause marked disfigurement particularly when located in visible areas of the head and neck.

Disclosure Statement: The authors have nothing to disclose.
Otolaryngology Head and Neck Surgery, Children's National Health System, George Washington University, 111 Michigan Avenue Northwest, Washington, DC 20817, USA
* Corresponding author.
*E-mail address:* nbauman@cnmc.org

Otolaryngol Clin N Am 51 (2018) 99–110
https://doi.org/10.1016/j.otc.2017.09.018
oto.theclinics.com

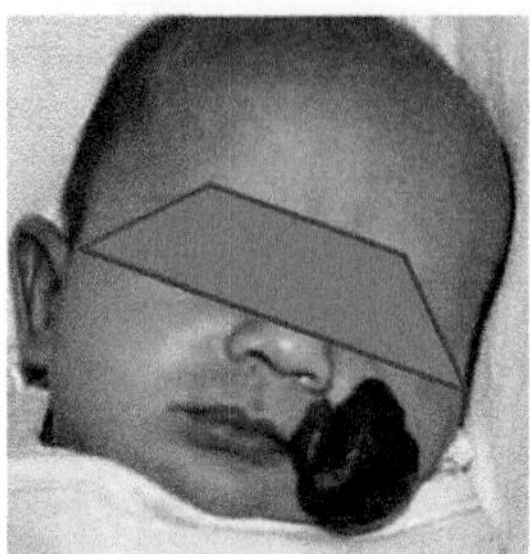
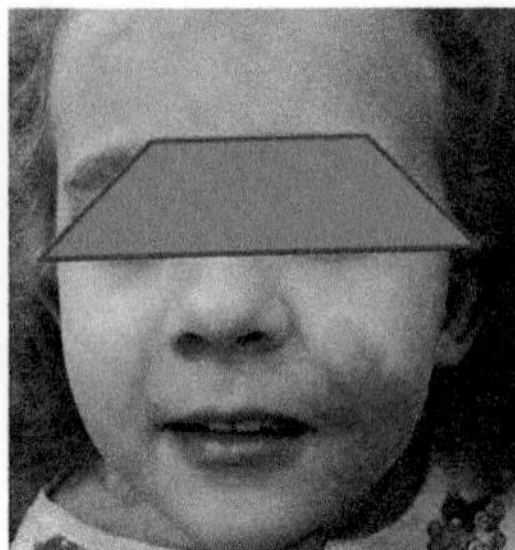
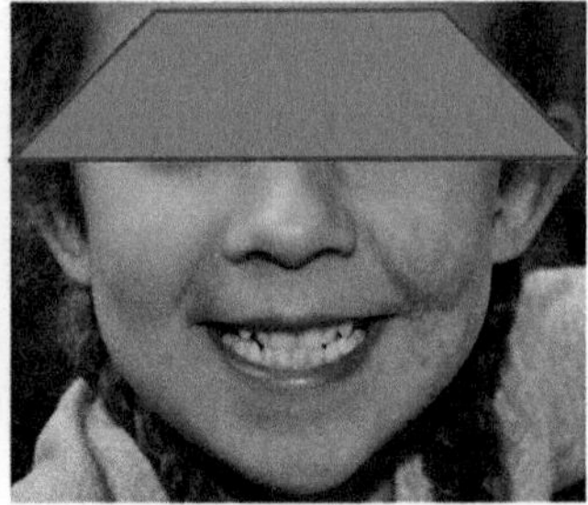

**Fig. 1.** Proliferating left-cheek IH in 1-month-old female infant (*left*) and same involuted lesion in a 4-year-old girl (*middle*). Despite marked involution, the family sought treatment options for residual fibrofatty tissue, skin discoloration, dimpling, and telangiectasias. Significant improvement in skin appearance post–serial pulsed dye laser treatments and fractionated $CO_2$ laser therapy (*right*).

The clinical manifestations of head and neck vascular anomalies are extremely varied. Treatment is reserved for vascular anomalies that are symptomatic or cosmetically disfiguring, and surgical and nonsurgical treatment options are widely varied with variable outcomes. Unlike other vascular anomalies, treatment of IHs is age dependent, with better responses reported for treatment during the proliferative phase of growth in early infancy. Anticipated involution of asymptomatic but cosmetically deforming IHs can delay critical early referral to vascular anomalies specialists for treatment. Deferring treatment of IHs in cosmetically sensitive areas, such as the nose, lip, and periorbital region, can convert a lesion easily treated during infancy into a lesion that is more difficult to treat in the older child. The paradigm shift among primary caregivers to refer patients with IHs in cosmetically sensitive areas early in infancy is occurring slowly.

Depending on the child, the site and size of the deformity, vascular anomalies, or scars from vascular anomalies may potentially have a detrimental effect on a child's psychosocial development, particularly if untreated.[2] Recognizing the impact of facial vascular anomalies on psychosocial development is critical in evaluating treatment options and timing of treatment to achieve the best possible outcome. This article defines psychosocial impact, presents inherent difficulties and relevant studies assessing its occurrence in patients with vascular anomalies, and discusses treatment considerations, particularly the optimal age of intervention when warranted.

## PSYCHOSOCIAL IMPACT

Psychosocial impact is defined as "the effect caused by environmental and/or biological factors on an individual's social and/or psychological aspects."[3] In cases of facial vascular lesions, patients are faced with the anomaly as a biological factor as well as how others react to the lesion as an environmental factor. The psychosocial effects vary because vascular anomalies have a wide range of manifestations and severity. Although young children are not aware of body image, they perceive how social interactions may differ from others based on any obvious abnormalities. In a society that places great importance on physical appearance, sustaining a facial vascular anomaly can significantly influence the psychosocial development of children and thus have lifelong effects.[4]

Negative psychosocial consequences are known to occur in some, but not all, children with craniofacial abnormalities, such as cleft lip and palate and craniosynostosis, but psychosocial challenges of vascular anomalies in cosmetically sensitive areas are not well described.[5] Masnari and colleagues[6,7] concluded that all children who look different, regardless of the cause, face similar problems. In adults with disfiguring acquired or congenital facial lesions, there is no linear relationship between the degree of deformity and the degree of distress experienced from the deformity.[8]

Based on cleft lip and palate literature, vascular anomalies in cosmetically sensitive areas that also affect speech, ability to breathe, and ability to eat are more likely to have a greater impact on psychosocial development compared with those that cause only a facial deformity alone.[9] Patients with treated vascular malformations of the tongue report the most pain and psychological distress postoperatively compared with those with treated vascular malformations of other head and neck sites. This is because even small residual changes can impede speech and swallowing.[10] Furthermore, many social and environmental factors besides lesion appearance and/or functional deficits play a role in distress caused by the lesion. In some cases, more advanced lesions garner greater support from medical professionals and families and patients develop better coping skills than those with less significant appearing lesions who may lack strong support systems.[8]

Psychosocial effects of facial vascular anomalies manifest in the teenage years as difficulties with public appearances and making new friends.[1,11] Additionally, teenagers with facial differences are found to have poorer overall health-related quality of life (HRQOL) with impaired physical, psychological, and school functioning. They are at risk for internalizing anxiety, depression, and social withdrawal. These factors place teens at risk in social situations and may result in avoiding potentially harmful social encounters, causing loneliness and social isolation.[6,12] Despite these difficulties, teenagers do not have difficulties with close friendships once they overcome the initial obstacles of confronting the unknown and turning strangers into friends.[6,7]

## CHALLENGES IN MEASURING PSYCHOSOCIAL IMPACT

Cosmetic, functional, and psychosocial challenges associated with cleft lip and palate are predictable and well described. Disfiguring vascular anomalies of the face are also thought to have a significant impact on a child's psychological adjustment but are less well described. Understanding the psychosocial impact of vascular anomalies of cosmetically sensitive areas is difficult for several reasons, including the following:

1. All vascular lesions are different and behave differently.

   Every vascular lesion behaves differently, thus making treatment plans, treatment effectiveness, and psychosocial impact unique to each patient. The range of physical deformity and functional deficiency differs with size, location, and type of lesion. A small deformity of the lip or nasal tip may have a greater impact on psychosocial issues than a larger deformity of the cheek. Despite involution in cases of hemangiomas or treatment with respect to all vascular lesions, permanent deformity, asymmetry, or functional impairment can be particularly devastating when involving the face. Reports of psychosocial impact often pool findings from a heterogeneous group of patients making interpretation of results difficult and nongeneralizable. Because the treatment is specific to the lesion and location, treatment effect also varies. This diversity makes it difficult to predict or quantify results of the lesion on overall psychosocial well-being
2. There is no validated questionnaire to specifically measure the psychosocial impact of vascular anomalies, rendering interpretation of study results difficult.

   Patient-reported outcome (PRO) and parent-reported outcome measures to assess psychosocial impact have generally not been validated for vascular anomalies. Tapia and colleagues[13] performed a systemic review of HRQOL instruments used for pediatric patients with diverse facial deformities that sometimes included vascular anomalies. From a pool of 155 articles, 120 different HRQOl tools were used to analyze physical, psychological, and social function. Of 60 of these articles using the top 10 most frequently used PRO measures, several were validated for cleft lip and palate but only 1, the Craniofacial Experiences Questionnaire, was validated for use in pediatric patients with many different craniofacial conditions, including hemangiomas. Closer review of this article disclosed hemangiomas in only 2 participants, suggesting results may not be generalizable to vascular anomalies. The lack of an appropriate measurement tool makes it difficult to draw conclusions based on collected data and to pool data collected from multiple studies because each investigator uses as different tool.

3. Studies addressing this topic are limited by small sample sizes.

   Recruiting participants for PRO studies to assess psychological impact can be difficult. Patients with vascular anomalies may be seen frequently during infancy but may be difficult to locate, or less motivated to participate, years later when psychological impact is best assessed. As previously discussed, it is impossible to pool data from multiple studies for a meta-analysis. Therefore, we are forced to accept the small numbers in each individual study and interpret conclusions with caution.

4. Studies are flawed by selection bias

   All of the studies assessing impact of facial abnormalities are prone to selection bias because participation suggests awareness of the lesion. Therefore, all studies may overestimate the psychosocial effects because those who are unaware or unaffected by the lesions are less likely to participate.

## CURRENT KNOWLEDGE OF PSYCHOSOCIAL IMPACT OF HEMANGIOMAS ON PARENTS AND CHILDREN

Despite significant limitations, data are emerging to guide understanding of the psychosocial impact of facial vascular lesions, mostly regarding IHs.

Infants and children cannot always express their emotional concerns and many may be unaware of facial abnormalities. In contrast, parents are acutely aware of their child's appearance and perceptions from others and are often asked to gauge the psychosocial impact of vascular anomalies. In some cases parents are asked to reply based on their own emotions whereas in others they serve as a proxy for their child.

Fortunately, normal attachment patterns exist between babies and parents indicating no discrimination by parents despite the presence of a vascular anomaly in their baby.[4] Nevertheless, many parents of infants with facial hemangiomas report personally experiencing loss, grief, and guilt with respect to their child's hemangioma.[14,15] They also experience panic and disbelief,[11,14] accusations of child abuse,[16] sense of isolation, negative stares, and lifestyle changes, including less recreation, avoidance of public places, and avoidance of enrolling their child into daycare.[5,11,12,14–19] Parents of children with hemangiomas have significantly more emotional distress when compared with the unaffected population and the degree of distress is directly related to the size of the hemangiomas and potential complications.[17]

Worse than a parent's personal grief is their fear of impending psychosocial complications for their child. Parents report sensitivity to reactions from strangers, which makes their children more aware and sensitive to the hemangioma and forces them to confront aspects of social stigmatization.[11,14] They believe their child's life would be different without the hemangioma and express concern for social functioning if the lesion is left untreated.[11,18] Parents worry that their child will be bullied and in 1 study, 9 of 19 parents wanted the hemangioma removed before the child started school.[16] Parents believe the children are too young to appreciate their own condition or any benefit from treatment at the time but believe older children will have less embarrassment and higher self-esteem if treated when they are young.[18] This belief can force parents to make treatment decisions sometimes against the will of their young child.

Physicians must provide anticipatory guidance and support to parents of children with vascular lesions, recognizing that their greatest fear is long-term effects on self-esteem.

In a review published prior to 2012 assessing the psychosocial impact of IHs on children and parents, Zweegers and colleagues[19] identified 7 studies, each using different tools of assessment. The studies used nonvalidated, hemangioma-specific questionnaires as well as validated nonhemangioma specific ones. Studies show mixed results with some reporting significant psychosocial impacts of facial hemangiomas whereas others report no significant effect. Most studies have some degree of skewing and bias. When overall well-being is assessed, it is difficult to determine what is related to the lesion as opposed to other environmental factors, including a parent's ability to help a child cope with a disfiguring lesion. Herein, salient features of these studies are summarized. Although each study used at least 1 validated questionnaire, none of the questionnaires was specific for vascular lesions and at most addressed psychosocial concerns as 1 domain of the questionnaire. Although pertinent positive concerns are highlighted in this review, it is important to recognize that not all studies show concerns of negative effects of IHs.

Dieterich-Miller and colleagues16 reported PRO data from a small pilot study of 19 children, ages 3 years to 5 years, with untreated hemangiomas of the face, head, or neck. Children completed the Joseph Pre-School and Primary Self-concept Screeing Test, and parents completed the Achenbach Child Behavior Checklist as well as nonvalidated open-ended questionnaires. Results were compared with age-matched and socioeconomic-matched control children. No differences were found for behavioral problems and the only difference noted between controls and subjects was that the latter had a lower view of how others value them. The investigators concluded that waiting to treat hemangiomas until patients are at least age 5 is not associated with problems in psychosocial development. This conclusion was determined by open-ended questions not specified in the article.[16]

Kunkel and colleagues[17] surveyed parents of children, 8 months to 9 years of age, with treated hemangiomas of the face and other sites using the Mental Health Inventory and a nonvalidated open-ended questionnaire. Their findings include that parents of children with hemangiomas seem very emotionally distressed compared with the general population; this distress is not correlated with the location of the hemangioma but rather with larger lesions or complications from them. This study was limited by a small sample size and selection bias.

Tanner and colleagues[14] used nonvalidated, in-depth interviews to evaluate 25 children, ages 0 to 8 years, with facial hemangiomas. Half were treated with steroids, laser, or surgery, indicating more severe lesions in the prepropranolol era. Their findings include that parents have negative feelings of disbelief, fear, and mourning, particularly during the hemangioma's growth phase. Approximately half the parents were dissatisfied with their child's care. Based on their findings, the investigators concluded that children may be aware of their hemangioma as early as 18 months of age but do not perceive it negatively until age 4. This study was also limited by small sample size and possible selection bias because more than half the patients required treatment.

Williams and colleagues[18] conducted telephone interviews with 39 parents of children with treated hemangiomas of all sites. Treatment included laser (31), surgery (22), steroid injection (7), and oral steroids (6). A nonvalidated questionnaire using a Likert scale was used. The investigators concluded that parents bear the burden of distress in young children, and earlier treatment may protect from psychosocial repercussions. This study was also limited by small sample size and selection bias of more severe cases because all patients had lesions disfiguring enough to warrant treatment.

Hoornweg and colleagues'[11] retrospective study of 140 parents and 61 children (ages 1–15 years) with facial and nonfacial hemangiomas concluded that it does not seem necessary for early treatment to prevent psychological damage. This study used age-specific, validated HRQOL questionnaires compared with age-adjusted controls as well as a nonvalidated hemangioma specific questionnaire. Although the majority of parents expressed feeling of panic during the growing phase of the hemangioma, a majority of children of all ages and their parents believed that children with hemangiomas can live a good life. They believed most problems, should they exist, would be related to public reaction. No differences were seen in quality of life (QOL) in patients with hemangiomas in visible locations or having a complicated course compared with those with uncomplicated course or lesions that were not readily visible. Children ages 12 to 15 with hemangiomas actually reported significantly more positive emotions than controls, indicating a better QOL score for that domain. Also, mothers of 6-year-old to 11year-old children with hemangiomas reported significantly fewer negative emotions than controls. The findings are limited by possible selection bias, not specifying if patients were treated, measurement tools used, and possible cultural differences of the Netherlands but nevertheless did not show negative psychosocial impacts of hemangiomas.

Sandler and colleagues[15] used a nonvalidated open-ended questionnaire for parents of 16 children with a mean age at presentation of 25 months with hemangiomas of the face and other sites, to conclude that health providers should be aware of the clinical and social consequences of hemangiomas because parents are most stressed by the uncertainty.[15] This was limited by the sample size and measurement tool.

Synder and Pope[5] evaluated more than 200 children with a large range of craniofacial abnormalities and found no difference on the Child Behavior Checklist scores in 2-year-old to 3-year-old children with hemangiomas. Although this study has a large sample size overall, only 13 patients had hemangiomas therefore limiting its generalizability to vascular anomalies.[5]

Cohen-Barak and colleagues[20] evaluated the QOL of patients ages 5 to 8 with head and neck hemangiomas to find no negative effect on QOL or self-esteem from the hemangioma. Half the patients in the hemangioma group, however, had been treated. Those with scars or residual treatment effects reported lower QOL than those without hemangioma. Similar results were found in children ages 4 to 12 with treated port-wine stains (PWSs).[21] These results suggest the protective effect of treatment on QOL and self-esteem.

Reports since Zweegers and colleagues'[19] review have attempted to study a better-defined population of patients with facial anomalies. Two pertinent reports are presented in this article.

Cohen-Barak and colleagues[20] compared QOL scores in 21 5-year-old to 8 year-old children with face, scalp, and/or neck hemangiomas measuring greater than or equal to 2 cm with normal, age-matched controls and found no difference in the validated nonspecific Pediatric Quality of Life Inventory scores of the children.[20] Parents of children with hemangiomas reported higher HRQOL scores for their children compared with scores reported by parents of nonaffected children. Furthermore, the Harter scale of self-esteem showed no difference in scores between affected and nonaffected children. The investigators conclude that a conservative approach for treatment is reasonable for head and neck hemangiomas. Although these findings are encouraging, almost half the patients in their series had treatment, which may have blunted the hemangioma impact on HRQOL, Furthermore, 15% of their patients had neck or scalp lesions, which are more easily concealed, and may have less psychosocial impact than facial lesions alone.

Costa and colleagues[2] studied psychosocial impact of involuted facial IHs in preteen children more systematically by excluding scalp and neck lesions and enrolling only those with an IH in a cosmetically sensitive facial area defined as the nose, lip, cheek, ear, forehead, or periorbital area. The Social Anxiety Scale–Revised was completed by children and parents as well as the Social Competence Inventory by parents. Both surveys were validated to assess social anxiety only and are more specific than generalized HRQOL anxiety scales although not specific for cosmetically disfiguring lesions. Participants scores were compared with pre-established normative data; 144 of the eligible 236 children could be reached since their initial encounter approximately a decade earlier. Thirty 10-year-old children (5.4–12.9 years) participated, two-thirds of whom had received some form of therapy prior to the propranolol era.[2]

Findings disclosed that treatment may significantly affect a child's psychosocial scores. Overall, participants showed lower fear of negative evaluation and reported better social avoidance and social distress scores compared with controls. When separating treated versus untreated lesions, however, only those with treated lesions had better scores. Similarly, prosocial orientation scores (reflecting a child's voluntary social behavior, like helping or sharing) were no different for participants versus controls. Participants without treatment, however, had significantly poorer scores compared with both control data and those receiving treatment. Similar to other studies,[20,21] these findings suggest a protective effect of treatment.

Parent and child Social Anxiety Scale–Revised scores showed good concordance, indicating that parents were a good proxy for their children. Approximately 45% of participants had attended college and another 45% graduate school. Because better educated parents may have greater ability to seek coping strategies for their children, it is possible that selection bias underestimates the social impact of facial IH.

Of 11 participants who elected to send photos, 4 were judged by a panel of surgeons as having major residual scars worthy of offering cosmetic surgery and 7 were minor. Although too small to analyze statistically, it the median social anxiety scores of those with minor lesions were actually worse than those with major residual lesions that had been treated early in life. This finding deserves further reinvestigation because it suggests a psychological benefit of treatment beyond the cosmetic outcome.[21]

## PSYCHOSOCIAL IMPACT OF FACIAL PORT-WINE STAINS

Psychosocial impact of facial PWS was studied in the late 1990s. Although the surveys used were less refined than newer surveys, the participants represent a relatively homogenous group. Van der Horst and colleagues[21] reported data from 41 parents of affected children (mean age 6.4 years) who completed the Child Behavior Checklist and 41 affected adults and adolescents over 13 (mean age 19.2) who completed a validated general health survey modified with additional nonvalidated questions regarding psychosocial, vitality, and energy concerns. Similar to IH data, behavioral problems were not noted in children with PWS. Parents of affected children and affected participants, however, had statistically more negative psychosocial consequences regarding new contacts, entering a public place, visits with relatives and finding a friend/partner. Because all participants were seeking laser treatment of their lesion, the data may be skewed but nevertheless show significant impact of facial PWS.

Other studies have confirmed that participants with PWS and congenital vascular malformations report poorer QOL and sense of well-being compared with a healthy general population predisposing them to increased anxiety and depression.[21,22] As expected, congenital vascular malformation patients report that physical symptoms are less burdensome than the psychological stresses of lack of effective treatment, delay in diagnosis, or uncertain prognosis.[22]

In another interesting study, children ages 8 to 11 rated photographs of other children with and without PWS. Participants clearly discriminated against children based on the presence of PWS and believed the lesion would attract teasing and staring. They personally did not rate these children as less attractive, however, or report they would be less likely to befriend them.[23]

## PSYCHOSOCIAL IMPACT AND AGE OF TREATMENT

Although most children with facial vascular lesions can live a happy and productive life, many children have psychosocial implications for which treatment would be beneficial and earlier treatment of disfiguring lesions may lessen such repercussions later in life.

Both lesions and children's self-image evolve with time. In children with aesthetic, not functional, facial differences, parents perceived significantly more stigmatization of older children because lack of self-awareness in younger children protects from these deleterious effects.[7] Discrimination and teasing early in life can impair psychological development, leading to negative self-perceptions and emotional problems that in adulthood can manifest as difficulties in social situations, particularly new and unfamiliar ones.[12] A supportive home environment can be somewhat protective against social withdrawal but cannot entirely prevent it.[4]

The ideal timing of treatment is dependent on the nature of the lesion, the severity of the disfigurement, the safety and efficacy of available treatment options, and the patient's support system. Most vascular lesions present during infancy or early childhood during which time self-awareness is developing. Toddlers are generally too young to be aware of conditions that make them visibly different.[6,7] Tanner and colleagues[14] report that children with hemangiomas are aware of them as early as 18 months of age but do not perceive themselves as different because of them until age 4. Treatment of disfiguring vascular lesions has consequently historically been recommended by the age of 4 or 5. Beginning at age 7, parents note impaired physical, psychological, and school function that they did not report for younger ages, supporting intervention during preschool age or earlier.[7]

Laser treatment to lighten facial PWS and possibly reduce thickening is generally recommended during infancy.[24] Despite attempts,[25] the ideal age of intervention has not been adequately determined by a prospective randomized study.

Both pharmacologic and surgical treatments are used for cosmetically challenging IH. Pharmacologic treatment is most effective when administered during the proliferative phase of hemangioma growth and, when indicated, should be started in infancy. Although both propranolol and corticosteroids are equally effective in hastening involution, propranolol has fewer serious adverse effects than corticosteroids and has become the mainstay of early pharmacologic treatment.[26,27] To date, propranolol use in infants has not been implicated in causing neurodevelopmental problems although theoretic concerns exist.[28] The human significance of impaired short-term memory in propranolol-treated mice[29] will likely be addressed by long term neurodevelopmental studies assessing propranolol use in early infancy. Such studies are anticipated to appear in the next several years. Like corticosteroids, response to propranolol can be very dramatic or in some cases minimal. It is unclear how often propranolol improves the outcome of hemangioma involution versus merely hastening involution onset.[26] Despite the lack of generalizable outcome knowledge, if not contraindicated, early treatment with propranolol for cosmetically disfiguring lesions seems safe and is indicated at this time.

Surgical excision is also a useful option in managing cosmetically disfiguring IH and may be performed early in infancy for proliferating lesions or delayed until later in childhood for involuted or involuting lesions. Surgical excision of unsightly, poorly involuted IH is generally recommended at approximately ages 4 years to 5 years, before self-awareness develops. Early excision of proliferating IH is more controversial. Early excision during infancy offers advantages of rapid treatment and obviates prolonged pharmacologic treatment and its potential theoretic risks, discussed previously. Early surgical intervention may be particularly useful for small IHs, such as eyelid and nasal tip lesions, where compression of underlying structures may cause long-term abnormalities (Teresa O, MD, FACS, personal communication, 2017). Concerns of early anesthetic exposure on neurodevelopment have been raised[28] and may influence this approach. Although this concern requires further research, 2 recent studies show no differences in specific outcome measures for children undergoing early anesthetic exposure. The Pediatric Anesthesia NeuroDevelopment Assessment study found no difference in IQ scores nor other domain-specific neurocognitive functions, including memory and attention in 105 8-year-old to 15-year-old healthy sibling pairs (95% boys), 1 of whom had been exposed to a short general anesthetic for hernia repair before the age of 3 (mean age 17.3 months).[30] A Canadian retrospective matched cohort study compared standardized government educational scores between 4500 children receiving 1 or more general anesthetics to 13,000 age-matched controls to assess neurodevelopment.[31] There were no differences in scores in subjects exposed between infancy and 2 years of age to single or multiple general anesthetics compared with controls not undergoing anesthesia. Communication and language deficits were noted for those undergoing single general anesthetics between 2 years to 4 years of age but not for those undergoing multiple anesthetic exposure. Outcome data comparing propranolol treated lesions versus surgically excised lesions would be useful to determine whether early surgical intervention during infancy is superior to pharmacologic treatment for some lesions.

Surgical excision of unsightly, poorly involuted IH is generally recommended around age of 4 to 5, before self-awareness develops.

## EFFECT OF SIZE, SEVERITY, AND LOCATION OF FACIAL DIFFERENCES ON PSYCHOSOCIAL DEVELOPMENT

When children with facial differences were evaluated, there was no correlation between the size or type of facial difference and psychological adjustment or HRQOl. Based on these findings, several investigators have concluded that all children who look different face similar problems.[4,6–8]

The closer a lesion is to the central facial triangle, the more noticeable it is to others. Patients with facial anomalies are sensitive to how strangers evaluate them as they are scanned to assess the facial difference. The severity of the lesion can have an impact on how patients adapt to these encounters. Those with minor lesions are the most sensitive and can misinterpret glances from others. They feel ashamed when comparing themselves to others. Major differences force patients to predict social reactions and explain their abnormality given the constant social reactions. Patients with moderate disfigurement have the greatest problems as strangers stare to make sense of the facial difference as opposed to looking away when major differences are present.[8] The goals of health care providers should be to minimize disfigurement and its resulting psychosocial impact.

## SUMMARY

Society has a long history of stigmatizing facial disfigurement, which can cause discrimination and bullying early in life impairing psychosocial development. Symmetry is associated with health, whereas asymmetry can provoke distress in others. The modern-day culture emphasizing appearance and sharing of photographs across the digital universe increases the pressure on those who look different.[7] Drawing conclusions about the psychosocial impact of facial vascular anomalies can be daunting; however, it can be concluded that they do occur for many patients and most often affect social interactions, particularly in new situations. Effects begin to be seen in adolescence and show no correlation with the size or severity of the lesion. Patients also suffering from functional deficits have more troubles than those without. Treatment may be protective against the development of psychosocial problems, in some cases regardless of how aesthetically effective it is. It is important for health care providers to be aware of these psychosocial aspects when managing patients and their families with facial vascular lesions.

## REFERENCES

1. Bauland CG, Luning TH, Smit JM, et al. Untreated hemangiomas: growth pattern and residual lesions. Plast Reconstr Surg 2011;127:1643–8.
2. Costa AV, Haimowitz R, Cheng YI, et al. Social impact of facial infantile hemangiomas in preteen children. JAMA Otolaryngol Head Neck Surg 2016;142(1):13–9.
3. Martini de Oliveria A, Buchain PC, Vizzotto ADB, et al. Psychochosocial impact. In: Gellman MD, Turner JR, editors. Encyclopedia of behavioral medicine. New York: Springer; 2013. p. 1583–4.
4. Rumsey N, Harcourt D. Visible differences amongst children and adolescents: issues and interventions. Dev Neurorehabil 2007;10(2):113–23.
5. Snyder H, Pope AW. Psychosocial adjustment in children and adolescents with craniofacial anomaly: diagnosis-specific patterns. Cleft Palate Craniofac J 2010;47:264–72.
6. Masnari O, Schiestl C, Rossler J, et al. Stigmatization predicts psychological adjustment and quality of life in children and adolescents with a facial difference. J Pediatr Psychol 2013;38:162–72.
7. Masnari O, Landolt MA, Roessler J, et al. Self- and parent-perceived stigmatization in children and adolescents with congenital or acquired facial differences. J Plast Reconstr Aesthet Surg 2012;65(12):1664–70.
8. Bradbury E. Meeting the psychological needs of patients with facial disfigurement. Br J Oral Maxillofac Surg 2012;50(3):193–6.

9. Millard T, Richman LC. Different cleft conditions, facial appearance, and speech: relationship to psychological variables. Cleft Palate Craniofac J 2001;38(1): 68–75.
10. Kenny SA, Majeed N, Zhand N, et al. Psychological comorbidities and compliance to interventional treatment of patients with cutaneous vascular malformations. Interv Neuroradiol 2016;22(4):489–94.
11. Hoornweg MJ, Grootenhuis MA, van der Horst CMAM. Health-related quality of life and impact of haemangiomas on children and their parents. J Plast Reconstr Aesthet Surg 2009;62:1265–71.
12. Weinstein JM, Chamlin SL. Quality of life in vascular anomalies. Lymphat Res Biol 2005;3:256–9.
13. Tapia VJ, Epstein S, Tolmach OS, et al. Health-related quality of life instruments for pediatric patients with diverse facial deformities: a systematic literature review. Plast Reconstr Surg 2016;138(1):175–87.
14. Tanner JL, Dechert MP, Frieden IJ. Growing up with a facial hemangioma: parent and child coping and adaptation. Pediatrics 1998;101(3 Pt1):446–52.
15. Sandler G, Adams S, Taylor C. Paediatric vascular birthmarks the psychological impact and the role of the GP. Aust Fam Physician 2009;38(3):169–71.
16. Dieterich-Miller CA, Cohen BA, Liggett J. Behavioral adjustment and self-concept of young children with hemangiomas. Pediatr Dermatol 1992;9:241–5.
17. Kunkel EJ, Zager R, Hausman CL, et al. An interdisciplinary group for parents and children with hemangiomas. Psychosomatics 1994;35:524–32.
18. Williams EF III, Hochman M, Rodgers BJ, et al. A psychological profile of children with hemangiomas and their families. Arch Facial Plast Surg 2003;5(3):229–34.
19. Zweegers J, van der Vleuten CJM. The psychosocial impact of an infantile haemangioma on children and their parents. Arch Dis Child 2012;97:922–6.
20. Cohen-Barak E, Rozenman D, Shani Adir A. Infantile haemangiomas and quality of life. Arch Dis Child 2013;98:676–9.
21. Van der Horst CM, de Borgie CA, Knopper JL, et al. Psychosocial adjustment of children and adults with port wine stains. Br J Plast Surg 1997;50(6):463–7.
22. Fahrni JO, Cho EY, Engelberger RP, et al. Quality of life in patients with congenital vascular malformations. J Vasc Surg Venous Lymphat Disord 2014;2(1):46–51.
23. Demellweek C, Humphris GM, Hare M, et al. Children's perceptions of, and attitude towards, unfamiliar peers with facial port-wine stains. J Pediatr Psychol 1997;22(4):471–85.
24. Ashinoff R, Geronemus RG. Flashlamp-pumped pulsed dye laser for port-wine stains in infancy: earlier versus late treatment. J Am Acad Dermatol 1991;24: 467–72.
25. van der Horst CM, Koster PH, de Borgie CA, et al. Effect of the timing of treatment of port-wine stains with the flash-lamp-pumped pulsed-dye laser. N Engl J Med 1998;338:1028–33.
26. Bauman NM, McCarter RJ, Guzzetta PC, et al. Propranolol vs prednisolone for symptomatic infantile hemangiomas: a randomized clinical trial. JAMA Otolaryngol Head Neck Surg 2014;140:323–30.
27. Leaute-Labreze C, Boccara O, Degrugillier-Chopinet C, et al. Safety of oral propranolol for the treatment of infantile hemangioma: a systematic review. Pediatrics 2016;138(4) [pii:e20160353].
28. Stratman G, Lee J, Sall JW, et al. Effect of general anesthesia in infancy on long-term recognition memory in humans and rats. Neuropsychopharmacology 2014; 39:2275–87.

29. Sun H, Mao Y, Wang J, et al. Effects of beta-adrenergic antagonist, propranolol, on spatial memory and exploratory behavior in mice. Neurosci Lett 2011;498: 133–7.
30. Sun LS, Guohua L, Miller TL, et al. Association between a single general anesthesia exposure before age 36 months and neurocognitive outcomes in later childhood. JAMA 2016;315:2312–20 (PANDA study).
31. Graham MR, Bronwell M, Chateau DG, et al. Neurodevelopmental assessment in kindergarten in children exposed to general anesthesia before the age of 4 years: a retrospective matched cohort study. Anesthesiology 2016;125:667–77.

# Outcome Measurement for Vascular Malformations of the Head and Neck

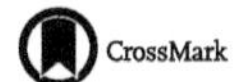

Sophie E.R. Horbach, MD[a,b,*], Amber P.M. Rongen, MD[a], Teresa M. O, MD, MArch[b], Milton Waner, MBBCh(Wits), FS(SA), MD[b], Chantal M.A.M. van der Horst, MD, PhD[a]

**KEYWORDS**

• Vascular anomalies • Outcomes • Outcome measures • Core outcome set
• Measurement instruments

**KEY POINTS**

- Patients with peripheral vascular malformations of the head and neck vary greatly in clinical symptoms, cosmetic appearance, and perceived impairment in psychological and physical well-being.
- There are multiple treatment modalities for vascular malformations; therefore, it is important that a standardized evaluation of outcome data is performed so that study data can be compared and aggregated into meta-analyses and treatment guidelines.
- A consensus-derived set of core outcome domains has recently been developed by a large group of experts on vascular anomalies, including patients and parents of patients.
- Although various outcome instruments have previously been developed and tested to measure these constructs, it is not yet clear what the best available outcome instruments are for measuring these core outcome domains in clinical trials.

## INTRODUCTION

Vascular malformations are abnormally developed blood vessels or lymphatic vessels that are caused by an erroneous embryologic development of the vascular system. In the classification of the International Society for the Study of Vascular Anomalies,[1,2] vascular malformations are categorized based on the types of vessels involved, into

Disclosure Statement: The authors have nothing to disclose.

[a] Department of Plastic, Reconstructive and Hand Surgery, Academic Medical Center, University of Amsterdam, Meibergdreef 9, Amsterdam 1100 DD, The Netherlands; [b] Department of Otolaryngology–Head and Neck Surgery, Vascular Birthmark Institute of New York, Facial Nerve Center, Manhattan Eye, Ear and Throat Hospital, 210 East 64th Street, 7 Floor, New York, NY 10065, USA

* Corresponding author. Department of Plastic, Reconstructive and Hand Surgery, Academic Medical Center (AMC), PO Box 22660, Amsterdam 1100 DD, The Netherlands.
*E-mail address:* s.e.horbach@amc.uva.nl


https://doi.org/10.1016/j.otc.2017.09.014

simple and combined vascular malformations. Only 1 type of vessel is affected in simple vascular malformations: capillary malformations (CM), venous malformations (VM), lymphatic malformations (LM), arteriovenous malformations (AVM), and arteriovenous fistulas. Multiple types of blood vessels and/or lymphatic vessels are present in the malformation in combined vascular malformations.[2] Vascular malformations can occur sporadically or as part of a syndrome.

Each malformation type has characteristic clinical signs and symptoms. There are many factors that contribute to the effect a specific type of vascular malformation has on an individual patient. It is important to consider the type of the malformation and the size, extent, and location of the lesion in determining the disease burden.

Some vascular malformations can cause aesthetic and functional disability. Vascular malformations located in the head and neck may distort facial features and, therefore, can drastically alter the facial appearance of a patient. The mass effect of the vascular malformation on adjacent body structures can also cause functional impairment or other specific complaints associated with the affected body part, such as speaking difficulties in patients with vascular malformations in the tongue or oropharynx. This in turn may limit patients in their study and/or work, sports, and hobby activities. Thus, despite the benign character of the disease, vascular malformations often cause significant burden that can interfere with patients' daily lives. Consequently, vascular malformations can have a great impact on a patient's psychosocial and physical functioning, as also pointed out in Alexandra G. Espinel and Nancy M. Bauman's article, "Psychosocial Impact of Vascular Anomalies on Children and Their Families," in this issue.

## HOW TO CHOOSE BETWEEN AN INCREASING NUMBER OF TREATMENT OPTIONS?

There are numerous treatment options for the different types of vascular malformations. For CMs, the most common therapeutic intervention is laser therapy using the pulsed dye laser.[3–5] The treatment of VMs and LMs ranges from a wait-and-see policy to minimally invasive interventions, such as sclerotherapy (eg, with bleomycin or ethanol), laser and surgery. More recent additions to the therapeutic armamentarium are systemic therapies, such as sirolimus[6] and sildenafil,[7] which primarily focus on relieving symptoms, such as pain, swelling, and bleeding. AVMs are usually treated with arterial embolization, surgery, or a combination of these modalities.

To differentiate between the large number of available therapeutic modalities, it is important to gain detailed information about the efficacy and safety of these interventions. Therefore, it is of utmost importance that prospective comparative effectiveness studies are conducted, so that outcomes of the available treatment strategies can be compared.

Investigators who have attempted to perform meta-analyses and systematic reviews in this field,[8–11] however, have been hindered by the lack of high-quality evidence. This was not only due to the fact that the number of prospective studies in this field are scarce but also because of the heterogeneity in outcome reporting across the published clinical studies.[9] Overall, clinical research studies on vascular malformations vary greatly in what is measured to evaluate treatment outcome (outcome domains) and how these measurements were performed (outcome instruments).

## OUTCOME MEASURES

As a result of the heterogeneity in outcome domains and outcome instruments that are used in clinical studies, comparing and pooling of study data of different clinical trials are nearly impossible. Ideally, outcome measures for vascular malformations should be standardized, so that study outcomes of different trials can be aggregated into systematic reviews and meta-analyses, which can facilitate the development of evidence-based guidelines.

To date, however, it is unknown which outcomes are a good reflection of the treatment success of an intervention. As discussed previously, vascular malformations can cause numerous different symptoms that may (or may not) impair a patient's physical or psychological well-being. Because of the clinical heterogeneity of the disease, the reasons why patients desire treatment may differ greatly as well. Consequently, the desired treatment outcomes may also vary between individual patients. This makes it challenging to determine which outcomes are most important to investigate when conducting a clinical trial. Omitting outcome data, however, that are not deemed important for 1 individual patient, but may be important for another, results in an incomplete data set when comparing study results for different treatment strategies or patient subgroups.

### *Core Outcome Set*

The development of a core outcome set (COS) could possibly address the issues (discussed previously) in outcome reporting. A COS is a consensus-derived standardized set of the most important outcomes for a certain health condition that should be measured as a minimum in all clinical trials investigating treatment outcome in that specific health condition.[12] With the ongoing Outcome Measures for Vascular Malformations (OVAMA) project, a group of international researchers and experts on vascular anomalies is attempting to create a COS for clinical research on vascular malformations (LM, VM, and AVM). This COS should include recommendations for the outcome domains that should be measured and which outcome instruments should be used. COSs are currently being developed for a broad variety of diseases, such as skin diseases,[13,14] cancer,[15,16] and disorders of the musculoskeletal system.[17] The need for a COSs has been advocated by disease-specific research groups, such as the Harmonizing Outcome Measures for Eczema initiative[18–20] and Outcome measures in Rheumatology.[21] COS development is relatively new but rapidly growing. The Core Outcome Measures in Effectiveness Trials initiative maintains a database with the aim of including all registered and ongoing COS projects. Furthermore, the Cochrane Skin Group – Core Outcome Set Initiative is a research working group within the international Cochrane Skin Group, which has the mission of developing and implementing COSs in dermatology. The increasing importance of COSs is noticeable, for example, the National Institute for Health Research Health Technology Assessment program, requires COSs to be considered in the funding applications of clinical trials, and the use of COSs in reviews and clinical practice guidelines is being encouraged by the Cochrane and the Grading of Recommendations Assessment, Development and Evaluation.[12]

### *Core Outcome Domains*

As determined in the ongoing OVAMA consensus project[22], the COS for vascular malformations should at least include outcome domains of radiological assessment of the vascular malformation, patient-reported and parent-reported pain, overall severity of symptoms, physician-assessed location-specific signs of disease, quality of life, patient satisfaction with treatment and outcome, and adverse events. Signs and symptoms that are specific for the type of vascular malformation should only be assessed when appropriate. It is recommended, but not (yet) considered essential, to additionally measure the appearance of the vascular malformation and whether or not there was recurrence of disease after the treatment intervention. Many physicians and patients agreed that recurrence and appearance were important domains but consensus was not yet reached because of disagreements concerning the domain definitions. These domains will be reappraised in a future meeting of the OVAMA consensus group of experts on vascular anomalies.

### *Core Outcome Instruments*

Ideally the set of core outcome instruments for vascular malformations should cover all relevant core outcome domains that were agreed on in the consensus project. This means that multiple instruments may have to be used to assure that all domains are measured in a clinical trial. It is also possible that some instruments included in a COS have the potential to measure multiple core domains (eg, a questionnaire covering both disease symptoms and quality of life). There is no consensus yet, however, on which instruments should be included in the COS. The selection of the core outcome instruments will be based on how well the available outcome instruments are validated in patients with vascular malformations. In general, it is preferred to use outcome instruments that have been developed and validated using appropriate methodology, which can be evaluated using a methodological checklist of the COnsensus-based Standards for the selection of health Measurement INstruments working group.[12,23] Overall, there is a choice between instruments that have been developed and validated specifically for vascular malformations (condition-specific instruments), those that have been validated for other diseases or conditions that resemble the symptoms and disease burden of vascular malformations, and instruments that have been developed to measure a certain construct in a general population without a specific health condition (generic instruments). Systematic reviews to inform the instrument selection process are under way and an international consensus meeting will be necessary to reach a final consensus on the core outcome instruments for the COS.

### *Disease-Specific Outcome Instruments*

So far, there is only 1 outcome measurement instrument specifically developed and validated for vascular malformations. The Lymphatic Malformation Function (LMF) instrument was developed by Balakrishnan and colleagues[24,25] and validated by Kirkham and colleagues.[26] This outcome instrument focuses on functional and clinical signs of disease and subsequent impact on daily life in LMs in the head and neck region in pediatric patients. It is a parent-reported outcome instrument, which asks parents to indicate on a 5-point Likert scale the frequency of disease-related signs and functional impacts over the previous 30 days. The questionnaire consists of 7 questions about signs (mouth bleeding, tongue swelling, difficulty chewing, difficulty swallowing, drooling, difficulty vocalizing, and difficulty breathing) and 5 questions about the impacts of the disease on the patient's life (missing out on things a patient wanted to do, avoiding going out in public, appearing sad or angry, appearing to be in pain, and difficulty sleeping). Preliminary validation studies have been carried out in parents of a group of patients aged from 0.5 year to 15 years old.[26] Internal consistency, test-retest reliability, content validity (face validity), and construct validity of the LMF have been investigated.

The LMF is only validated, however, for a very specific subgroup of pediatric patients.

### *Condition-Specific Outcome Measurement Instruments for Related Conditions*

Regarding the paucity of condition-specific instruments for vascular malformations, it may also be interesting to investigate the applicability of outcome instruments that were not specifically developed for vascular malformations but for other conditions that are relatable in terms of physical symptoms and disease burden. For example, instruments validated for chronic venous insufficiency, such as the 20-item Chronic Venous Insufficiency Quality of Life Questionnaire, could in theory also be relevant for patients VMs of the lower extremities, because these conditions are similar in terms of disease symptoms. To assure that this instrument is truly applicable in vascular malformations, however, further validation studies in this patient population are mandatory. Another outcome instrument is the FACE-Q Kids, a patient self-reported questionnaire currently being developed by the same research group that has developed the FACE-Q for measuring facial appearance in adults undergoing aesthetic procedures.[27] The FACE-Q Kids will specifically focus on congenital facial anomalies in pediatric patients. Although this instrument will be validated for various congenital facial anomalies, such as congenital nevi and other congenital skin conditions, it may also be tested in patients with vascular anomalies and, therefore, can be a useful instrument for this patient group in the future.

### *Generic Outcome Instruments*

Various health-related quality-of-life questionnaires have been developed and validated to measure any impairment in general health, including physical and psychological well-being. Well-known questionnaires, such as the 36-Item Short Form Health Survey and the EuroQoL-5D, have also been used in a few studies on vascular malformations[28,29]. It is, however, uncertain if these questionnaires have the potency to capture slight changes in health status, because generic questionnaires are usually crude and not sufficiently tailored to the disease burden caused by a specific health condition.

## SUMMARY

The large variety in clinical disease characteristics, for example, type, size, extent, and location of vascular malformations, makes this condition heterogeneous and challenging to treat. Although numerous treatment options are available and many have been investigated in the literature, therapeutic decision making is still mostly based on expert opinions because strong scientific evidence is lacking. It is difficult to combine and compare study results in evidence-based guidelines, because clinical research studies vary in outcomes that are measured and outcome instruments that are used to perform these measurements. Standardizing outcome measurement is thus an important step toward the evidence-based management for vascular malformations of the head and neck. A standardized COS for vascular malformations is under development. So far, there is a consensus on what should be measured in clinical trials. Although there are few condition-specific and possibly relevant generic outcome instruments available to measure desired treatment outcome in vascular malformations of the head and neck, a consensus-derived set of instruments that should be used to perform these measurements is not yet readily available.

## REFERENCES


1. Dasgupta R, Fishman SJ. ISSVA classification. Semin Pediatr Surg 2014;23(4): 158–61.
2. Wassef M, Blei F, Adams D, et al. Vascular anomalies classification: recommendations from the International Society for the Study of Vascular Anomalies. Pediatrics 2015;136(1):e203–14.

3. Brightman LA, Geronemus RG, Reddy KK. Laser treatment of port-wine stains. Clin Cosmet Investig Dermatol 2015;8:27–33.
4. Chen JK, Ghasri P, Aguilar G, et al. An overview of clinical and experimental treatment modalities for port wine stains. J Am Acad Dermatol 2012;67(2):289–304.
5. van der Horst CM, Koster PH, de Borgie CA, et al. Effect of the timing of treatment of port-wine stains with the flash-lamp-pumped pulsed-dye laser. N Engl J Med 1998;338(15):1028–33.
6. Adams DM, Trenor CC 3rd, Hammill AM, et al. Efficacy and safety of sirolimus in the treatment of complicated vascular anomalies. Pediatrics 2016;137(2): e20153257.
7. Danial C, Tichy AL, Tariq U, et al. An open-label study to evaluate sildenafil for the treatment of lymphatic malformations. J Am Acad Dermatol 2014;70(6):1050–7.
8. Horbach SE, Lokhorst MM, Saeed P, et al. Sclerotherapy for low-flow vascular malformations of the head and neck: a systematic review of sclerosing agents. J Plast Reconstr Aesthet Surg 2016;69(3):295–304.
9. Horbach SE, Rigter IM, Smitt JH, et al. Intralesional bleomycin injections for vascular malformations: a systematic review and meta-analysis. Plast Reconstr Surg 2016;137(1):244–56.
10. van der Vleuten CJ, Kater A, Wijnen MH, et al. Effectiveness of sclerotherapy, surgery, and laser therapy in patients with venous malformations: a systematic review. Cardiovasc Intervent Radiol 2014;37(4):977–89.
11. Gurgacz S, Zamora L, Scott NA. Percutaneous sclerotherapy for vascular malformations: a systematic review. Ann Vasc Surg 2014;28(5):1335–49.
12. Prinsen CA, Vohra S, Rose MR, et al. How to select outcome measurement instruments for outcomes included in a "Core Outcome Set" - a practical guideline. Trials 2016;17(1):449.
13. Thorlacius L, Ingram JR, Garg A, et al. Protocol for the development of a core domain set for hidradenitis suppurativa trial outcomes. BMJ Open 2017;7(2): e014733.
14. Eleftheriadou V, Thomas K, van Geel N, et al. Developing core outcome set for vitiligo clinical trials: international e-Delphi consensus. Pigment Cell Melanoma Res 2015;28(3):363–9.
15. McNair AG, Whistance RN, Forsythe RO, et al. Core outcomes for colorectal cancer surgery: a consensus study. PLoS Med 2016;13(8):e1002071.
16. MacLennan S, Bekema HJ, Williamson PR, et al. A core outcome set for localised prostate cancer effectiveness trials: protocol for a systematic review of the literature and stakeholder involvement through interviews and a Delphi survey. Trials 2015;16(1):76.
17. Chiarotto A, Deyo RA, Terwee CB, et al. Core outcome domains for clinical trials in non-specific low back pain. Eur Spine J 2015;24(6):1127–42.
18. Chalmers JR, Simpson E, Apfelbacher CJ, et al. Report from the fourth international consensus meeting to harmonize core outcome measures for atopic eczema/dermatitis clinical trials (HOME initiative). Br J Dermatol 2016;175(1): 69–79.
19. Schmitt J, Langan S, Stamm T, et al. Core outcome domains for controlled trials and clinical recordkeeping in eczema: international multiperspective Delphi consensus process. J Invest Dermatol 2011;131(3):623–30.
20. Schmitt J, Apfelbacher C, Spuls PI, et al. The Harmonizing Outcome Measures for Eczema (HOME) roadmap: a methodological framework to develop core sets of outcome measurements in dermatology. J Invest Dermatol 2015;135(1): 24–30.

21. Boers M, Kirwan JR, Wells G, et al. Developing core outcome measurement sets for clinical trials: OMERACT filter 2.0. J Clin Epidemiol 2014;67(7):745–53.
22. Horbach SER, van der Horst CMAM, Blei F, et al; The OVAMA consensus group. Development of an international core outcome set for peripheral vascular malformations (OVAMA project). Br J Dermatol. Accepted Author Manuscript. http://dx.doi.org/10.1111/bjd.16029.
23. Mokkink LB, Terwee CB, Patrick DL, et al. The COSMIN checklist for assessing the methodological quality of studies on measurement properties of health status measurement instruments: an international Delphi study. Qual Life Res 2010; 19(4):539–49.
24. Balakrishnan K, Edwards TC, Perkins JA. Functional and symptom impacts of pediatric head and neck lymphatic malformations: developing a patient-derived instrument. Otolaryngol Head Neck Surg 2012;147(5):925–31.
25. Balakrishnan K, Bauman N, Chun RH, et al. Standardized outcome and reporting measures in pediatric head and neck lymphatic malformations. Otolaryngol Head Neck Surg 2015;152(5):948–53.
26. Kirkham EM, Edwards TC, Weaver EM, et al. The lymphatic malformation function (LMF) instrument. Otolaryngol Head Neck Surg 2015;153(4):656–62.
27. Klassen AF, Cano SJ, Schwitzer J, et al. FACE-Q scales for health-related quality of life, early life impact and satisfaction with outcomes and decision to have treatment: development and validation. Plast Reconstr Surg 2014;135(2):375–86.
28. Ono Y, Osuga K, Takura T, et al. Cost-effectiveness analysis of percutaneous sclerotherapy for venous malformations. J Vasc Interv Radiol 2016;27(6):831–7.
29. Wohlgemuth WA, Muller-Wille R, Teusch V, et al. Ethanolgel sclerotherapy of venous malformations improves health-related quality-of-life in adults and children - results of a prospective study. Eur Radiol 2017;27(6):2482–8.

# The Role of Surgery in the Management of Infantile Hemangiomas: What is the Best Timing?

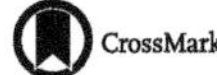

Marcelo Hochman, MD

**KEYWORDS**

• Surgery • Infantile hemangioma • Self-image • Timing • Developmental milestones

**KEY POINTS**

- Surgery can effect total removal of infantile hemangiomas.
- The aim of surgery, as with any other modality of treatment, is to obtain the best possible result for a given patient.
- Tumor size, location, and phase of the natural history in which the tumor presents for treatment have an impact on treatment options.

Surgery can effect total removal of infantile hemangiomas (IHs), set the stage for further multimodality treatment, or treat sequelae and complications of a tumor's natural history. Surgical techniques for removing IHs of specific anatomic locations can be found[1–3]; however, little has been written about the timing of surgery in the overall management of these tumors. The aim of surgery, as with any other modality of treatment, is to obtain the best possible result for a given patient. To successfully achieve that aim, defining what is meant by *best possible result* and by when to achieve that result is needed. Perhaps more important than defining the best possible result is to make a determination of what is an *acceptable result*. The visual impact of a 1-cm IH of the nasal tip is different from that of the same exact lesion on the thigh. The functional import of a 5-mm IH involving the oral commissure is potentially very different from the same lesion involving the upper eyelid. These examples highlight that variables, such as size and location, are important. What is considered acceptable as a result of treatment of the nasal tip and eyelid IH likely is different from that for the corresponding thigh and oral commissure lesions. To recap, IHs are true neoplasms that typically appear within the first few weeks of life and undergo rapid proliferation in the first 2 months. The rate of endothelial tumor cell hyperplasia slows down by approximately the sixth month and is overcome by apoptosis and regression of the tumor volume, mostly over the next 2 years to 3 years and even more slowly after that. This

Disclosure: M. Hochman has nothing to disclose.
The Hemangioma and Malformation Treatment Center, Charleston, SC, USA
*E-mail address:* DrHochman@FacialSurgeryCenter.com

Otolaryngol Clin N Am 51 (2018) 119–123
https://doi.org/10.1016/j.otc.2017.09.010

involution is characterized by slow replacement of the tumor burden by fibrofatty scar. Thus, during proliferation, the tissue that the clinician observes is quite different from that in involution and likewise variably responsive to different therapeutic modalities.

Thin, superficial, proliferating tumors may be amenable to laser or topical medical therapy. Thicker, larger, or functionally threatening proliferating lesions may require systemic medical therapy. During involution, when surgery is most useful, the type of IH (as defined by the depth of cutaneous involvement) determines the type of persistent tissue – thin superficial IHs may involute with no residuum whereas a compound IH may leave expanded, dystrophic, telangiectatic skin and a deep IH a mass underlying perfectly normal skin. Each scenario requires different potential medical, laser, and surgical options and combinations, which are discussed throughout this issue. Thus, tumor size, location, and phase of the natural history in which the tumor presents for treatment have an impact on treatment options. The choice of treatment options, however, cannot be based exclusively on the tumor qualities. Patients carrying the tumor need to be taken into account. This may seem an explicit concept when dealing with patients who can speak for themselves and make decisions and value judgements on their own behalf. Because the patients affected by IH are infants and young children, however, the burden of this decision making falls on parents and clinicians. Beyond relying on the characteristics of the tumor, as previously discussed, the best course of action can be further determined by considering the data on development of consciousness of self and on the value of restoration of appearance.

Self-awareness is a fundamental issue in developmental psychology that, in my opinion, is germane to the issue of when to strive to obtain the best possible result. Humans are a uniquely self-conscious species – caring how they look with others in mind. It is through the gaze of others that humans measure how securely accepted by others they are. Furmark[4] has shown that there is no more dreadful phobia than that of being socially rejected and alienated from others, which explains why people rank public speech as the most common, greatest fear. A review of the entire sequence of development of self-awareness,[5] although fascinating, is beyond the scope of this article. There is a general consensus, however, on a few major landmarks that are pertinent.[6] Infants between 3 months and 12 months old tend to treat their own image in a mirror as a playmate, an other. They are oblivious that a sticker or rouge has surreptitiously been placed on their forehead and is visible on the image in the mirror. By the end of the first year, children demonstrate enhanced curiosity of the specular image by touching or looking behind the mirror but still do not recognize their selves. It is only by 18 months that infants begin to look for the sticker or red blemish on their own bodies to remove it. This is the literal beginning of identity. At approximately 2 years of age, children begin to express embarrassment – the first signs of awareness of their public appearance. A stranger pointing at the hemangioma on a 2-year old's to 3-year old's face is recognized by the child as being about "me," that there is something that others see in them. Over time, this sense of self becomes rooted and by 3 years children begin to grasp the temporal dimension of the self – that their selves endure beyond what can be seen in the mirror or a photo. The cognitive ability of running a simulation of others' minds (what others are thinking of "me") is clearly established by age 3 years to 4 years. The basic fear and embarrassment that the red mark on the cheek that they see on themselves in the mirror persists and is visible to others at all times becomes ingrained by 4 years to 5 years of age.

A psychological profile survey of children with hemangiomas and their families[7] showed that given earlier intervention, affected children did not seem to experience significant emotional trauma from their condition; their families, however, experienced appreciable emotional and psychological distress in dealing with a child with a facial difference. That the presence of facial lesions induces a significant social penalty, specifically that observers are less comfortable communicating with people who have facial defects, has been demonstrated.[8] Other studies have shown that people with facial deformities are perceived as less attractive and are ascribed emotionally negative labels.[9] Another study showed that casual observers perceive that facial defects significantly decrease quality of life, an effect improved by reconstructive surgery. The value of the reconstruction, although highly valued by society,[10] is valued even more so by the affected patient. Patients' perceived improvement in appearance and function is greater than that of objective observers,[11] reiterating humans' concern about how they look.

The reviewed current knowledge of the biology of the IHs, the data on the development of self, and on the value of restoration of appearance can be used to help inform the role of surgery in the management of these tumors. If the known timelines about the biology of IH are superimposed on developmental milestones in the determination of self-image, important considerations appear (**Fig. 1**). By the time 85% of tumors have ceased proliferating (6 months), an infant has not met any psychological milestones pertinent to this discussion. The maximum rate of involution occurs between 12 months and 24 months of age.[12] Beyond that, the rate of regression of the tumor slows remarkably, to the point that by 4 years to 5 years it is barely clinically detectable. The replacement by fat and scar may continue at a reduced rate for some time but not in an asymptotic fashion, as depicted in most diagrams in the literature.

As discussed previously, a child's ability to pass the mirror sticker test occurs at approximately 18 months — during the fastest rate of involution. By 24 months to

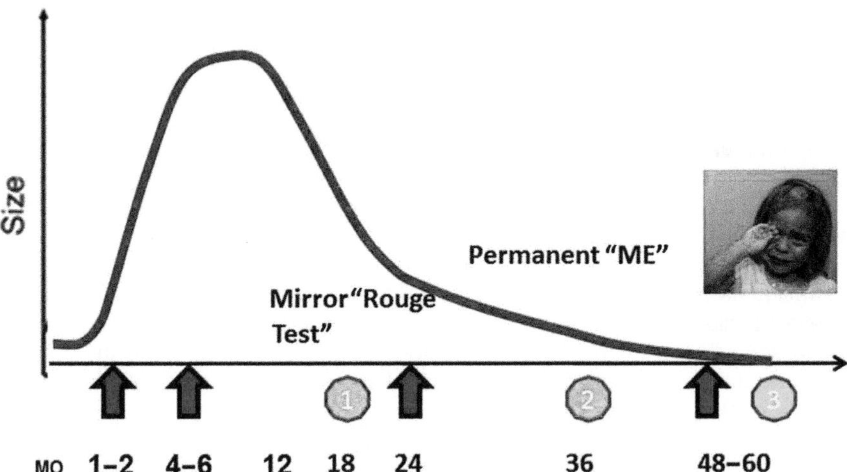


**Fig. 1.** Natural history of IH versus developmental milestones. The figure shows the natural history of IH (*blue curve*) with proliferation and involution (size) over time. The maximum rate of proliferation occurs at approximately 2 months (*first arrow*) and is complete in more than 85% of tumors by 6 months (*second arrow*). The maximum rate of involution occurs by 24 months (*third arrow*), coinciding with the infant's recognition of the sticker or rouge in the specular image (1) as being on her own body (development of identity). The rate of apoptosis and involution decreases over time (2), coinciding with further development of self-consciousness evidenced by embarrassment and avoidance behavior (3). By 4 years to 5 years of age, the rate of involution has decreased to a clinically insignificant level (*fourth arrow*). Surgical excision prior to this time is warranted to avoid the psychological trauma of facial difference.

36 months, a sense of me is established and the realization that "there is something on my face" coincides with the dramatic decrease in rate of involution. By late involution, 5 years to 6 years of age, a child's sense of self-image is ingrained. By then, most children are getting ready to enter formal schooling, with its attendant peer pressures from the other 5-year olds to 6-year olds who are comparing their appearances with that of the affected child because they are all on the same developmental timetable of self-recognition.

Synthesizing the previous discussions, if an acceptable result for a given IH can be obtained by surgery during involution but within the timeframe of specified developmental milestones, it is reasonable to propose it as an option. The collective experience of surgery for IH at various locations shows that acceptable results are achievable. In addition, these results are achievable with a limited number of procedures by the time a child is aware of the impact of these on his self.

Surgery in the proliferative phase of IHs is not usual because the tumor needs to be completely removed lest the remnant continue to proliferate as destined. Additionally, it may be too early to determine the final extent of the tumor. Exceptions for early surgery during the proliferative phase may include functional issues, such as threat to vision or the airway; refractory ulceration; and possibly very large lesions, which under special circumstances allow in toto removal of the tumor with primary closure and without deformation of anatomic entities.

Surgery during involution has become common when a procedure can achieve a result that is at least as good as waiting for involution to be complete. Focal tumors are more likely to benefit from single-stage, definitive excisions whereas segmental, diffuse, and/or large lesions can be addressed in serial fashion.[13]

Sequelae of involution and complications, such as scarring, distended skin, and distortion of anatomic features, fall into the surgical realm without much dissent. The key judgment is in the timing of the surgical interventions. In my opinion, as much as possible, the goal of surgery is to obtain the best possible result by the age of 3 years so the child's image of self is not affected. If this is not possible because of the complexity of the excision and reconstruction or timing of presentation to the surgeon, then the best effort should be made to finalize the result by the time the affected child is entering formal schooling, at approximately 5 years to 6 years of age. The concept of intervening by this age for elective otoplasties to avoid the stigma of facial difference has been applied for decades.

Surgery, as part of multimodality therapy for IH, is now commonplace and can achieve excellent results as demonstrated in the literature. It is the timing of the surgery in accord with developmental milestones that now needs to be the focus to give these children the best chance to literally face the world without adverse psychological sequelae.

## REFERENCES

1. Hochman M, Mascareño A. Management of nasal hemangiomas. Arch Facial Plast Surg 2005;7:295–300.
2. O TM, Schneidermann-Poley C, Tan M, et al. Distribution, clinical characteristics and surgical treatment of lip infantile hemangiomas. JAMA Facial Plast Surg 2013;15(4):292–304.
3. Cho YK, Ryu DW, Chung HY, et al. Surgical management of scalp infantile hemangiomas. J Craniofac Surg 2015;26(4):1169–72.
4. Furmark T. Social phobia: overview of community surveys. Acta Psychiatr Scand 2002;105(2):84–93.

5. Rochat P. Five levels of self-awareness as they unfold early in life. Conscious Cogn 2013;12:717–31.
6. Amsterdam BK, Levitt M. Consciousness of self and painful self-consciousness. Psychoanal Stud Child 2006;35:67–83.
7. Williams EF, Hochman M, Rodgers BJ, et al. A psychological profile of children with hemangiomas and their families. Arch Facial Plast Surg 2003;5:229–34.
8. Dey JK, Ishii LE, Byrne PJ, et al. The social penalty of facial lesions. New evidence supporting high quality reconstruction. JAMA Facial Plast Surg 2015; 17(2):90–6.
9. Godoy A, Ishii M, Dey J, et al. How facial lesions impact attractiveness and perception. Laryngoscope 2011;121(12):2542–7.
10. Dey JK, Ishii LE, Joseph AW, et al. The cost of facial deformity. A health utility and valuation study. JAMA Facial Plast Surg 2016;18(4):241–9.
11. Byrne M, Chan JCY, O'Broin E. Perceptions and satisfaction of aesthetic outcome following secondary cleft rhinoplasty: evaluation by patients versus health professionals. J Craniomaxillofac Surg 2014;42:1062–70.
12. Razon MJ, Kräling BM, Mulliken JB, et al. Increased apoptosis coincides with onset of involution in infantile hemangioma. Microcirculation 1998;5(2–3):189–95.
13. Kulbersh J, Hochman M. Serial excision of facial hemangiomas. Arch Facial Plast Surg 2011;13(3):199–202.

# The Surgical Management of Infantile Hemangiomas

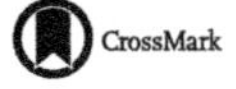

Milton Waner, MBBCh(Wits), FCS(SA), MD

**KEYWORDS**

- Nasal infantile hemangiomas • Eyelid infantile hemangiomas
- Cheek infantile hemangiomas • Lip infantile hemangiomas
- Forehead infantile hemangiomas • Segmental infantile hemangiomas

**KEY POINTS**

- Surgery remains an important modality in the management of infantile hemangiomas (IH).
- The aim of the surgeon should be to remove the hemangioma and to restore normal facial features.
- As a rule, hemangiomas do not invade adjacent tissues as they proliferate.

It would be ideal if all patients were treated early enough to obviate the need for surgery. Unfortunately, this is not the case, and not all patients respond well to beta blocker therapy (ie, propranolol).[1,2] Surgery therefore remains an important modality in the management of infantile hemangiomas (IHs), and although the role and the timing of surgery can and should be debated, there is no other way to accomplish what an experienced surgeon can do. By the same token, there is no way to undo the travesty of poorly planned and executed surgery. The surgical management of facial hemangiomas presents a unique challenge. The aim of the surgeon should be to remove the hemangioma and to restore normal facial features. Each of the facial zones has its own special features and challenges. The surgeon should always bear in mind the fact that the child started out with normal anatomy and that as the hemangioma proliferated, it displaced and thinned these normal structures and in many cases, expanded adjacent tissue. Hemangiomas do not as a rule, invade adjacent tissues as they proliferate. These facts will help in planning the various surgical approaches. Lastly, when discussing the surgery of IH, it is fortunate that the distribution of hemangiomas is nonrandom.[3] They occur in sites of predilection, and their effects are therefore predictable.

---

Disclosure Statement: The author has nothing that he wishes to disclose.
Lenox Hill and Manhattan Eye, Ear, and Throat Hospitals, Vascular Birthmark Institute of New York, Department of Otolaryngology–Head and Neck Surgery, 210 East 64th Street, 7th Floor, New York, NY 10065, USA
*E-mail address:* mwmd01@gmail.com

Otolaryngol Clin N Am 51 (2018) 125–131
https://doi.org/10.1016/j.otc.2017.09.011

## NASAL INFANTILE HEMANGIOMAS

Nasal IHs are common, representing 15% of all hemangiomas.[3] Most of these are midline and involve the nasal tip, although any zone of the nose can be affected. Several techniques have been described, but each of these has not stood the test of time. The modified subunit approach, first described in 2005,[4] has been adopted by several experienced surgeons and can be used as an approach to all of the nasal zones.[5] This approach enables the surgeon to expose the IH as well as the cartilaginous and bony nasal framework, and at the same time, resect any excess skin while redraping the nose. The incisions are made between the subunits of the nose and can be modified and limited to the needs of the case at hand (**Fig. 1**). Most nasal tip IHs originate between the lower lateral nasal cartilages and as they proliferate, displace the cartilages and widen the nasal tip. It is therefore important that this be corrected with dome binding sutures (**Fig. 2**). The surgeon should always bear in mind that the child started out with a normal nose and that as the IH proliferated, it displaced the normal nasal structures. Once the IH has been removed, this normal nasal anatomy can usually be restored. It should therefore only be necessary to rely on replacement techniques such as forehead flaps if there has been ulceration with extensive tissue destruction.

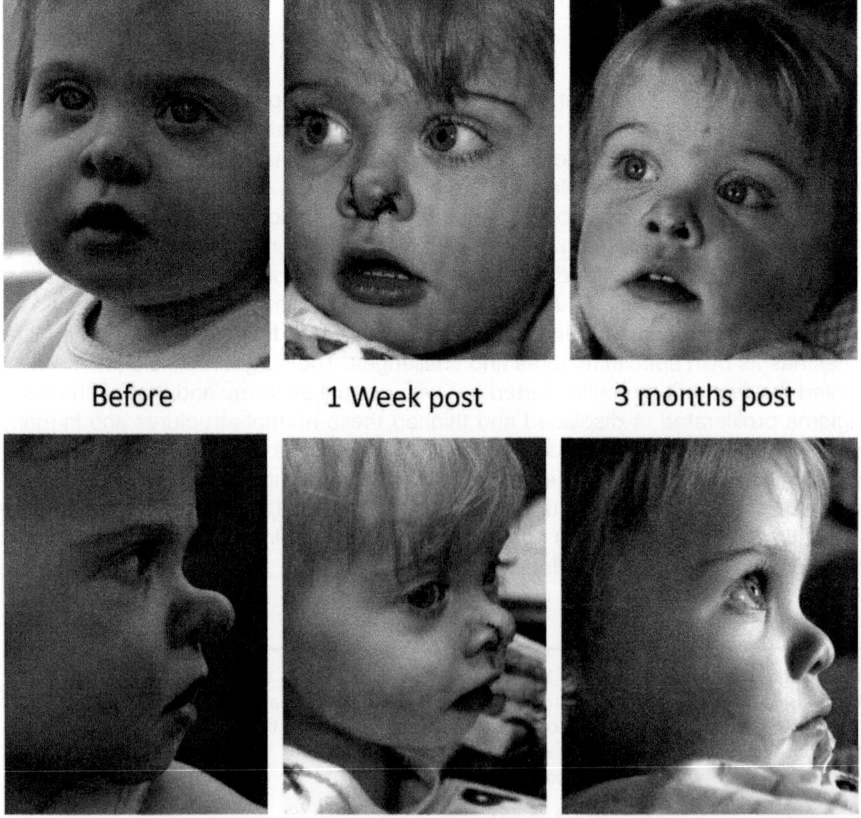


**Fig. 1.** A child with a nasal tip hemangioma before removal, 1 week after removal, and 3 months later. The modified subunit approach was used.

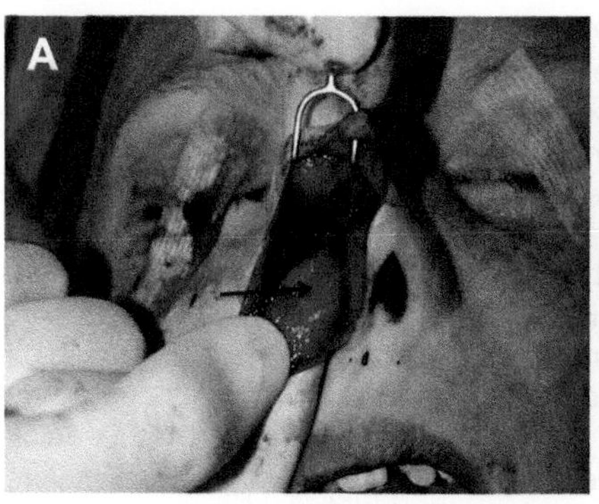


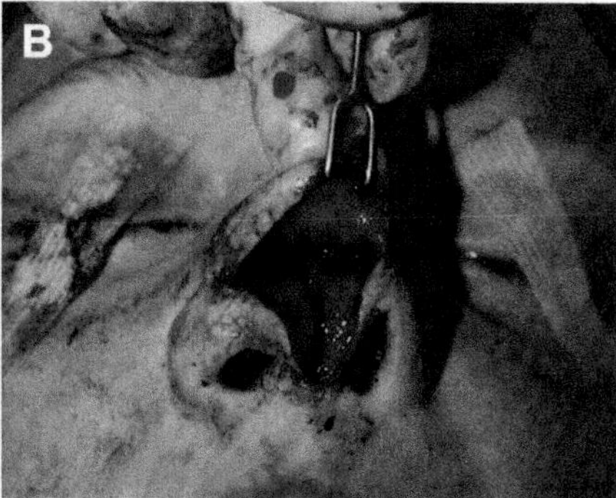


**Fig. 2.** The lower lateral cartilage marked by the arrow in (*A*), before correction, and after medialization with dome binding sutures (*B*).

## EYELID INFANTILE HEMANGIOMAS

The urgency of treating eyelid IHs cannot be overemphasized. Unilateral astigmatism and amblyopia are completely preventable, but despite this, cases are still encountered.[6] The common error made by some physicians is that reversing or correcting the problems caused by a proliferating IH is extremely time sensitive. The author has found that unilateral astigmatism can be reversed if the hemangioma is removed either medically or surgically by 8 months of age. If appropriate treatment is delayed and the effect of the IH is corrected between 8 and 13 months of age, some improvement will take place, but complete reversal of the astigmatism is unusual. After 13 months of age, the astigmatism is permanent.[7,8]

A lid crease incision is the most common approach to an upper eyelid lesion, and a subciliary incision is the most common approach to a lower eyelid lesion (**Fig. 3**). Most IHs are cutaneous and/or subcutaneous tumors and do not typically infiltrate the levator muscle. It should therefore be possible to remove the IH without disrupting levator function. Unfortunately, IHs that have been present for several months and are large will stretch and thin the levator muscle, leaving a ptotic eyelid even after adequate resection. This ptosis is then secondarily addressed.

## CHEEK INFANTILE HEMANGIOMAS

Large bulky infantile hemangiomas of the cheek will displace the ipsilateral oral commissure inferiorly.[9] Even if the IH responds favorably to propranolol or natural

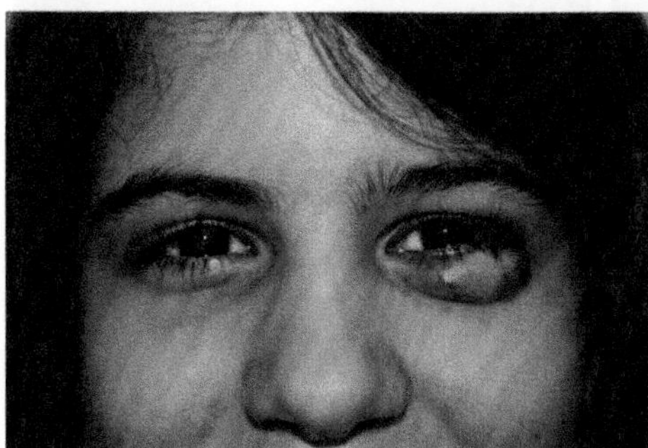

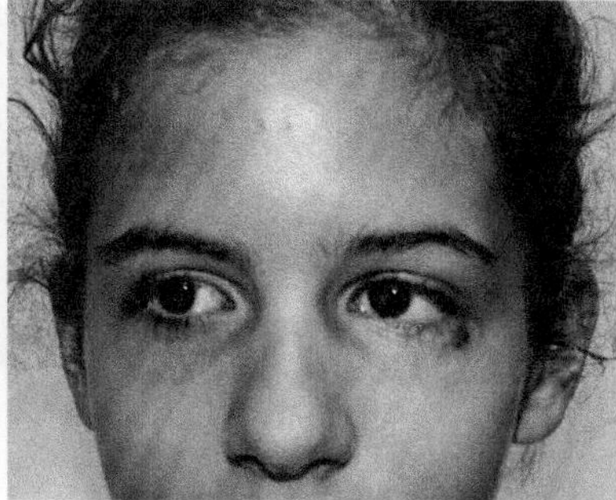

**Fig. 3.** A lower eyelid lesion removed through a subcilliary incision. A small portion of the cutaneous component remains. This can be removed with a pulsed dye laser.

involution, this ptosis of the commissure will remain, giving rise to facial asymmetry and a crooked smile. If it becomes necessary to remove the IH, this should be addressed. The surgeon should follow relaxed skin tension lines in planning the incision (**Fig. 4**). This will also enable correction of commissure ptosis.

The timing of surgery is critical. Surgical resection before 1 year of age is more likely to result in a favorable scar. Infants produce less type 2 collagen and are less likely to end up with a hypertrophic scar. Although delaying surgery beyond 18 months is sometimes unavoidable, the resultant scar is usually suboptimal. There is a tendency among nonsurgical colleagues to delay definitive surgical correction in the hope that it will become unnecessary. This is unfortunately a double-edged sword. Although some cases will be spared, those that do need surgery are poorly served by this delay. Although predictions are not foolproof, one should bear this in mind when making these decisions and surgically correct those that are unlikely to involute completely instead of uniformly waiting until 3 to 4 years of age before deciding which cases require surgery.

## LIP INFANTILE HEMANGIOMAS

Lower lip hemangiomas are usually lateral to the midline and typically spare the oral commissure.[10] In most cases, a considerable degree of tissue expansion has resulted in a ptotic lip. The most common surgical approach is a wedge resection. When planning a wedge resection, it is possible to remove more than the customary 30% without the risk of microstomia (**Fig. 5**); this is caused by the natural tissue expander effect created by IH proliferation.[11] Lesions of the vermillion can sometimes be resected through a horizontal incision, thereby avoiding an external scar.

Upper lip infantile hemangiomas can either be midline, in which case they are segmental lesions and are part of a frontonasal segmental lesion, or focal IHs which are lateral to the midline.[10] Focal IHs will usually expand the upper lip in 2 dimensions. The length of the lip is usually increased, and the vertical height is also often increased (**Fig. 6**). The behavior of upper lip focal IHs thus present a unique approach in which

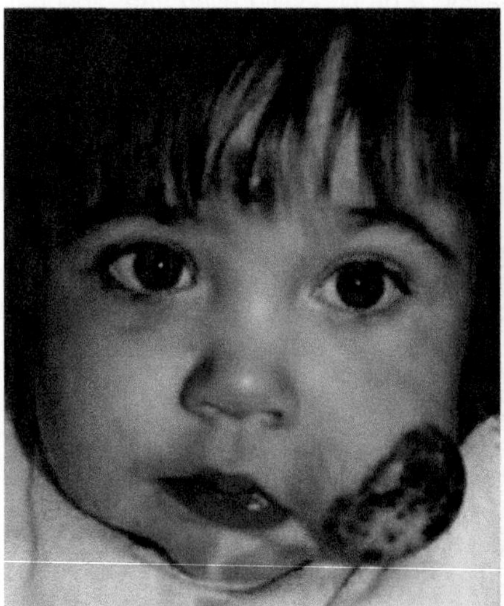

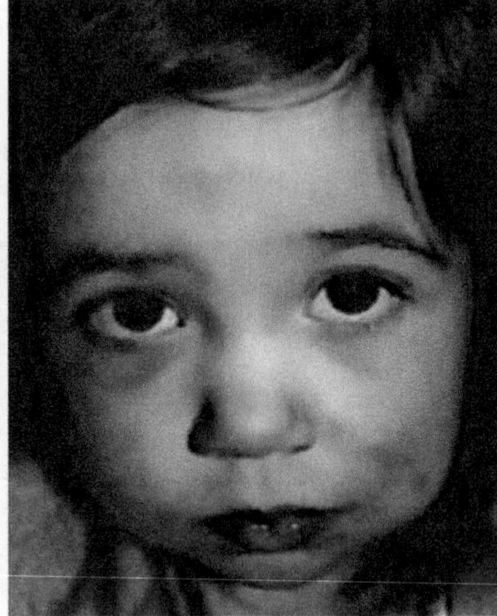

**Fig. 4.** A cheek hemangioma removed using an incision parallel to the relaxed tension lines of the cheek.

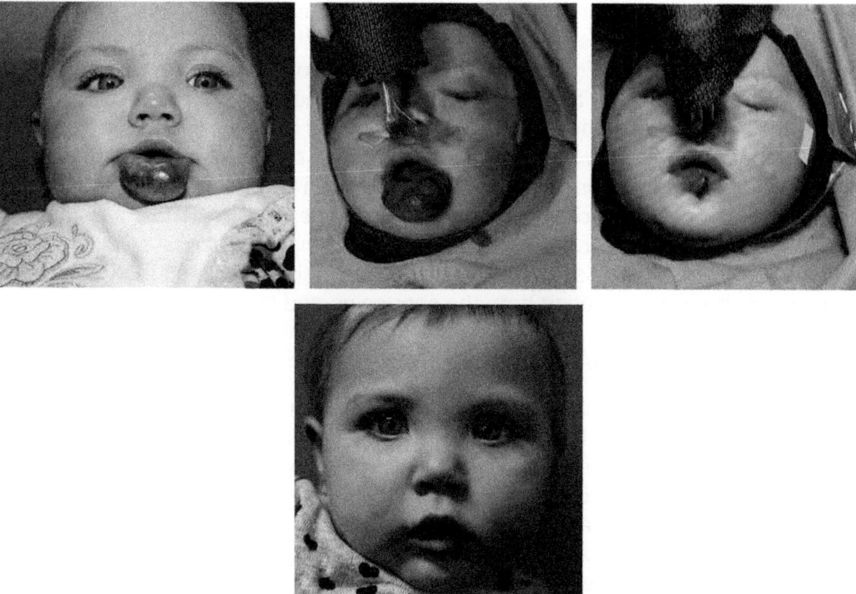

**Fig. 5.** A child with a lower lip hemangioma before, immediately after resection, and 3 months later. The tissue expansion effect of the hemangioma prevented microstomia despite such an extensive resection.

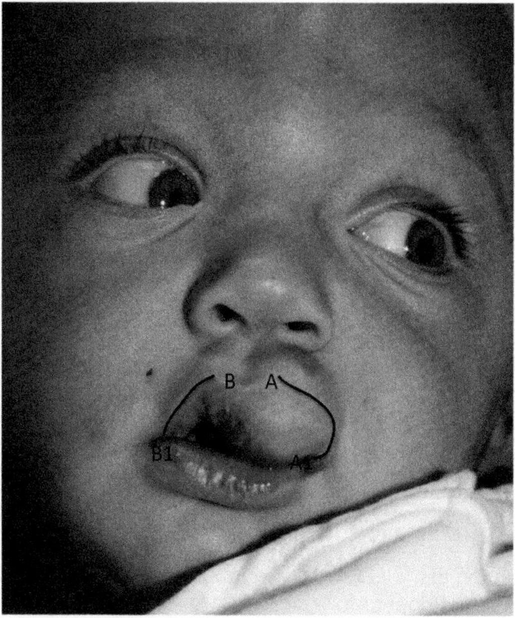


**Fig. 6.** A child with a large upper lip hemangioma. Note the increase in lip length A, A1 versus B, B1.

both of these dimensions can be corrected in 1 procedure. The most important feature to preserve in the upper lip is the philtrum. The initial incision will usually run parallel to the pillar of the philtrum. From here, the incision follows the nasal sill and curves around in the alar crease. The second incision is placed lateral to the first by the amount the horizontal length needs to be reduced. This incision will be placed parallel to the first but will run below the nasal sill at a distance determined by the measure of vertical height disparity. From here, the incision will run parallel to the alar crease but lateral at a distance equal to the degree of horizontal expansion. The 2 incisions will meet at the apex of the alar crease and at the labiogingival mucosal sulcus midway between the 2 vertical incisions on the outside. The incisions will run through muscle and mucosa, thereby correcting both the shortening and lifting the lip.

## FOREHEAD INFANTILE HEMANGIOMAS

The 2 most important principles one needs to adhere to in approaching forehead lesions is that the position of the eyelid should not be altered, and the frontalis muscle should not be resected. Where possible, the incision should be horizontal; however, if too much skin needs to be resected, this will displace the eyebrow superiorly, and this must be avoided. In such cases, a vertical incision should be made. This in turn may displace the eyebrow inferiorly. Burrows triangle in the suprabrow crease will prevent this. The underlying frontalis muscle must be preserved even though the IH will often infiltrate this muscle.

## SEGMENTAL INFANTILE HEMANGIOMAS

The primary treatment of segmental IH is also medical. However, affected areas may not completely respond to medical or laser therapy. For example, the lip, nose, or upper eyelid may require soft tissue debulking. Segmental IHs have a more aggressive growth pattern, and ulceration is much more common. Ulceration adjacent to fibrocartilage will often result in tissue loss. In these cases, cartilage grafting and local soft tissue reconstruction may be necessary. Similar surgical principles of incision placement are utilized.

## REFERENCES

1. Buckmiller LM, Munson PD, Dyamenahalli U, et al. Propranolol for infantile hemangiomas: early experience at a tertiary vascular anomalies center. Laryngoscope 2010;120(4):676–81.
2. Coulie J, Coyette M, Moniotte S, et al. Has propranolol eradicated the need for surgery in the management of infantile hemangioma? Plast Reconstr Surg 2015;136(4 Suppl):154.
3. Waner M, North PE, Scherer KA, et al. The nonrandom distribution of facial hemangiomas. Arch Dermatol 2003;139(7):869–75.
4. Waner M, Kastenbaum J, Scherer K. Hemangiomas of the nose: surgical management using a modified subunit approach. Arch Facial Plast Surg 2008; 10(5):329–34.
5. Keller RG, Stevens S, Hochman M. Modern management of nasal hemangiomas. JAMA Facial Plast Surg 2017;19(4):327–32.
6. Schwartz SR, Kodsi SR, Blei F, et al. Treatment of capillary hemangiomas causing refractive and occlusional amblyopia. J AAPOS 2007;11(6):577–83.
7. Waner M, O TM. The role of surgery in the management of congenital vascular anomalies. Tech Vasc Interv Radiol 2013;16(1):45–50.

8. Slaughter K, Sullivan T, Boulton J, et al. Early surgical intervention as definitive treatment for ocular adnexal capillary haemangioma. Clin Exp Ophthalmol 2003;31(5):418–23.
9. Waner M, O TM. Congenital vascular anomalies of the head and neck. In: Cheney ML, Hadlock T, editors. Facial surgery: plastic and reconstructive. Boca Raton (FL): CRC Press; 2014. p. 1037–75.
10. O TM, Scheuermann-Poley C, Tan M, et al. Distribution, clinical characteristics, and surgical treatment of lip infantile hemangiomas. JAMA Facial Plast Surg 2013;15(4):292–304.
11. Brennan TE, Waner M, O TM. The tissue expander effect in early surgical management of select focal infantile hemangiomas. JAMA Facial Plast Surg 2017;19(4):282–6.

# Management of Infantile Hemangiomas of the Airway

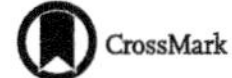

David H. Darrow, MD, DDS

**KEYWORDS**

• Airway • Subglottic • Hemangioma • Propranolol • Surgery • Management • Laser

**KEY POINTS**

- Symptoms of airway hemangioma mimic those of croup, often resulting in a delay in diagnosis.
- Distribution of airway infantile hemangiomas may be focal or segmental. Segmental airway IHs are associated with cutaneous segmental IHs.
- Propranolol has largely supplanted steroids and surgical intervention in the management of airway hemangiomas.
- There is still a role for multimodality therapy for airway hemangiomas depending on the size of the lesion, location of the patient at the time of diagnosis, and response to medical therapy.

## INTRODUCTION

Although infantile hemangiomas (IHs) are a common tumor of infancy, their occurrence in the airway is uncommon. When present, they may affect any portion of the airway; however, they most frequently involve the narrowest portion of the pediatric airway, namely the subglottis, often resulting in symptoms of stridor and respiratory distress. Unrecognized or untreated, the rapid growth of airway IHs may result in complete obstruction of the airway. As a result, otolaryngologists who treat children should be familiar with the diagnosis and management of these lesions (**Fig. 1**).

## EPIDEMIOLOGY AND PATHOGENESIS

The incidence of airway IHs has not been determined in any formal study. An analysis of the 37-hospital Pediatric Health Information System database over the 5-year

Disclosure: The author has no financial relationships with commercial interest(s) that produce health care products or services discussed in this article nor any relationships or activities that present a potential conflict of interest.
Department of Otolaryngology–Head and Neck Surgery, Eastern Virginia Medical School, 600 Gresham Drive, Norfolk, VA 23507, USA
*E-mail address:* David.Darrow@chkd.org

Otolaryngol Clin N Am 51 (2018) 133–146
https://doi.org/10.1016/j.otc.2017.09.001
0030-6665/18/

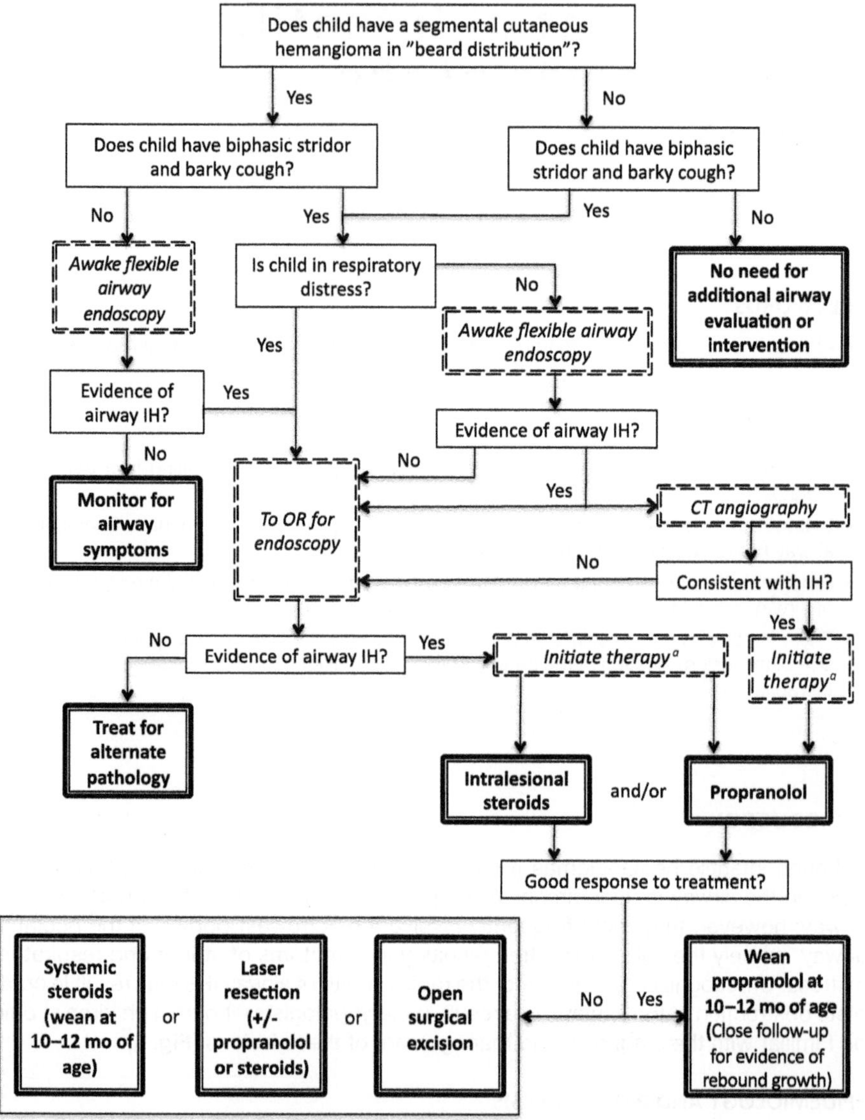


**Fig. 1.** Algorithm for evaluation and management of IH of airway. [a] In rare cases in which expert medical or surgical management is not readily accessible and symptoms are severe, placement of a temporary tracheotomy may be most expedient. OR, operating room.

period from 2001 to 2005 found that, of 2890 admissions for a primary or secondary diagnosis of IH, 337 (12%) underwent an airway procedure during at least 1 admission.[1] Thus, on average, pediatric hospitals in this cohort likely treated fewer than 3 symptomatic airway IHs each year. In a 1967 series, IHs of the airway accounted for 1.5% of congenital laryngeal anomalies.[2] As with IHs in general, airway IHs involving the subglottis have been reported more frequently in girls, with a 2:1 female-to-male preponderance.[3–7] It is unknown if the other risk factors associated with IHs in general apply equally to the subset of IHs of the airway.

The pathogenesis of IH of the airway remains incompletely established but is likely similar to that in IHs of other locations. A popular theory suggests that circulating endothelial progenitor cells find their way to certain locations that provide conditions favorable for growth into placenta-like tissues. The predilection for growth of IH in the airway and in the subglottis in particular has not been explained. Once endothelial progenitor cells are established in such tissues, they may encounter cellular signals and local tissue factors that stimulate their development. Such factors may include angiogenic and vasculogenic factors within the IH.[8–10] It is also theorized that disturbances causing placental hypoxia trigger a vascular response that increases the likelihood of IH.[11–13] In utero hypoxia is also the most common cause of low birth weight and may explain the association seen with premature delivery. Etiology and pathogenesis of IH are discussed in greater detail by Dr Denise M. Adams and Kiersten W. Ricci's article, "Infantile Hemangiomas in the Head and Neck Region", in this issue.

## CLINICAL PRESENTATION

Airway IHs, similar to cutaneous IHs, may be described as focal or segmental (diffuse). Segmental airway lesions (**Fig. 2**) are typically associated with cutaneous segmental disease distributed along the mandible and chin (beard distribution). They may involve multiple mucosal subsites within the airway as well as paratracheal extension.[14] Such lesions, as well as focal IHs involving the oral cavity and pharynx, may remain asymptomatic unless there is significant involvement of the larynx. Focal IHs of the larynx (**Fig. 3**), as

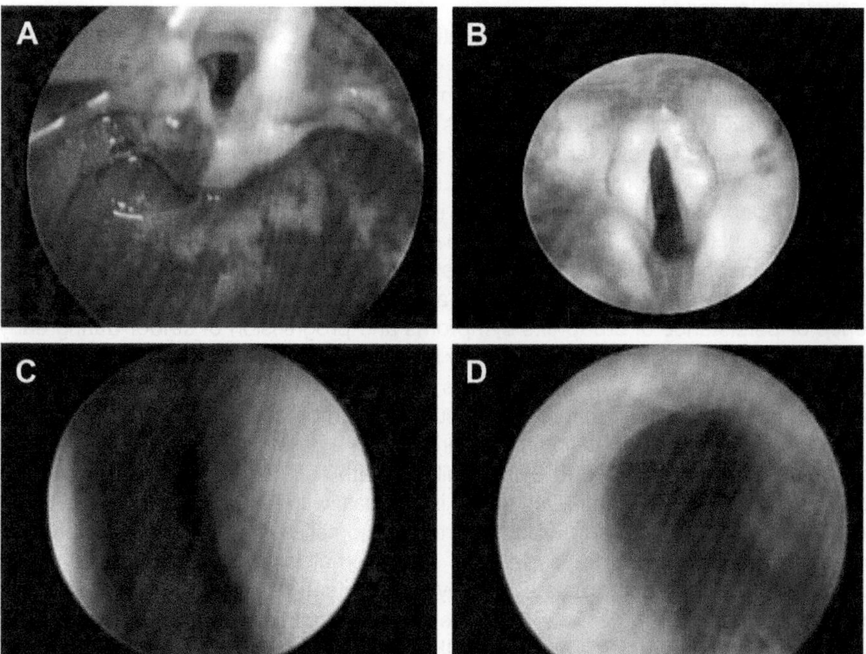


**Fig. 2.** Segmental IH of airway. (*A*) Involvement of posterior pharyngeal wall, epiglottis, aryepiglottic fold, and arytenoid. (*B*) Involvement of left vestibular fold. True vocal folds are unaffected. (*C*) Right subglottic hemangioma. (*D*) Posterior membranous tracheal wall involvement. (*From* O TM, Alexander RE, Lando T, et al. Segmental hemangiomas of the upper airway. Laryngoscope 2009;119:2245; with permission.)

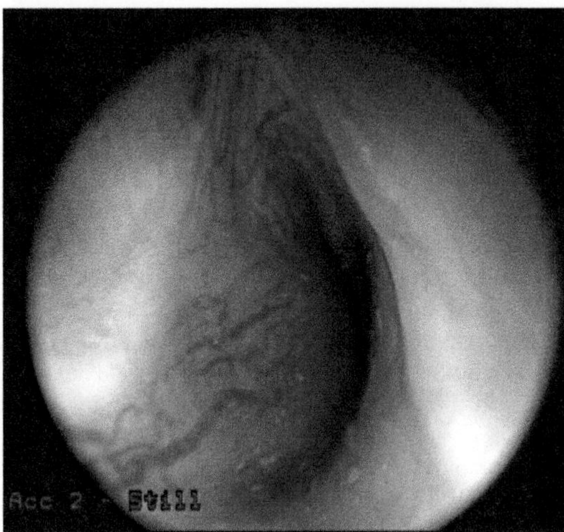

**Fig. 3.** Hemangioma on left lateral wall of subglottis. (*Courtesy of* Ian Jacobs, MD, Children's Hospital of Philadelphia.)

well as segmental lesions with laryngeal involvement, generally present with symptoms due to involvement of the subglottis; as a result, investigators have traditionally referred to these lesions as "subglottic hemangiomas". Many of the latter have been shown to be transglottic lesions.[14]

Airway IHs are not generally symptomatic at birth but develop as the lesion proliferates during early infancy; 80% to 90% of affected babies present within the first 6 months of life, with a mean age of 3.6 months at diagnosis.[3,15] As is the case with most masses of the subglottis, symptoms typically include biphasic stridor and barky cough in the absence of dysphonia. The symptoms may, therefore, be mistaken for those seen in more common disorders, such as infectious or inflammatory croup, especially because they typically worsen in the presence of upper respiratory illness. Furthermore, IHs respond to many of the same treatments used for croup, including racemic epinephrine and nebulized and systemic steroids. As a result, children may be symptomatic for several weeks before a definitive diagnosis is made. It is the recurrence or persistence of croup-like symptoms and progression of stridor during early infancy that suggest a diagnosis of airway IH and the need for additional investigation. Swallowing in children with airway IHs is usually normal; however, feeding may be affected as an infant tries to coordinate sucking with breathing.

Approximately one-half of infants diagnosed with an airway IH also have a cutaneous IH, although only 1% to 2% of children with cutaneous IHs also have airway IHs.[16,17] The risk is substantially higher in individuals with PHACE (posterior fossa defects, hemangiomas, cerebrovascular arterial anomalies, cardiovascular anomalies including coarctation of the aorta, and eye anomalies) syndrome, among whom more than 50% have demonstrated airway involvement.[18] Even in asymptomatic children, the presence of cutaneous IH in the beard distribution (parotid area, lips, chin, and neck [**Fig. 4**]) may be a predictor of IH in the airway, the highest risk associated with lesions in the median distribution (lower lip, lower gingiva, chin, and anterior neck).[19–21] Such cases likely represent segmental IHs.[14,22] IHs with a telangiectatic pattern seem to have the highest risk of airway involvement.[21]

Once the proliferative phase is completed (6–12 months of age), respiratory symptoms tend to slowly resolve. Gradual spontaneous involution or regression of

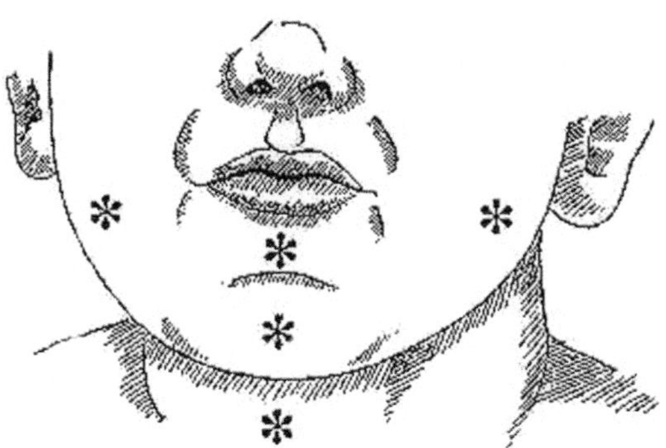

**Fig. 4.** Subsites of IHs in beard distribution, denoted by asterisks. (*From* Orlow S, Isakoff M, Blei F. Increased risk of symptomatic hemangiomas of the airway in association with cutaneous hemangiomas in a "beard" distribution. J Pediatr 1997;131:644; with permission.)

cutaneous IHs starts by 1 year of age,[16,23–29] and airway IHs generally follow this timeline as well. Although the duration of the involution process is variable, growth of a child over time allows the airway to better accommodate the IH, resulting in diminished frequency and severity of symptoms.

## DIAGNOSIS

Because many congenital and inflammatory processes of the airway can mimic IH during the early months of infancy, diagnosis of airway IH begins with a high index of suspicion. The persistence or recurrence of croup-like symptoms and the presence of cutaneous lesions, especially involving the lower face, are important clues. When airway IH is suspected, diagnosis may be confirmed by either performing an imaging study or proceeding directly to laryngoscopy and bronchoscopy. Advocates of imaging prefer to make a presumptive diagnosis based on flexible airway endoscopy and confirm the diagnosis and assess the extent of the lesion by CT scan with angiography.[30] This approach avoids the need for general anesthesia, especially because most airway IHs are now treated medically rather than surgically, but has the disadvantage of exposure to ionizing radiation at an early age. In most cases, the uncertainty of the diagnosis or the severity of symptoms necessitates a trip to an operating room, where the pathology may be visualized directly and treated surgically if necessary. This approach avoids the risks associated with radiation exposure. Office flexible endoscopy alone has also been successful in evaluating the airway below the vocal folds for IH in a cohort of high-risk patients.[31]

When endoscopy is performed, symptomatic airway IHs are usually found to involve the subglottis, but bulk and blush may be present at adjacent and distant sites as well. Bulky lesions are smooth, submucosal, compressible, and pink or blue in color, often with surface telangiectasias (see **Fig. 3**). A left-sided predominance has been reported, but airway IHs may be bilateral, circumferential, or multiple. Biopsy is not usually necessary to establish the diagnosis; however, when the diagnosis is in doubt, specimens from true IHs stain positively for glucose transporter protein isoform 1 (GLUT1).[32,33] The most useful and widely used immunohistochemical marker for the diagnosis of IH, GLUT1 is strongly expressed by IH endothelial cells and not by other benign vascular anomalies and has been validated for the identification of IHs of the airway.[34]

On CT imaging, IHs demonstrate an intensely staining, well-circumscribed mass with lobular architecture. MR imaging, although often diagnostic, is less advantageous because the duration of the study generally often requires general anesthesia. Fluoroscopy or anterior-posterior radiographs of the neck may demonstrate an asymmetric subglottic narrowing; however; these studies do not definitively establish the diagnosis.

A staging system for airway IHs has been proposed by Perkins and colleagues.[30] IH stage is determined from CT angiography based on location, percentage of laryngeal airway obstruction, and estimated total volume of the IH (**Table 1**). This staging system is limited to lesions of the larynx and is not yet correlated with need for treatment or prognosis.

## MANAGEMENT

Once the diagnosis of airway IH has been established, the clinician must determine whether intervention is required urgently and what type of intervention is most appropriate. Because involution is the ultimate fate of nearly all infantile IHs, watchful waiting is reasonable for patients who are minimally symptomatic. For those patients with more significant symptoms whose caretakers prefer no intervention for the lesion itself, tracheotomy with observation is highly successful.[5] This approach, however, requires a high level of maintenance to avoid tube occlusion, accidental decannulation, exposure of the airway to water, and delayed communication skills.

As a result, in most cases, some sort of intervention for the IH itself is generally more desirable. Lesions causing severe airway obstruction may require urgent surgical reduction or intubation while awaiting pharmacologic therapy to take effect. In less severe cases diagnosed by endoscopy in the operating room, intralesional steroids might be considered to augment planned pharmacotherapy. Thus, the degree of airway obstruction and the location of the patient at the time of diagnosis as well as the extent of extralaryngeal IH, the experience of the treating physician, and the preferences of the caretaker, are all considerations in determining the best course of action.

### *Pharmacotherapy*

Over the past several years, propranolol has become the mainstay of pharmacologic therapy for all IHs. In 2008, Léauté-Labrèze and colleagues[35] first reported their serendipitous observation that involution of IHs may be accelerated with the administration of propranolol. At doses of 2 mg/kg/d to 3 mg/kg/d used to treat cardiac complications of their IHs, 2 children experienced marked and rapid involution of their IHs. The following year, these same investigators reported additional treatment successes using propranolol in 32 patients with IH.[36] The efficacy of propranolol in treating cutaneous IH is now well established in systematic reviews and meta-analyses of clinical

**Table 1**
**Proposed airway infantile hemangioma staging system and treatment protocol**

| Stage[a] | Unilateral Airway Hemangioma | Circumferential or Bilateral Airway Hemangioma | Percent Laryngeal Airway Obstruction | CT Angiography or MR Imaging Extralaryngeal Hemangioma Volume ($mm^3$) |
|---|---|---|---|---|
| 1 | Yes | No | ≤50 | <4000 |
| 2 | Yes | Yes | >50–90 | 4001–10,000 |
| 3 | No | Yes | >90 | >10,000 |

[a] Stage based on lowest stage in a row with two or more positive findings.

*From* Perkins JA, Chen EY, Hoffer FA, et al. Proposal for staging airway hemangiomas. Otolaryngol Head Neck Surg 2009;141:519; with permission.

reports,[37,38] large cohort studies,[39] and randomized clinical trials.[40,41] Propranolol has also been used successfully in the management of airway IHs.[42–56] Response is not universal, however, and symptoms may recur while on the medication or during weaning, with reported symptom recurrence rates as high as 50%.[52–54,57,58] An oral formulation free of alcohol, sugar, and paraben (Hemangeol; Pierre Fabre; Castres, France) has been approved by the US Food and Drug Administration for use in children.[41]

Proposed mechanisms by which propranolol inhibits IH growth include inhibition of vasculogenesis, blocking of proangiogenic signals (vascular endothelial growth factor, basic fibroblast growth factor, and matrix metalloproteinases 2 and 9), inactivation of the renin-angiotensin system, vasoconstriction due to decreased release of nitric oxide, and induction of apoptosis in proliferating endothelial cells.[36,59–61] It has also been suggested that propranolol may prevent the differentiation of IH stem cells into endothelial cells or pericytes[62] or that it may hasten the differentiation of progenitor cells into adipocytes.[42]

The pretreatment assessment, optimal dose, and appropriate duration of propranolol therapy vary considerably in the literature. Contraindications to use of the drug include cardiogenic shock, sinus bradycardia, hypotension, heart block greater than first degree, heart failure, bronchial asthma, and known hypersensitivity to the drug. Once these disorders are ruled out, most clinicians perform a cardiac evaluation, assess baseline heart rate and blood pressure, and determine whether additional input from a cardiologist is indicated. Pretreatment cardiac screening seems of limited value in patients with an unremarkable cardiac history and examination.[63,64] Pretreatment electrocardiography is recommended, however, for patients considered at high risk for potential cardiac complications.[60] Special precautions have been suggested for children diagnosed with PHACE syndrome and significant intracranial vascular anomalies because of the theoretically increased risk of acute ischemic stroke.[60] In most series, the drug is started at a dose of 1 mg/kg/d to 2 mg/kg/d divided 2 to 3 times a day and then increased over several days to a week to 2 mg/kg/d to 3 mg/kg/d. Heart rate and blood pressure are checked each hour for the first 2 hours after the initial dose and with each dosage increase. The drug is usually administered throughout most of the first year of life. Although a consensus multidisciplinary protocol has been published,[60] protocols for propranolol initiation authored by otolaryngologists have also been published in the otolaryngology literature.[65,66] There is a single report of successful use of intravenous propranolol for airway obstruction in a critically ill neonate with a large cervicofacial IH.[67] It has been suggested that propranolol should become the standard for initial management of all airway IHs.[68]

Propranolol has a well-established safety profile based on years of use for control of high blood pressure and cardiac pathology. Additional safety information specifically regarding the use of propranolol in IH comes from the adverse effect data from the Hemangeol trial[41] as well as a recent systematic review.[69] The most common propranolol-related adverse effects are diarrhea (approximately 19%), peripheral coldness (approximately 7%–8%), and a variety of sleep disorders (approximately 2%–6% each).[41] Other potentially significant adverse effects include bronchospasm, bronchiolitis, and asymptomatic hypotension. Rare but potentially serious side effects include bradycardia, exposure of an undiagnosed atrioventricular block, and hypoglycemia.[41,69] Temporary discontinuation of oral propranolol therapy is recommended in cases of poor oral feeding, diarrhea, and obstructive bronchitis. Rebound growth after discontinuation of therapy has been observed in 6% to 25% of children, often well after their first birthday, leading some clinicians to wean propranolol over weeks to months.[70–74]

Although propranolol has largely supplanted systemic corticosteroids as first-line pharmacotherapy, the latter are occasionally useful in refractory cases. Steroid medications inhibit growth of the lesion during the proliferative phase, by inhibiting vasculogenesis and promoting adipogenesis. These drugs lose their effectiveness once involution begins.[75] Doses of prednisolone at 2 mg/kg/d to 3 mg/kg/d are generally necessary to control growth of the mass and should be maintained for one to 2 weeks before starting a 2-week to 4-week taper. Response rates reported in the literature vary between 30% and 93%, although there is little consistency among dosing regimens.[68,76] Long-term management on steroids carries a significant risk of complications, including gastroesophageal reflux, gastritis, immune suppression, cushingoid changes, hyperglycemia and glycosuria, hypertension, fluid and electrolyte disturbances, and growth retardation. IH patients on maintenance steroids should concomitantly receive courses of $H_2$-receptor blockers and trimethoprim-sulfamethoxazole as prophylaxis against gastritis and pneumocystis carinii infection, respectively. Live vaccinations should also be avoided while a child is taking high-dose steroids.

Interferon $\alpha$-2A is mentioned for historical reasons because it has been used with success in treating IHs, but this drug should only be considered when all other traditional modalities fail.[77–80] Potential side effects associated with this therapy include fever, myalgia, transient elevation of hepatic transaminase levels, transient neutropenia, anemia, and spastic diplegia.[81,82]

### *Surgical Intervention*

Indications for surgical management of airway IH have become few since the efficacy of propranolol was established. Surgery is a reasonable consideration when (1) the obstruction found at operative endoscopy is severe and likely requires a lengthy intubation while medical therapy is initiated and (2) the patient remains severely symptomatic despite an adequate trial of medical therapy.

Operative intervention may include intralesional injection of corticosteroids and/or partial ablation of the IH or complete surgical excision of the portion of the lesion within the airway. In most cases, the patients remain on medical therapy postoperatively to reduce the likelihood of recurrence. This is of particular importance in segmental airway lesions with known extension outside of the airway.

Intralesional steroids should be considered for patients whose IHs have necessitated a trip to the operating room for endoscopy or endoscopic resection. Although repeated injections are usually necessary as single-modality therapy,[83] these medications may be effective adjuvant therapy for patients whose lesions are being observed, treated pharmacologically, or partially resected. In most cases, triamcinolone, 40 mg/mL, is administered at a dose of 3 mg/kg to 5 mg/kg either alone or supplemented by betamethasone, 6 mg/mL, dosed at 0.5 mg/kg to 1.0 mg/kg.[75] Total volume delivered may be limited by the size of the lesion, and care must be taken to avoid depositing the steroid medication deep enough to affect the underlying cartilage. Patients usually require at least overnight intubation due to the increased volume of the lesion after injection. Cure rates of 77% to 87% using intralesional steroids have been reported.[15,83]

Airway IHs causing focal obstruction may be addressed surgically by a subtotal endoscopic approach using a microscope or telescope or by total excision through an open approach, dividing the thyroid and cricoid cartilages in the midline. Subtotal resection, more often than total excision, carries the risk of growth of the residual lesion during the proliferative phase, potentially resulting in additional surgical procedures unless combined with pharmacologic therapy. Endoscopic excision is usually performed using an apneic anesthesia technique, intermittently interrupting the surgery for reinsertion of the tube and ventilation of the patient. Alternatively, the procedure may be performed under spontaneous ventilation with anesthetic insufflation or Venturi jet ventilation.

The laser has been the most popular endoscopic surgical modality,[15] with the carbon dioxide ($CO_2$),[4,6,17,84–86] potassium titanyl phosphate (KTP),[87,88] and Nd:YAG[89,90] lasers all demonstrating some effectiveness. All these lasers are currently available for airway use through fiber delivery systems; however, only $CO_2$ is used by direct beam. $CO_2$ lasers are preferentially absorbed by water, whereas KTP and Nd:YAG lasers take advantage of absorption peaks that approximate those of hemoglobin and are thought to penetrate more deeply. All of these lasers, however, cause destruction by ablation rather than selective photothermolysis. As a result, in addition to the risk of recurrence, laser treatment carries a risk of subglottic stenosis of 5% to 25% that is likely greatest with deeper resections and in cases of bilateral or circumferential disease.[6,23,91] Debulking of the lesion using rotary powered instrumentation (microdébrider, or shaver) has also been reported.[92,93] Postoperatively, patients are observed in an intensive care setting. Some clinicians recommend face tent humidification to prevent airway obstruction due to eschar formation.

Although the first open surgical excision of a focally obstructing airway IH was reported in 1949, the procedure did not gain popularity until the 1990s, after complications of laser therapy became increasingly apparent.[94–99] Over the 15 years prior to the discovery of effects of propranolol, open resection seemed to be emerging as the intervention of choice for airway IHs. The procedure is of greatest advantage in patients with bilateral or circumferential lesions that may otherwise have been at risk for postoperative stenosis, recurrence, or tracheotomy. Some investigators have found the procedure useful for their propranolol failures, which may be as high as 50%.[58] Open surgical excision may be more difficult, however, in cases involving significant extralaryngeal extension, and the procedure may potentially result in some degree of dysphonia.

After initial intubation through the obstructed portion of the airway, the lesion is approached through the anterior neck via laryngofissure. After the tube has been relocated to the inferior aspect of the incision, the IH is removed submucosally under the operating microscope. At the conclusion of the dissection, the patient is intubated; in some cases, a thyroid cartilage graft may be placed to enlarge the subglottic laryngeal framework. After the neck is closed, the patient is transported to the ICU where intubation is maintained for 3 days to 7 days.

## REFERENCES

1. Perkins JA, Oliaei S, Garrison MM, et al. Airway procedures and hemangiomas: treatment patterns and outcome in U.S. pediatric hospitals. Int J Pediatr Otorhinolaryngol 2009;73:1302–7.
2. Holinger PH, Brown WT. Congenital webs, cysts, laryngoceles and other anomalies of the larynx. Ann Otol Rhinol Laryngol 1967;76:744–52.
3. Shikhani AH, Marsh BR, Jones MM, et al. Infantile subglottic hemangiomas: an update. Ann Otol Rhinol Laryngol 1986;95:336–47.
4. Sherrington CA, Sim DK, Freezer NJ, et al. Subglottic haemangioma. Arch Dis Child 1997;76:458–9.
5. Feuerstein SS. Subglottic hemangioma in infants. Laryngoscope 1973;83:466–75.
6. Chatrath P, Black M, Jani P, et al. A review of the current management of infantile subglottic haemangioma, including a comparison of CO2 laser therapy versus tracheostomy. Int J Pediatr Otorhinolaryngol 2002;64:143–57.

7. Hughes CA, Rezaee A, Ludemann JP, et al. Management of congenital subglottic hemangioma. J Otolaryngol 1999;28:223–8.
8. Greenberger S, Adini I, Biscolo E, et al. Targeting NF-kB in infantile hemangioma-derived stem cells reduces VEGF-A expression. Angiogenesis 2010;13:327–35.
9. Chang J, Most D, Bresnick S, et al. Proliferative hemangiomas: analysis of cytokine gene expression and angiogenesis. Plast Reconstr Surg 1999;103:1–9 [discussion: 10].
10. Razon MJ, Kräling BM, Mulliken JB, et al. Increased apoptosis coincides with onset of involution in infantile hemangioma. Microcirculation 1998;5:189–95.
11. Colonna V, Resta L, Napoli A, et al. Placental hypoxia and neonatal haemangioma: clinical and histological observations. Br J Dermatol 2010;162:208–9.
12. Drolet BA, Frieden IJ. Characteristics of infantile hemangiomas as clues to pathogenesis: does hypoxia connect the dots? Arch Dermatol 2010;146:1295–9.
13. Kleinman ME, Blei F, Gurtner GC. Circulating endothelial progenitor cells and vascular anomalies. Lymphat Res Biol 2005;3:234–9.
14. Perkins JA, Duke W, Chen E, et al. Emerging concepts in airway infantile hemangioma assessment and management. Otolaryngol Head Neck Surg 2009;141:207–12.
15. Bitar MA, Moukarbel RV, Zalzal GH. Management of congenital subglottic hemangioma: trends and success over the past 17 years. Otolaryngol Head Neck Surg 2005;132:226–31.
16. Bivings L. Spontaneous regression of angiomas in children: twenty-two years' observation covering 236 cases. J Pediatr 1954;45:643–7.
17. Sie KC, McGill T, Healy GB. Subglottic hemangiomas: 10 years experience with the carbon dioxide laser. Ann Otol Rhinol Laryngol 1994;103:167–72.
18. Durr ML, Meyer AK, Huoh KC, et al. Airway hemangiomas in PHACE syndrome. Laryngoscope 2012;122:2323–9.
19. Orlow S, Isakoff M, Blei F. Increased risk of symptomatic hemangiomas of the airway in association with cutaneous hemangiomas in a "beard" distribution. J Pediatr 1997;131:643–6.
20. Uthurriague C, Boccara O, Catteau B, et al. Skin patterns associated with upper airway infantile haemangiomas: a retrospective multicentre study. Acta Derm Venereol 2016;2(96):963–6.
21. Piram M, Hadj-Rabia S, Boccara O, et al. Beard infantile hemangioma and subglottic involvement: are median pattern and telangiectatic aspect the clue? J Eur Acad Dermatol Venereol 2016;30:2056–9.
22. O TM, Alexander RE, Lando T, et al. Segmental hemangiomas of the upper airway. Laryngoscope 2009;119:2242–7.
23. Lister WA. Natural history of strawberry nevi. Lancet 1938;231(5991):1429–30.
24. Margileth AM, Museles M. Current concepts in diagnosis and management of congenital cutaneous hemangiomas. Pediatrics 1965;36:410–6.
25. Moroz B. Long-term follow-up of hemangiomas in children. In: Williams HB, editor. Symposium on vascular malformations and melanotic lesions. St Louis (MO): CV Mosby; 1982. p. 27–35.
26. Mulliken JB. Diagnosis and natural history of hemangiomas. In: Mulliken JB, Young AE, editors. Vascular birthmarks: hemangiomas and malformations. Philadelphia: WB Saunders; 1988. p. 41–62.
27. Esterly NB. Cutaneous hemangiomas, vascular stains and malformations, and associated syndromes. Curr Probl Pediatr 1996;26:3–39.
28. Bowers RE, Graham EA, Tominson KM. The natural history of the strawberry nevus. Arch Dermatol 1960;82:667–70.

29. Chang LC, Haggstrom AN, Drolet BA, et al. Growth characteristics of infantile hemangiomas: implications for management. Pediatrics 2008;122:360–7.
30. Perkins JA, Chen EY, Hoffer FA, et al. Proposal for staging airway hemangiomas. Otolaryngol Head Neck Surg 2009;141:516–21.
31. Chun RH, McCormick ME, Martin T, et al. Office-based subglottic evaluation in children with risk of subglottic hemangioma. Ann Otol Rhinol Laryngol 2016; 125:273–6.
32. North PE, Waner M, Mizeracki A, et al. GLUT1: a newly discovered immunohistochemical marker for juvenile hemangiomas. Hum Pathol 2000;31:11–22.
33. North PE, Waner M, Mizeracki A, et al. A unique microvascular phenotype shared by juvenile hemangiomas and human placenta. Arch Dermatol 2001;137:559–70.
34. Badi AN, Kerschner JE, North PE, et al. Histopathologic and immunophenotypic profile of subglottic hemangioma: multicenter study. Int J Pediatr Otorhinolaryngol 2009;73:1187–91.
35. Léauté-Labrèze C, Dumas de la Roque E, Hubiche T, et al. Propranolol for severe hemangiomas of infancy. N Engl J Med 2008;358:2649–51.
36. Sans V, de la Roque ED, Berge J, et al. Propranolol for severe infantile hemangiomas: follow-up report. Pediatrics 2009;124:e423–31.
37. Marqueling AL, Oza V, Frieden IJ, et al. Propranolol and infantile hemangiomas four years later: a systematic review. Pediatr Dermatol 2013;30:182–91.
38. Chinnadurai S, Fonnesbeck C, Snyder KM, et al. Pharmacologic interventions for infantile hemangioma: a meta-analysis. Pediatrics 2016;137:e20153896.
39. Wedgeworth E, Glover M, Irvine AD, et al. Propranolol in the treatment of infantile haemangiomas: lessons from the European Propranolol in the Treatment of Complicated Haemangiomas (PITCH) taskforce survey. Br J Dermatol 2016; 174:594–601.
40. Hogeling M, Adams S, Wargon O. A randomized controlled trial of propranolol for infantile hemangiomas. Pediatrics 2011;128:e259.
41. Léauté-Labrèze C, Hoeger P, Mazereeuw-Hautier J, et al. A randomized, controlled trial of oral propranolol in infantile hemangioma. N Engl J Med 2015; 372:735–46.
42. Mistry N, Tzifa K. Use of propranolol to treat multicentric airway haemangioma. J Laryngol Otol 2010;124(12):1329–32.
43. Truong MT, Chang KW, Berk DR, et al. Propranolol for the treatment of a life-threatening subglottic and mediastinal infantile hemangioma. J Pediatr 2010; 156:335–8.
44. Maturo S, Hartnick C. Initial experience using propranolol as the sole treatment for infantile airway hemangiomas. Int J Pediatr Otorhinolaryngol 2010;74:323–5.
45. Buckmiller LM, Munson PD, Dyamenahalli U, et al. Propranolol for infantile hemangiomas: early experience at a tertiary vascular anomalies center. Laryngoscope 2010;120:676–81.
46. Manunza F, Syed S, Laguda B, et al. Propranolol for complicated infantile haemangiomas: a case series of 30 infants. Br J Dermatol 2010;162:466–8.
47. Jephson CG, Manunza F, Syed S, et al. Successful treatment of isolated subglottic haemangioma with propranolol alone. Int J Pediatr Otorhinolaryngol 2009;73: 1821–3.
48. Buckmiller L, Dyamenahalli U, Richter GT. Propranolol for airway hemangiomas: case report of novel treatment. Laryngoscope 2009;119:2051–4.
49. Leboulanger N, Fayoux P, Teissier N, et al. Propranolol in the therapeutic strategy of infantile laryngotracheal hemangioma: a preliminary retrospective study of French experience. Int J Pediatr Otorhinolaryngol 2010;74:1254–7.

50. Anderson de Moreno LC, Matt BH, Montgomery G, et al. Propranolol in the treatment of upper airway hemangiomas. Ear Nose Throat J 2013;92:209–14.
51. Mahadevan M, Cheng A, Barber C. Treatment of subglottic hemangiomas with propranolol: initial experience in 10 infants. ANZ J Surg 2011;81:456–61.
52. Rosbe KW, Suh KY, Meyer AK, et al. Propranolol in the management of airway infantile hemangiomas. Arch Otolaryngol Head Neck Surg 2010;136:658–65.
53. Broeks IJ, Hermans DJ, Dassel AC, et al. Propranolol treatment in life-threatening airway hemangiomas: a case series and review of literature. Int J Pediatr Otorhinolaryngol 2013;77:1791–800.
54. Elluru RG, Friess MR, Richter GT, et al. Multicenter evaluation of the effectiveness of systemic propranolol in the treatment of airway hemangiomas. Otolaryngol Head Neck Surg 2015;153:452–60.
55. Li XY, Wang Y, Jin L, et al. Role of oral propranolol in the treatment of infantile subglottic hemangioma. Int J Clin Pharmacol Ther 2016;54:675–81.
56. Vlastarakos PV, Papacharalampous GX, Chrysostomou M, et al. Propranolol is an effective treatment for airway haemangiomas: a critical analysis and meta-analysis of published interventional studies. Acta Otorhinolaryngol Ital 2012;32:213–21.
57. Raol N, Metry D, Edmonds J, et al. Propranolol for the treatment of subglottic hemangiomas. Int J Pediatr Otorhinolaryngol 2011;75:1510–4.
58. Siegel B, Mehta D. Open airway surgery for subglottic hemangioma in the era of propranolol: is it still indicated? Int J Pediatr Otorhinolaryngol 2015;79:1124–7.
59. Greenberger S, Bischoff J. Infantile hemangioma-Mechanism(s) of drug action on a vascular tumor. Cold Spring Harb Perspect Med 2011;1:a006460.
60. Drolet BA, Frommelt PC, Chamlin SL, et al. Initiation and use of propranolol for infantile hemangioma: report of a consensus conference. Pediatrics 2013;131: 128–40.
61. Ji Y, Chen S, Xu C, et al. The use of propranolol in the treatment of infantile haemangiomas: an update on potential mechanisms of action. Br J Dermatol 2015; 172:24–32.
62. Frieden IJ, Drolet BA. Propranolol for infantile hemangiomas: promise, peril, pathogenesis. Pediatr Dermatol 2009;26:642–4.
63. Raphael MF, Breugem CC, Vlasveld FA, et al. Is cardiovascular evaluation necessary prior to and during beta-blocker therapy for infantile hemangiomas?: a cohort study. J Am Acad Dermatol 2015;72:465–72.
64. Blei F, McElhinney DB, Guarini A, et al. Cardiac screening in infants with infantile hemangiomas before propranolol treatment. Pediatr Dermatol 2014;31:465–70.
65. Bajaj Y, Kapoor K, Ifeacho S, et al. Great Ormond Street Hospital treatment guidelines for use of propranolol in infantile isolated subglottic haemangioma. J Laryngol Otol 2013;127:295–8.
66. Parikh SR, Darrow DH, Grimmer JF, et al. Propranolol use for infantile hemangiomas: American Society of Pediatric Otolaryngology Vascular Anomalies Task Force practice patterns. JAMA Otolaryngol Head Neck Surg 2013;139:153–6.
67. Fernando SJ, Leitenberger S, Majerus M, et al. Use of intravenous propranolol for control of a large cervicofacial hemangioma in a critically ill neonate. Int J Pediatr Otorhinolaryngol 2016;84:52–4.
68. Denoyelle F, Garabédian EN. Propranolol may become first-line treatment in obstructive subglottic infantile hemangiomas. Otolaryngol Head Neck Surg 2010;142:463–4.

69. Léaute-Labrèze C, Boccara O, Degrugillier-Chopinet C, et al. Safety of oral propranolol for the treatment of infantile hemangioma: a systematic review. Pediatrics 2016;138:e20160353.
70. Braqazquoitia L, Hernandez-Martin A, Torrelo A. Recurrence of IH treated with propranolol. Pediatr Dermatol 2011;28:658–62.
71. Shehata N, Powell J, Dubois J, et al. Late rebound of infantile hemangioma after cessation of oral propranolol. Pediatr Dermatol 2013;30:587–91.
72. Shah SD, Baselga E, McCuaig C, et al. Rebound growth of infantile hemangiomas after propranolol therapy. Pediatrics 2016;137(4) [pii:e20151754].
73. Solman L, Murabit A, Gnarra M, et al. Propranolol for infantile haemangiomas: single centre experience of 250 cases and proposed therapeutic protocol. Arch Dis Child 2014;99:1132–6.
74. Giachetti A, Garcia-Monaco R, Sojo M, et al. Long-term treatment with oral propranolol reduces relapses of infantile hemangiomas. Pediatr Dermatol 2014;31:14–20.
75. Waner M, Suen JY. Treatment options for the management of hemangiomas. In: Waner M, Suen JY, editors. Hemangiomas and vascular malformations of the head and neck. New York: Wiley-Liss, Inc.; 1999. p. 233–62.
76. Waner M, Suen JY. Advances in the management of congenital vascular lesions of the head and neck. Adv Otorhinolaryngol 1996;10:31–54.
77. Ezekowitz RAB, Mulliken JB, Folkman J. Interferon alfa-2A therapy for life-threatening hemangiomas of infancy. N Engl J Med 1992;326:1456–63.
78. Ohlms LA, Jones DT, McGill TJ, et al. Interferon alfa2A therapy for airway hemangiomas. Ann Otol Rhinol Laryngol 1994;103:1–8.
79. Bauman MN, Burke DK, Smith RJH. Treatment of massive or life-threatening hemangiomas with recombinant $\alpha$ 2a-interferon. Otolaryngol Head Neck Surg 1997;117:99–110.
80. MacArthur CJ, Senders CW, Katz J. The use of interferon Alfa-2A for life-threatening hemangiomas. Arch Otolaryngol Head Neck Surg 1995;121:690–3.
81. Barlow CF, Priebe CJ, Mulliken JB, et al. Spastic diplegia as a complication of interferon Alpha-2a treatment of hemangiomas of infancy. J Pediatr 1998;132:527–30.
82. Michaud AP, Bauman NM, Burke DK, et al. Spastic diplegia and other motor disturbances in infants receiving interferon-alpha. Laryngoscope 2004;114:1231–6.
83. Hoeve LJ, Kuppers GLE, Verwoerd CDA. Management of infantile subglottic hemangioma: laser vaporization, submucous resection, intubation or intralesional steroids? Int J Pediatr Otorhinolaryngol 1997;42:179–86.
84. Walker P, Cooper D, MacDonald D. Subglottic haemangioma: controversies in management. J Paediatr Child Health 1999;35:392–5.
85. Re M, Forte V, Berardi C, et al. Role of endoscopic CO2 laser surgery in the treatment of congenital infantile subglottic hemangioma. Experience in the Department of Otolaryngology, "Sick Children Hospital", Toronto, Canada. Acta Otorhinolaryngol Ital 2003;23:175–9.
86. Clarós A, Fokouo JV, Roqueta C, et al. Management of subglottic hemangiomas with carbon dioxide laser: our 25-year experience and comparison with the literature. Int J Pediatr Otorhinolaryngol 2015;79:2003–7.
87. Madgy D, Ahsan SF, Kest D, et al. The application of the Potassium-Titanyl-Phosphate (KTP) laser in the management of subglottic hemangioma. Arch Otolaryngol Head Neck Surg 2001;127:47–50.

88. Kacker A, April M, Ward RF. Use of potassium titanyl phosphate (KTP) laser in management of subglottic hemangiomas. Int J Pediatr Otorhinolaryngol 2001; 59:15–21.
89. Fu CH, Lee LA, Fang TJ, et al. Endoscopic Nd:YAG laser therapy of infantile subglottic hemangioma. Pediatr Pulmonol 2007;42:89–92.
90. Azizkhan RG. Laser surgery: new applications for pediatric skin and airway lesions. Curr Opin Pediatr 2003;15:243–7.
91. Cotton RT, Tewfik T. Laryngeal stenosis following carbon dioxide laser in subglottic hemangioma. Ann Otol Rhinol Laryngol 1985;94:494–7.
92. Pransky SM, Canto C. Management of subglottic hemangioma. Curr Opin Otolaryngol Head Neck Surg 2004;12:509–12.
93. Jai H, Huang Q, Lü J, et al. Microdebrider removal under suspension laryngoscopy: An alternative surgical technique for subglottic hemangioma. Int J Pediatr Otorhinolaryngol 2013;77:1424–9.
94. Froehlich P, Stamm D, Floret D, et al. Management of subglottic hemangioma. Clin Otolaryngol 1995;4:336–9.
95. Wiatrak BJ, Reilly JS, Seid AD, et al. Open surgical excision of subglottic hemangioma in children. Int J Pediatr Otorhinolaryngol 1996;34:191–206.
96. Van Den Abbeele T, Triglia J-M, Lescanne E, et al. Surgical removal of subglottic hemangiomas in children. Laryngoscope 1999;109:1281–6.
97. Vijayasekaran S, White D, Hartley BEJ, et al. Open excision of subglottic hemangiomas to avoid tracheostomy. Arch Otolaryngol Head Neck Surg 2006;132: 159–63.
98. Bajaj Y, Hartley BEJ, Wyatt ME, et al. Subglottic haemangioma in children: experience with open surgical excision. J Laryngol Otol 2006;120:1033–7.
99. O-Lee TJ, Messner A. Open excision of subglottic hemangioma with microscopic dissection. Int J Pediatr Otorhinolaryngol 2007;71:1371–6.

# New Frontiers in Our Understanding of Lymphatic Malformations of the Head and Neck

## Natural History and Basic Research

Jonathan A. Perkins, DO[a,b,*]

**KEYWORDS**

- Lymphatic malformations • Head and neck • Natural history • Basic research

**KEY POINTS**

- Head and neck lymphatic malformation (HNLM) is not a result of disrupted vasculogenesis but arises from sporadic genetic abnormalities in specific cells.
- Clinical research into HNLM has focused on nomenclature, diagnosis, the assessment of natural history, and the evaluation of invasive treatment efficacy.
- Because of the rarity and clinical variability of HNLM, the evidence created by this research is low quality (levels 2–4), but the gap between experience-based decision-making and evidence-based practice is closing.

The future of head and neck lymphatic malformation (HNLM) evaluation and treatment is changing because of 2 decades of clinical research and the recent basic science investigation. HNLM is not a result of disrupted vasculogenesis but arises from genetic abnormalities in specific cells within the malformation.[1,2] Clinical research into HNLM has focused on nomenclature, diagnosis, assessment of natural history, and evaluation of invasive treatment efficacy.[3–8] Because of the rarity and clinical variability of HNLM, the evidence created by this research is low quality (levels 2–4); but the gap between experience-based decision-making and evidence-based practice is closing.[8] Basic science investigation using cellular biology and molecular genetics has revealed the genetic cause of some HNLMs, which has created the possibility of medical treatment specific to HNLM.[1,9] This

Disclosure Statement: J.A. Perkins has nothing he wishes to disclose.
Funded by NIH: grant numbers R01 NS092772, NIHMS-ID 905693.
[a] Otolaryngology/Head and Neck Surgery, University of Washington School of Medicine, 1959 Pacific Avenue NE, Box 366515, Seattle, WA 98195, USA; [b] Vascular Anomalies Program, Seattle Children's Hospital, 4800 Sand Point Way Northeast, Seattle, WA 98105, USA
* 4800 Sand Point Way Northeast, Seattle, WA 98105.
*E-mail address:* jonathan.perkins@seattlechildrens.org

Otolaryngol Clin N Am 51 (2018) 147–158
https://doi.org/10.1016/j.otc.2017.09.002
oto.theclinics.com

article summarizes the clinical and basic science research that will likely influence the future of HNLM assessment and treatment.

The nomenclature for all vascular anomalies (VAs) has slowly evolved based on clinical phenotypic observation and the availability of improved high-resolution imaging. The descriptive terms of *cystic hygroma* for large fluid-filled neck masses and *lymphangioma* for infiltrative lymphatic channels seen in oral and oropharyngeal lymphatic malformation (LM) have been changed to the more inclusive *common LMs* by the International Society for the Study of Vascular Anomalies (ISSVA) (See **Table 1** in Paula E. North's article, "Classification and pathology of congenital and perinatal vascular anomalies of the head and neck," in this issue for further details).[10,11] The ISSVA nomenclature for all VAs enabled providers to better distinguish different congenital vascular lesions, particularly congenital and acquired lymphatic disease. Careful categorization of VA and lymphatic diseases allowed for improvements in clinical research and provided a framework to direct basic science investigation. Categorization of HNLM based on anatomic location and laterality led to a staging/grading system for intraoral and head and neck lesions (**Fig. 1**).[12,13] Treatment outcomes have been measured comparing differences between HNLM stages.[5,7,14] Further refinement of our understanding of HNLM has been accomplished with radiographic imaging that categorizes these lesions as macrocystic and microcystic. This information often directs the type of invasive treatment.[15–17]

Prenatal diagnosis of HNLM is frequently made with in utero ultrasound imaging. Lucency in the soft tissue of the posterior/dorsal neck with nuchal thickening is still called cystic hygroma in obstetrics literature. Radiolucent lesions in the nuchal region indicate an increased risk for abnormal fetal karyotype, whereas radiolucent anterior or ventral neck lymphatic lesions do not confer this same risk (**Fig. 2**).[18] There are now highly sensitive and specific screening tests (noninvasive prenatal testing) that allow direct sampling of fetal DNA from maternal blood, without the need for invasive amniocentesis or chorionic villus sampling.[19] In utero characterization of HNLM can be further functionally assessed with in utero MRI and 3-dimensional duplex imaging of the upper aerodigestive tract in mothers with polyhydramnios to guide high-risk delivery planning and airway management.[4]

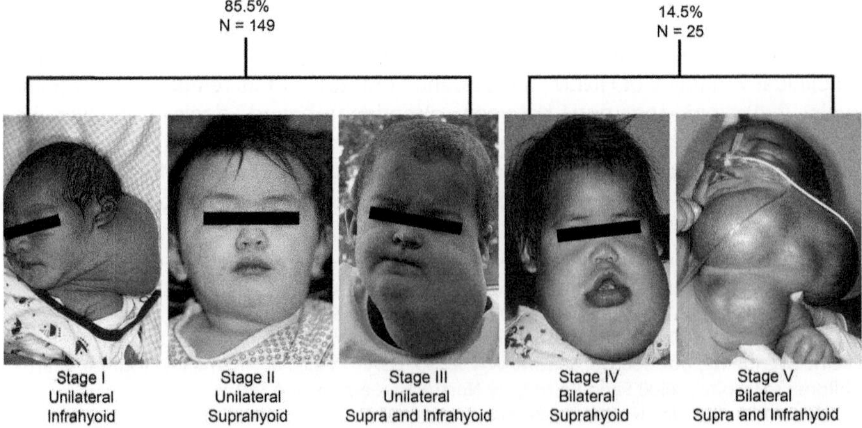


**Fig. 1.** The deSerres head and neck LM staging system used to improve treatment outcome measurement and allow for quantitative data analysis. In a series of 174 HNLMs, 85.5% were stages 1 to 3 and 14.5% were stages 4 or 5; in lower stage lesions, surgery and sclerotherapy had the same efficacy.

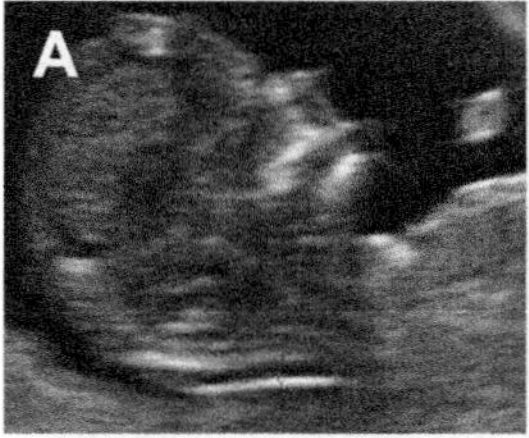


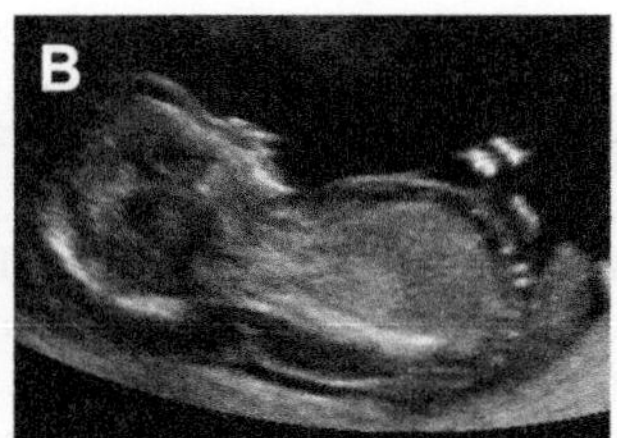


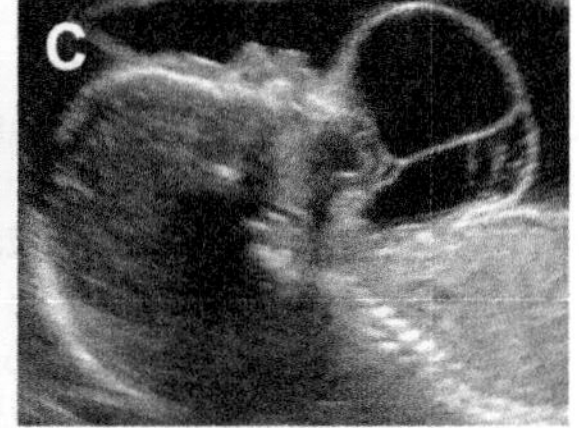


**Fig. 2.** In utero ultrasound images demonstrating (*A*) nuchal thickening, (*B*) dorsal lymphatic malformation, and (*C*) ventral lymphatic malformation.

Postnatal HNLM diagnosis is either anticipated through prenatal diagnosis or clinical examination and radiographic characterization when presented after infancy. If the diagnosis is in question, histologic assessment of the lymphatic endothelium by the identification of podoplanin (D2-40) can be used to clarify the diagnosis.[20] Of note, the radiographic distinction of macrocystic and microcystic is not apparent histologically.[21]

The evaluation of the natural history and treatment efficacy in specific HNLMs has been aided by staging or grading.[12,17] Determining the HNLM stage/grade has shown the normal distribution of these lesions. In a large 2-institution prospectively collected series whereby HNLMs were treated primarily, lower stage 1 to 3 HNLMs, lesions that are all unilateral, represented more than 80% of all HNLMs and had a similar response to surgery and sclerotherapy (see **Fig. 1**).[7] Interestingly, stage 1 and 2 lesions normally do not cause functional compromise (ie, airway obstruction, dysphagia) and have been reported to shrink without invasive therapy in up to 30% of cases (**Fig. 3**).[5] In contrast, higher stage 4 and 5 lesions cause functional

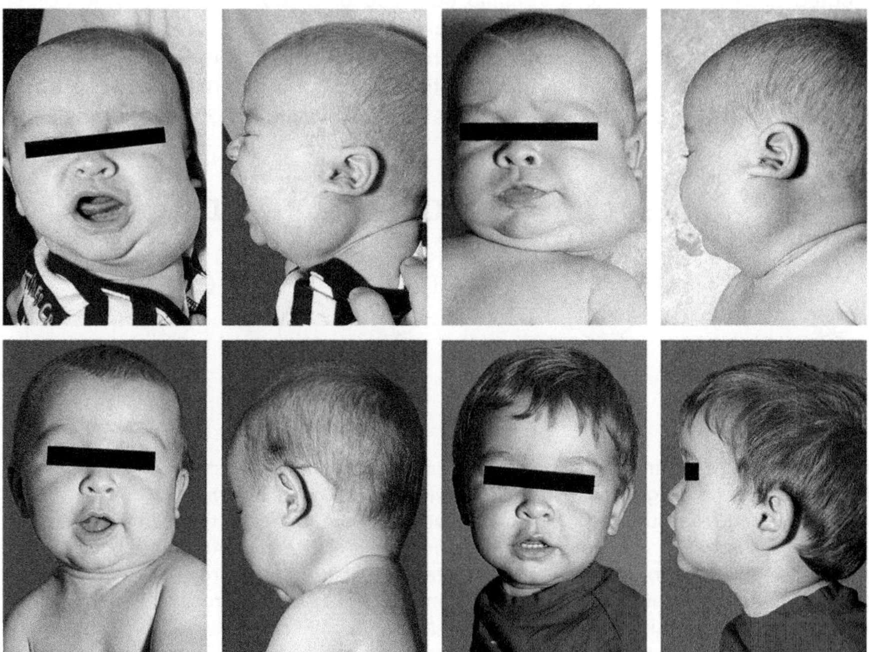

**Fig. 3.** Stage 1 HNLM demonstrating regression without therapy. From left to right top row: aged 2.5 months and 3.0 months. From left to right bottom row: aged 6 months and 17 months.

compromise, are bilateral, are usually predominately microcystic, possibly associated with lymphocytopenia and tertiary lymphoid organ formation, and are prone to persist and be recalcitrant to standard therapies.[7,9,22] The same use of lesion staging has been applied to the analysis of tongue LM natural history and treatment.[13,23] Smaller, lower stage tongue lesions have a different history and treatment response compared with transmural malformations involving mucosa, muscle, and multiple anatomic spaces in and adjacent to the tongue (**Fig. 4**).[23] The assessment of differences in invasive HNLM therapy (ie, surgery, sclerotherapy) efficacy is impossible based on the extensive systematic review of existing medical literature.[8] Determining differences between treatments is impossible due to the lack of consistent reporting of pretreatment LM findings, and undefined treatment end points. In response to this systematic review, a multidisciplinary group representing differing treatment philosophies has published reporting guidelines for future reports of HNLM treatment, which will help create higher levels of evidence for treatment decisions.[14]

Following the completion of the Human Genome Project, the development of massively parallel DNA sequencing technology has enabled detailed exploration of molecular genetics causing rare conditions and contributing to neoplasms, including HNLM and other VAs.[24–26] This new molecular genetic knowledge has resulted in the ISSVA classification of VA to include known molecular genotypes (**Table 1**).[27,28] In 2015, researchers discovered that most anterior or ventral HNLMs are caused by a gain-of-function postzygotic somatic gene mutation (phosphatyidylinositol-4,5-bisphosphate 3-kinase, catalytic subunit alpha [PIK3CA]).[1] Mutations in this gene have been detected in other types of tissue overgrowth.[24–26,29] Somatic mutations differ from germline mutations in that the affected area is isolated to a specific cell type or anatomic region, which gives rise to cellular and phenotypic mosaicism (**Fig. 5**). An important implication here is that the pathogenic mutations are not necessarily present in blood, the most frequently sampled tissue for genetic testing. In 3 different LMs, one being HNLM, the PIK3CA somatic mutation was detected in the lymphatic endothelium.[2]

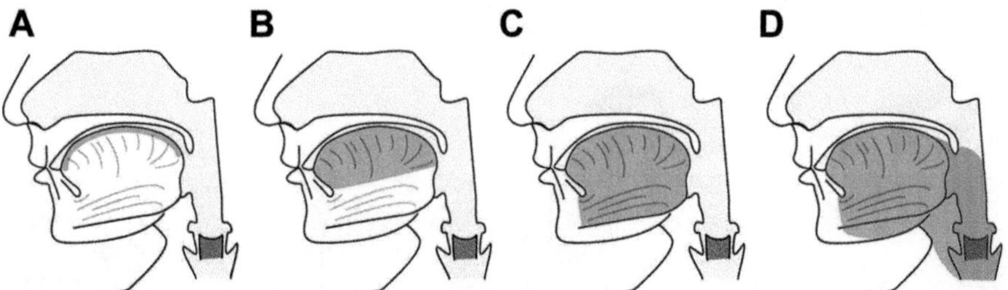


**Fig. 4.** Tongue LM staging used to describe treatment outcomes and strategies in malformations involving the tongue (*shaded area is involved with lymphatic malformation*). Malformations ranged from superficial to transmural. The more extensive the malformation, the poorer the treatment outcome and malformation persistence. (*A*) Isolated microcystic lymphatic malformation on tongue surface (Stage 1), (*B*) Isolated microcystic lymphatic malformation of the tongue with muscle involvement (Stage 2), (*C*) Microcystic lymphatic malformation of the tongue and floor of mouth (Stage 3), (*D*) Extensive microcystic lymphatic malformation of the tongue, floor of mouth and surrounding cervical structures (stage 4). (*From* Wiegand S, Eivazi B, Zimmermann AP, et al. Microcystic lymphatic malformations of the tongue: diagnosis, classification, and treatment. Arch Otolaryngol Head Neck Surg 2009;135(10):977; with permission.)

**Table 1**
**International Society for the Study of Vascular Anomalies' vascular anomalies classification scheme from 2015**

| | |
|---|---|
| Capillary Malformations | |
| Cutaneous and/or mucosal CM (port wine stain) | GNAQ |
| CM with bone and/or soft tissue hyperplasia | — |
| CM with CNS and/or eye anomalies (Sturge-Weber) | GNAQ |
| CM of CM-AVM | RASA1 |
| Telangiectasia | — |
| HHT | — |
| HHT1 | ENG |
| HHT2 | ACVRL1 |
| HHT3 | — |
| Others | — |
| CMTC | — |
| Nevus simplex/salmon patch | — |
| LM | |
| Primary lymphedema | — |
| Nonne-Milroy syndrome | FLT4/VEGRFR3 |
| Primary hereditary lymphedema | VEGFC |
| Primary hereditary lymphedema | GJC2/connexin 47 |
| Lymphedema-distichiasis | FOXC2 |
| Hypotrichosis-lymphedema-telangiectasia | SOX18 |
| Primary lymphedema with myelodysplasia | GATA2 |
| Primary generalized lymphatic anomaly | CCBE1 |
| Microcephaly with/without chorioretinopathy | KIF11 |
| Lymphedema or mental retardation syndrome | — |
| Lymphedema-choanal atresia | PTEN14 |
| VMs | |
| Common VM | TIE2 somatic |
| VMCM | TIE2 |
| Blue rubber bleb nevus (Bean) syndrome VM | — |
| Glomuvenous malformation (VM with glomus cells) | Glomulin |
| CCM | — |
| CCM1 | KRIT1 |
| CCM2 | Malcavernin |
| CCM3 | PDCD10 |
| AVMs | |
| Sporadic in HHT | — |
| *HHT1* | ENG |
| *HHT2* | ACVRL1 |
| JPHT | SMADA4 |
| CM-AVM | RASA1 |
| AVFs | |
| VMs associated with other anomalies | |
| Klippel-Trénaunay syndrome | — |
| Parkes Weber syndrome | RASA1 |
| Servelle-Martorell syndrome | — |

(*continued on next page*)

**Table 1**
**(*continued*)**

| | |
|---|---|
| Sturge-Weber syndrome | GNAQ |
| Limb CM + congenital nonprogressive limb overgrowth | — |
| Maffucci syndrome | — |
| MCAP | PIK3CA |
| MICCAP | STAMBP |
| CLOVES syndrome | PIK3CA |
| Proteus syndrome | AKT1 |
| Bannayan-Riley-Ruvalcaba syndrome | PTEN |
| Provisionally unclassified VAs | |
| Verrucous hemangioma | — |
| Multifocal lymphangioendotheliomatosis with thrombocytopenia/cutaneovisceral angiomatosis with thrombocytopenia | — |
| Kaposiform lymphangiomatosis | — |
| PTEN (type) hamartoma of soft tissue/angiomatosis of soft tissue | PTEN |

*Abbreviations:* AVFs, arteriovenous fistulas; AVM, arteriovenous malformations; CCM, cerebral cavernous malformation; CM, capillary malformations; CMTC, cutis marmorata telangiectatica congenita; CNS, central nervous system; HHT, hereditary hemorrhagic telangiectasia; JPHT, juvenile polyposis/hereditary hemorrhagic telangiectasia syndrome; MCAP, macrocephaly–capillary malformation; MICCAP, microcephaly–capillary malformations; PIK3CA, phosphatyidylinositol-4,5-bisphosphate 3-kinase, catalytic subunit alpha; VM, venous malformation.

*Data from* International Society for the Study of Vascular Anomalies.

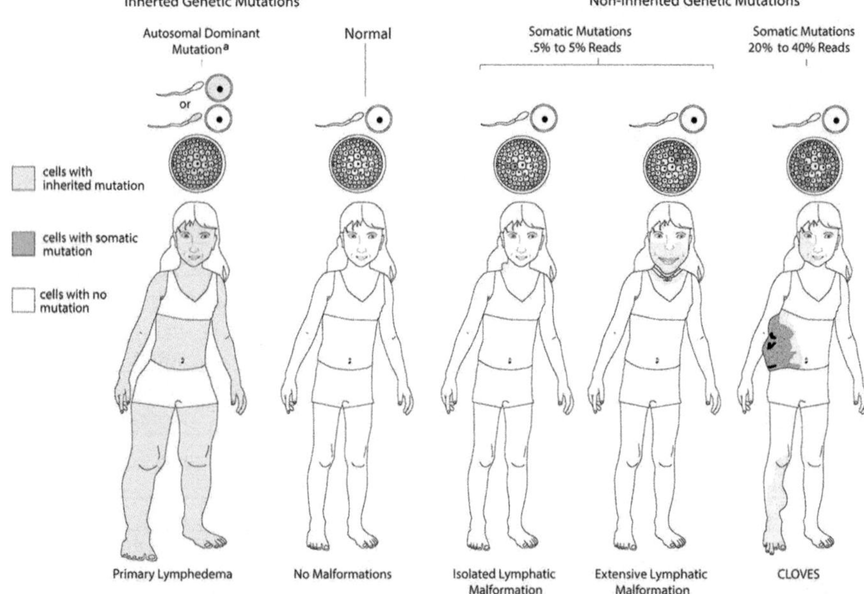


**Fig. 5.** Current theory of molecular genetics applied to germline and postzygotic somatic gene mutations creation of phenotype. On the left, a person without malformations has a normal genome in all cells. In autosomal dominant germline inheritance, all cells in the body have a mutation, shown as yellow. Somatic mutations occur after conception (ie, zygote formation) and affect a variable number of cells in the blastomere, shown as blue. Cells with somatic mutations, by unknown mechanisms, affect one portion of the body as seen in blue. When 5% to 10% of cells, assuming reads are a surrogate measure for affected cells, are affected, the involved area is small. The involved area becomes larger and more dysfunctional when more cells have that mutation. [a] At this time, there are no known autosomal recessive VAs.

Evidence is emerging that cells containing somatic mutations influence phenotypic changes in adjacent cells with normal genomes; this results in the abnormal histologic appearance of malformation tissue (**Fig. 6**). At this time, it is unclear how genetic mosaicism in a single cell induces phenotypic mosaicism in complex tissues or if it has not been discovered that multiple cell types are actually producing the histologic phenotype. PIK3CA gene mutations are associated with larger cell size, tissue overgrowth, and some malignant tumors.[30,31] This gain of function gene mutation explains the tissue overgrowth present in most HNLMs (**Fig. 7**). Exactly how these mutations induce tissue overgrowth and LM is unknown, but primary or adjunctive medical suppression of this gene and its pathway could be

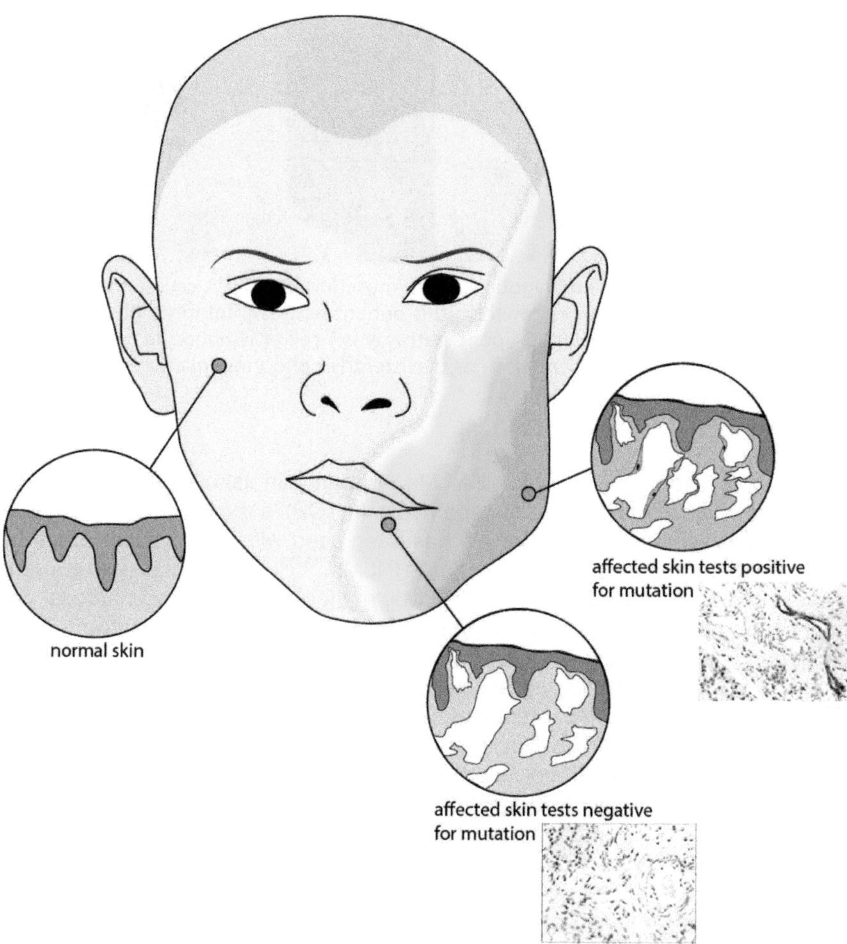


**Fig. 6.** Adjacent cells interact, through mobile genomic sequences (ie, transposable elements) and programmed cell death (ie, apoptosis), creating an environment in which cells with somatic mutations cause neighboring genetically normal cells to exhibit mutant histologic phenotype. This may explain the occurrence and persistence of large areas of histologically abnormal LM tissue, schematically depicted and mirrored with HNLM tissue sections (*top image*: lymphatic endothelium [*brown*] [D2-40 immunostain]), although not all cells in the region have detectable mutations.

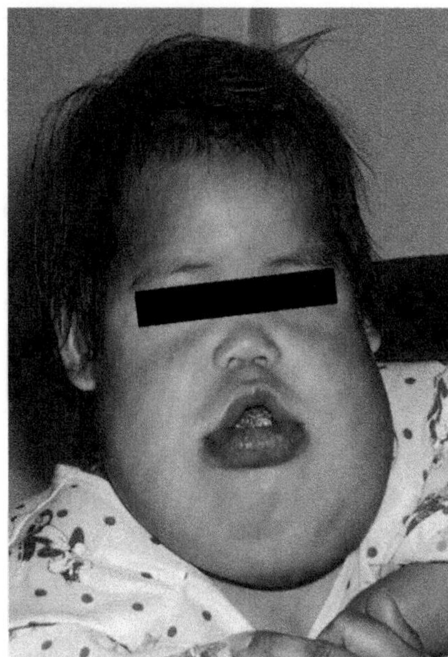

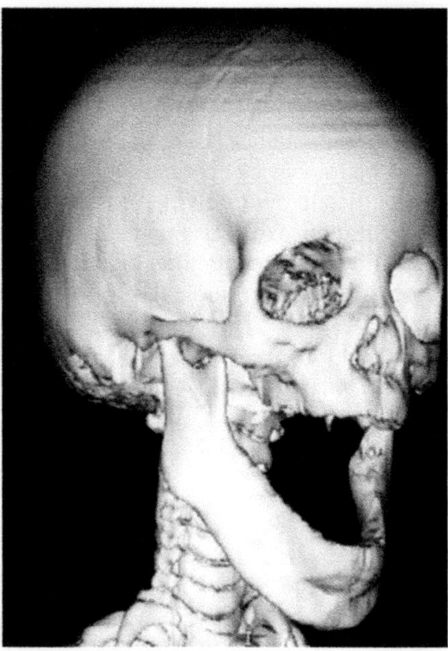

**Fig. 7.** The gain-of-function postzygotic somatic mutation in PIK3CA causes the persistent soft tissue and boney tissue overgrowth in this patient with LM. Interestingly, one of the other known functions of the PIK3CA gene pathway is T-cell or lymphocyte differentiation by the mTOR enzyme. This patient also has persistent lymphocytopenia, which is probably related to disordered PIK3CA function.

therapeutic for some recalcitrant HNLMs. Rapamycin (sirolimus), which suppresses the mammalian target of rapamycin (mTOR) enzyme, a component of the PIK3CA cellular signaling pathway, has been used with varied success for severe lymphatic conditions, including some HNLMs.[32,33] In presentations reporting the effect of sirolimus on unselected HNLMs, malformation-induced mucosal and skin changes have improved but reductions in HNLM size is inconsistent.[34] There has been no effect on tissue hypertrophy.

Future innovations in HNLM assessment hinge on much of the work summarized in preceding paragraphs. As prenatal imaging capabilities improve to accurately assess the fetal airway and swallowing function, planning of HNLM patient delivery will be perfected to reduce any need for extensive delivery interventions (ie, Ex utero intrapartum treatment [EXIT] procedure). Additionally, prenatal molecular genetic diagnosis will refine the characterization and predictions regarding HNLM clinical presentation and behavior. Genetic characterization of HNLM is in its infancy; as our understanding of and ability to detect somatic mutations improves, biological reasons for varied HNLM clinical behavior (ie, regression vs persistence), distribution (ie, stage or grade), and radiographic characteristics will be explained. Further study of the PIK3CA gene locus and other gene loci associated with lymphatic disease is warranted. Associating specific base pair rearrangements in this gene with the HNLM clinical phenotype, natural history, and treatment outcomes will probably change HNLMs and other lymphatic disease nomenclature as it is doing in other conditions of tissue overgrowth.[25,29,35] The cost of sophisticated and sensitive means of automated genetic testing is decreasing and moving into the clinical arena. New information derived from widely available testing will enable the development of treatment plans specific to an individual patient's HNLM. The detection of malformation-causing somatic mutations in specific cells raises the possibility of targeting treatment to the destruction of these affected cells to predictably improve therapeutic outcomes. For example, a localized HNLM may be best treated by complete removal followed by biologically driven therapy to eradicate remaining cells, whereas extensive infiltrative lesions may be best treated with medical therapy that suppresses PIK3CA activity. This treatment will be a complete shift in treatment philosophy and strategy. It is anticipated that medications that completely suppress the whole PIK3CA pathway, rather than a downstream target (ie, mTOR), will eliminate the possibility of treatment-induced feedback mechanisms, so that medical therapy will be more consistently effective (**Fig. 8**).[24,26] The possibility of HNLM chronic medical therapy, either primary or adjunctive, opens the possibility of more comparative treatment trials, which in turn necessitates careful assessment of treatment efficacy and value. Parent and self-report questionnaires will be essential in measuring treatment outcomes.[36] Function threatening HNLM would cause problems with breathing, eating and bleeding. These trials would also provide a basis for evidence-

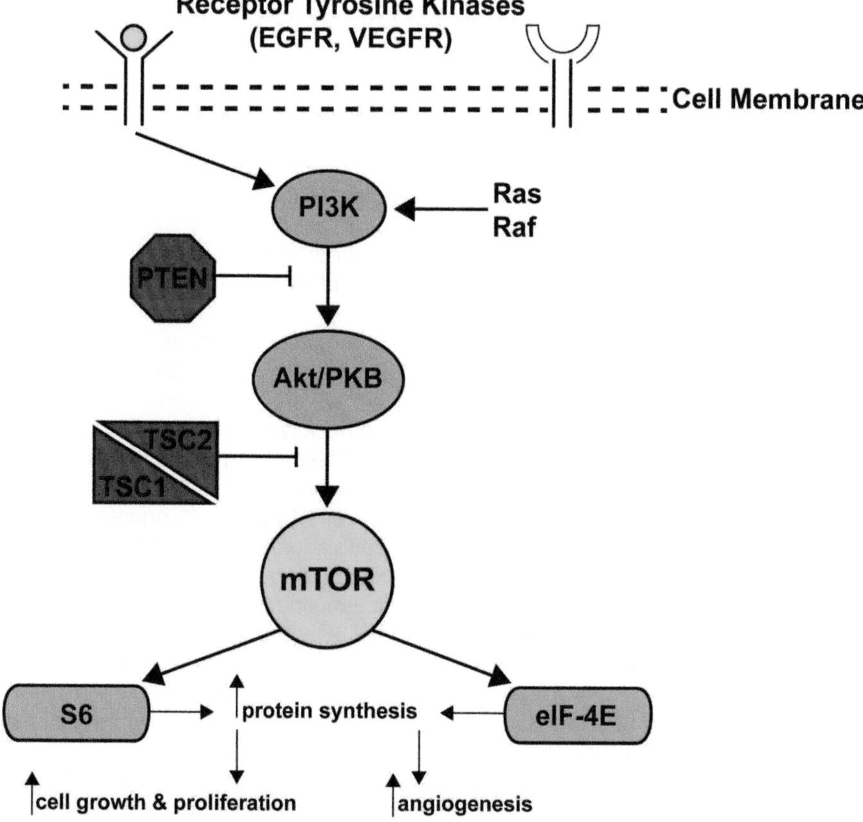


**Fig. 8.** PIK3CA cellular signaling pathway. Note, one of the principal functions of the mTOR enzyme is T-cell differentiation or programming.

driven treatment approaches. Investigation into other methods of cell-specific gene regulation (ie, epigenetics) has been reported in other VAs.[37] These biological mechanisms may reveal new relevant biomarkers for HNLM and reveal cell-specific targets for biological therapy.[26] In the next several decades, with further collaborative work, the treatment of HNLM will change significantly through the application of a new clinical investigation and cellular biological discovery translated to the clinic.

## ACKNOWLEDGMENTS

The author thanks Carrie Capri for article preparation and Eden Palmer for figure creation and assistance with figure preparation for publication.

## REFERENCES

1. Luks VL, Kamitaki N, Vivero MP, et al. Lymphatic and other vascular malformative/overgrowth disorders are caused by somatic mutations in PIK3CA. J Pediatr 2015;166(4):1048–54.e1-5.
2. Osborn AJ, Dickie P, Neilson DE, et al. Activating PIK3CA alleles and lymphangiogenic phenotype of lymphatic endothelial cells isolated from lymphatic malformations. Hum Mol Genet 2015;24(4):926–38.
3. Longstreet B, Bhama PK, Inglis AF Jr, et al. Improved airway visualization during direct laryngoscopy using self-retaining laryngeal retractors: a quantitative study. Otolaryngol Head Neck Surg 2011;145(2):270–5.
4. Dighe MK, Peterson SE, Dubinsky TJ, et al. EXIT procedure: technique and indications with prenatal imaging parameters for assessment of airway patency. Radiographics 2011;31(2):511–26.
5. Perkins JA, Maniglia C, Magit A, et al. Clinical and radiographic findings in children with spontaneous lymphatic malformation regression. Otolaryngol Head Neck Surg 2008;138(6):772–7.
6. Lee S, Finn L, Sze RW, et al. Gorham Stout syndrome (disappearing bone disease): two additional case reports and a review of the literature. Arch Otolaryngol Head Neck Surg 2003;129(12):1340–3.
7. Balakrishnan K, Menezes MD, Chen BS, et al. Primary surgery vs primary sclerotherapy for head and neck lymphatic malformations. JAMA Otolaryngol Head Neck Surg 2014;140(1):41–5.
8. Adams MT, Saltzman B, Perkins JA. Head and neck lymphatic malformation treatment: a systematic review. Otolaryngol Head Neck Surg 2012;147(4):627–39. Available at: http://KT8EW8CQ5H.search.serialssolutions.com/?sid=OVID: Ovid+MEDLINE%28R%29+%3C2011+to+June+Week+1+2015%3E&genre=article&id=pmid:22785242&id=doi:&issn=0194-5998&volume=147&issue=4&spage=627&pages=627-39&date=2012&title=Otolaryngology+-+Head+%26+Neck+Surgery&atitle=Head+and+neck+lymphatic+malformation+treatment%3A+a+systematic+review.&aulast=Adams&pid=%3Cauthor%3EAdams+MT%3C%2Fauthor%3E&%3CAN%3E22785242%3C%2FAN%3E. Accessed November 27, 2012.
9. Kirsh AL, Cushing SL, Chen EY, et al. Tertiary lymphoid organs in lymphatic malformations. Lymphat Res Biol 2011;9(2):85–92.
10. Adams D, Mulliken J, Azizkhan R, et al. Panel discussion on a consensus for lymphatic anomalies. International Society for the Study of Vascular Anomalies. Poster presentation at International Society for Study of Vascular Anomalies 2012(Poster abstracts). Sweden, June 16–19, 2012.

11. Garzon MC, Enjolras O, Frieden IJ. Vascular tumors and vascular malformations: evidence for an association. J Am Acad Dermatol 2000;42(2 Pt 1):275–9.
12. de Serres LM, Sie KC, Richardson MA. Lymphatic malformations of the head and neck. A proposal for staging. Arch Otolaryngol Head Neck Surg 1995;121(5): 577–82.
13. Wiegand S, Eivazi B, Zimmermann AP, et al. Microcystic lymphatic malformations of the tongue: diagnosis, classification, and treatment. Arch Otolaryngol Head Neck Surg 2009;135(10):976–83.
14. Balakrishnan K, Bauman N, Chun RH, et al. Standardized outcome and reporting measures in pediatric head and neck lymphatic malformations. Otolaryngol Head Neck Surg 2015;152(5):948–53.
15. Burrows PE, Mason KP. Percutaneous treatment of low flow vascular malformations. J Vasc Interv Radiol 2004;15(5):431–45.
16. Alomari AI, Karian VE, Lord DJ, et al. Percutaneous sclerotherapy for lymphatic malformations: a retrospective analysis of patient-evaluated improvement. J Vasc Interv Radiol 2006;17(10):1639–48.
17. Smith MC, Zimmerman MB, Burke DK, et al. Efficacy and safety of OK-432 immunotherapy of lymphatic malformations. Laryngoscope 2009;119(1):107–15.
18. Bingham MM, Saltzman B, Vo NJ, et al. Propranolol reduces infantile hemangioma volume and vessel density. Otolaryngol Head Neck Surg 2012;147(2):338–44.
19. Norton ME, Rink BD. Changing indications for invasive testing in an era of improved screening. Semin Perinatol 2016;40(1):56–66.
20. Arai E, Kuramochi A, Tsuchida T, et al. Usefulness of D2-40 immunohistochemistry for differentiation between kaposiform hemangioendothelioma and tufted angioma. J Cutan Pathol 2006;33(7):492–7.
21. Chen EY, Hostikka SL, Oliaei S, et al. Similar histologic features and immunohistochemical staining in microcystic and macrocystic lymphatic malformations. Lymphat Res Biol 2009;7(2):75–80.
22. Tempero RM, Hannibal M, Finn LS, et al. Lymphocytopenia in children with lymphatic malformation. Arch Otolaryngol Head Neck Surg 2006;132(1):93–7.
23. Kim SW, Kavanagh K, Orbach DB, et al. Long-term outcome of radiofrequency ablation for intraoral microcystic lymphatic malformation. Arch Otolaryngol Head Neck Surg 2011;137(12):1247–50.
24. Mei ZB, Duan CY, Li CB, et al. Prognostic role of tumor PIK3CA mutation in colorectal cancer: a systematic review and meta-analysis. Ann Oncol 2016;27(10): 1836–48.
25. Muller MF, Ibrahim AE, Arends MJ. Molecular pathological classification of colorectal cancer. Virchows Arch 2016;469(2):125–34.
26. Cai Y, Dodhia S, Su GH. Dysregulations in the PI3K pathway and targeted therapies for head and neck squamous cell carcinoma. Oncotarget 2017;8(13): 22203–17.
27. Kirkorian AY, Grossberg AL, Puttgen KB. Genetic basis for vascular anomalies. Semin Cutan Med Surg 2016;35(3):128–36.
28. ISSVA classification for vascular anomalies-2014.
29. Keppler-Noreuil KM, Rios JJ, Parker VE, et al. PIK3CA-related overgrowth spectrum (PROS): diagnostic and testing eligibility criteria, differential diagnosis, and evaluation. Am J Med Genet A 2015;167A(2):287–95.
30. Hutchins AP, Pei D. Transposable elements at the center of the crossroads between embryogenesis, embryonic stem cells, reprogramming, and long noncoding RNAs. Sci Bull (Beijing) 2015;60(20):1722–33.

31. Perez-Garijo A, Steller H. Spreading the word: non-autonomous effects of apoptosis during development, regeneration and disease. Development 2015; 142(19):3253–62.
32. Adams DM, Trenor CC 3rd, Hammill AM, et al. Efficacy and safety of sirolimus in the treatment of complicated vascular anomalies. Pediatrics 2016;137(2): e20153257.
33. Hammill AM, Wentzel M, Gupta A, et al. Sirolimus for the treatment of complicated vascular anomalies in children. Pediatr Blood Cancer 2011;57(6):1018–24.
34. Strychowsky J, Rahbar R, Padua H, et al. Sirolimus for the treatment of cervicofacial lymphatic malformations. Poster at Annual Meeting of the American Society of Pediatric Otolaryngology. Boston(MA), April 23–26, 2015.
35. Loconte DC, Grossi V, Bozzao C, et al. Molecular and functional characterization of three different postzygotic mutations in PIK3CA-related overgrowth spectrum (PROS) patients: effects on PI3K/AKT/mTOR signaling and sensitivity to PIK3 inhibitors. PLoS One 2015;10(4):e0123092.
36. Kirkham EM, Edwards TC, Weaver EM, et al. The lymphatic malformation function (LMF) instrument. Otolaryngol Head Neck Surg 2015;153(4):656–62.
37. Strub GM, Kirsh AL, Whipple ME, et al. Endothelial and circulating C19MC microRNAs are biomarkers of infantile hemangioma. JCI Insight 2016;1(14):e88856.

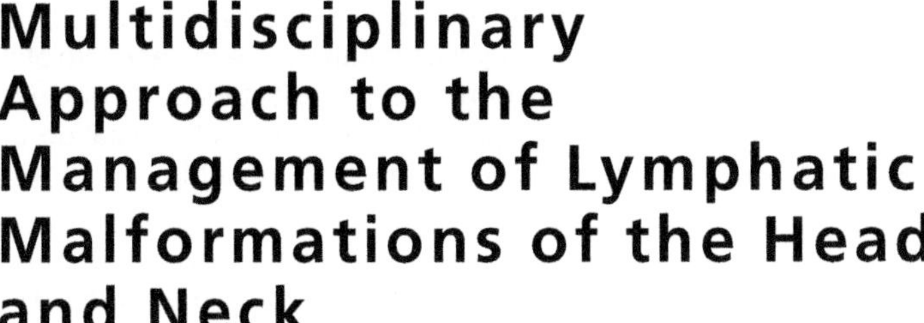

# Multidisciplinary Approach to the Management of Lymphatic Malformations of the Head and Neck

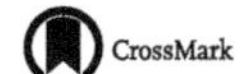

Milton Waner, MBBCh(Wits), FCS(SA), MD[a,*], Teresa M. O, MD, MArch[b]

**KEYWORDS**

- Lymphatic malformations • Head • Neck • Multimodal treatment • Sclerotherapy
- Surgery

**KEY POINTS**

- Lymphatic Malformations (LMs) may present clinically as low, intermediate, or high grade lesions.
- The typical presentation of a LM is a flesh colored or bluish noncompressible mass.
- They are characterized by episodes of exacerbation and remission.
- Multimodal treatment provides significantly improved outcomes for patients.

Lymphatic malformations (LMs) occur in 2.8 to 5:100,000 live births.[1,2] Most involve the head and neck and they are equally common in males and females.[3–5] They are developmental anomalies of unknown cause, although recent evidence suggests that an upregulation of the mammalian target of rapamycin (mTOR) pathway may be a causal factor leading to the overproduction of abnormal lymph vessels.[6] These vessels are likely dilated lymphatic sacs sequestered from the lymphatic and venous systems.[7,8] This overproduction results in the accumulation of lymph in dilated cystic spaces, which in turn results in the clinical features of a LM.

## CLINICAL PRESENTATION

In about 50% of cases, the condition is apparent at birth and, in 90% of cases, symptoms are present by 2 years of age.[9] Routine prenatal ultrasonography has led to a

Disclosure: The author has nothing to disclose.

[a] Lenox Hill Hospital, 210 East 64th Street, 7th Floor, New York, NY 10065, USA; [b] Department of Otolaryngology–Head and Neck Surgery, Vascular Birthmark Institute of New York, Facial Nerve Center, Manhattan Eye, Ear and Throat Hospital, 210 East 64th Street, 7 Floor, New York, NY 10065, USA
* Corresponding authors.
*E-mail address:* mwmd01@gmail.com

Otolaryngol Clin N Am 51 (2018) 159–172
https://doi.org/10.1016/j.otc.2017.09.012
oto.theclinics.com

higher incidence of prenatal diagnosis.[10,11] However, not all prenatally diagnosed LMs are present at birth. Some are associated with significant cardiac, renal, and skeletal deformities and do not proceed to parturition, aborting either spontaneously or electively. Longstreet and colleagues[12] recently proposed an anatomic classification of fetal nuchal lymphatic anomalies. They recognized 3 groups of fetal LMs.

### *Nuchal Thickening*

Nuchal thickening is a hypoechoic region exceeding the 95th percentile between skin and soft tissues bordered by the fetal spine and occiput. About 30% of these lesions are associated with chromosomal abnormalities, such as trisomy 21, trisomy 18, and Turner syndrome. A large percentage (80%) of these resolve by birth.

### *Dorsal Lymphatic Malformations*

Dorsal LMs are septated, fluid-filled, multilocular cavities extending along the entire dorsal length of the fetus. These cavities are associated with a high percentage of other abnormalities, such as cardiac, renal, and skeletal. Many of these abort spontaneously or electively. Of those that did survive to parturition, 50% had resolved spontaneously.

### *Ventral Lymphatic Malformations*

Ventral LMs were defined as those occurring on the anterior and/or lateral cervical region of the fetus. None of these were associated with other congenital anomalies and all were present at birth. Ventral LMs are at risk for airway obstruction and may necessitate an ex utero intrapartum treatment (EXIT) procedure.

The typical presentation of an LM is a noncompressible flesh-colored or bluish mass involving the head and/or neck (**Fig. 1**). The location and extent of involvement are

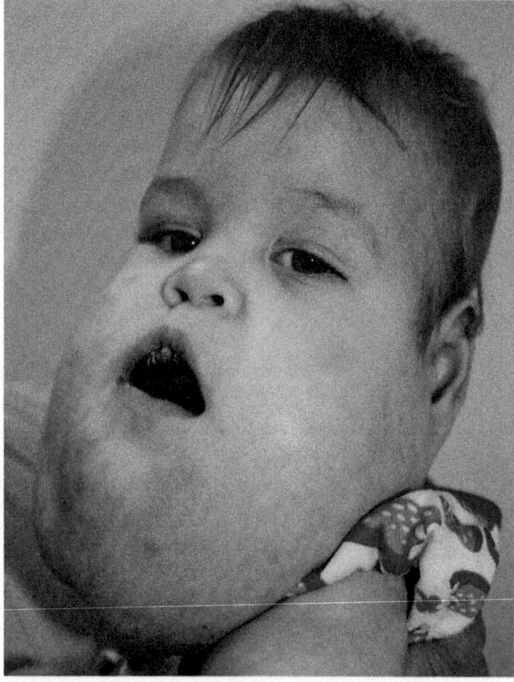

**Fig. 1.** A child with a large bilateral cervicofacial LM.

variable. The consistency of the mass varies according to the activity of the lesion. Active inflamed lesions are typically firm and, in an acute exacerbation, the overlying skin may be inflamed and tender, whereas inactive lesions are softer. The LM mass is composed of lymph-filled cysts, which may be very large. This condition is typically seen in cervical lesions, which can present with a small number of large cysts. The other extreme of this is a facial lesion made up of predominantly small cysts. The size of the cysts is relevant in the selection of a treatment.[13] A lesion comprising cysts greater than 2 cm in diameter is macrocystic, whereas a lesion with cysts less than 2 cm in diameter is microcystic.[13] Most lesions are mixed and have both macrocystic and microcystic components. de Serres and colleagues[1] described a classification of LMs based on their *anatomic location with respect to the hyoid*. They recognized that the location as well as the extent of the lesion plays a critical role in determining both the prognosis and the management of the lesion. The lesion may be below the hyoid, above the hyoid, or both. In addition to this, the lesion may be bilateral or unilateral. In general, unilateral infrahyoid lesions are typically macrocystic and respond best to treatment (**Fig. 2**). In contrast, suprahyoid lesions are more likely to be microcystic or mixed and are more difficult to treat effectively. This classification is useful in both choosing a treatment and prognostication.

Involvement of the overlying skin and/or mucosa produces lymph-filled vesicles. Blood products may also be found within some of these vesicles. The appearance

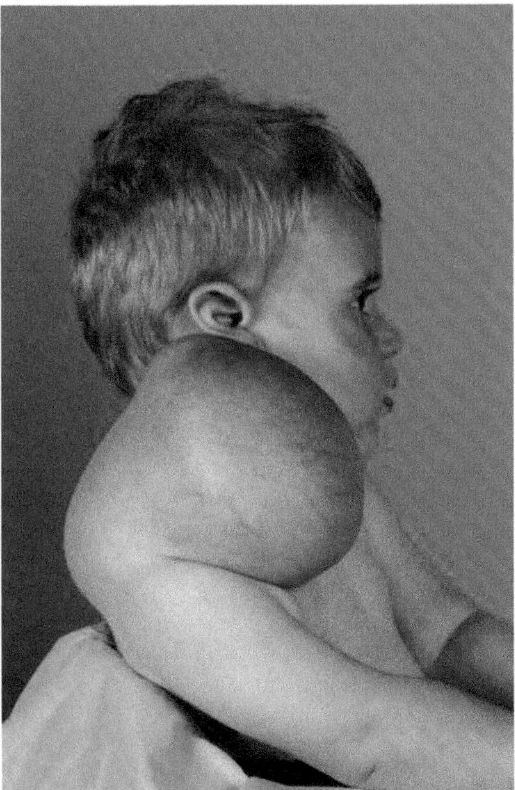

**Fig. 2.** A child with an infrahyoid macrocystic LM involving his lower cervical and supraclavicular area extending into the axilla.

of these vesicles may coincide with an exacerbation of the lesion. These vesicles are typically 2 to 3 mm in diameter and commonly involve the tongue and floor of mouth (**Fig. 3**). They often rupture resulting in a discharge of lymph or lymph mixed with blood, which is especially disturbing for the patient. These vesicles can also be found in the skin overlying an LM. Bleeding has been reported in as many as 11% of cases.[14]

The involved area commonly causes asymmetry of the face and/or head and neck with varying degrees of disfigurement (**Fig. 4**). The mass effect of an LM also deforms the underlying bony structures, giving rise to classic facial deformities.[15] A large cervical lesion can cause outward displacement or winging of the angles of the mandible. A large parotid lesion causes displacement of the ramus of the mandible and, in some cases, a pseudoarthrosis of the temporomandibular joint forms. Macroglossia with glossoptosis results in an open-bite deformity.[15]

Airway obstruction may result from mass effect involving structures adjacent to the airway and/or direct involvement of the airway.[16] Swelling of structures such as the base of tongue and the floor of the mouth can obstruct the airway. In addition, direct involvement of the supraglottic larynx can cause airway obstruction. O and colleagues[16] documented the site of airway obstruction in a large number of cases and found that, where direct laryngeal involvement was present, the disease always involved the supraglottic larynx. An omega-shaped epiglottis with extensive false vocal fold involvement was common (**Fig. 5**). High-grade LMs are often diagnosed during routine prenatal ultrasonography examinations. These LMs probably fit the classification of Longstreet and colleagues[12] as dorsal LMs. If airway obstruction is suspected, an EXIT procedure is planned and, if warranted, a tracheotomy is the final outcome. A child who undergoes a tracheotomy is unlikely to be decannulated for about 5 to 6 years. In addition, most also need a feeding gastrostomy.

The swelling can also cause other functional disturbances, such as visual obstruction leading to amblyopia, or macroglossia and glossoptosis, which cause speech and swallowing difficulties and dentofacial deformity[16,17] (**Figs. 6** and **7**). An open-bite

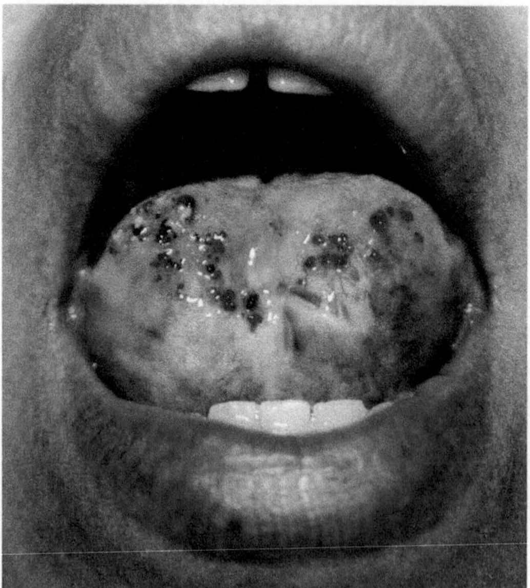

**Fig. 3.** A patient with LM of her tongue. Note the vesicles, many of which are hemorrhagic. The tongue is swollen from diffuse microcystic involvement.

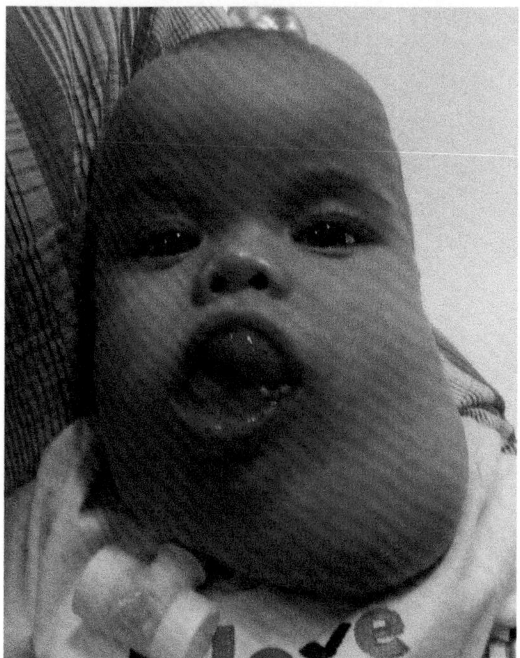

**Fig. 4.** An infant with a unilateral suprahyoid LM. This lesion has involvement of the floor of mouth with resultant glossoptosis and an anterior open-bite deformity.

deformity significantly affects the patient's speech intelligibility as well as the patient's caloric intake.

One of the clinical hallmarks of LMs is their tendency to exacerbate and then remit. Exacerbations usually occur in association with upper respiratory infections but they can also occur after trauma. During these episodes, the lesion becomes firm, inflamed, and swollen. These exacerbations can last 10 to 12 days.

In a review of a large series of cases, clinical symptoms included the following[14]:

- Asymmetry/disfigurement (48%)
- Pain and/or discomfort (20%)

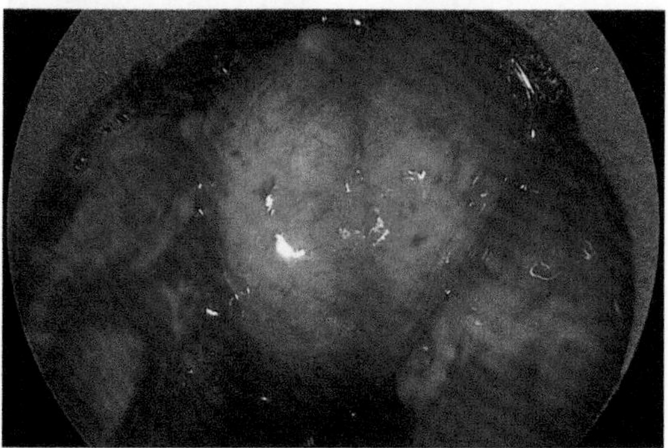

**Fig. 5.** The larynx of an infant with airway obstruction. Note the edematous omega-shaped epiglottis and base of tongue disease.

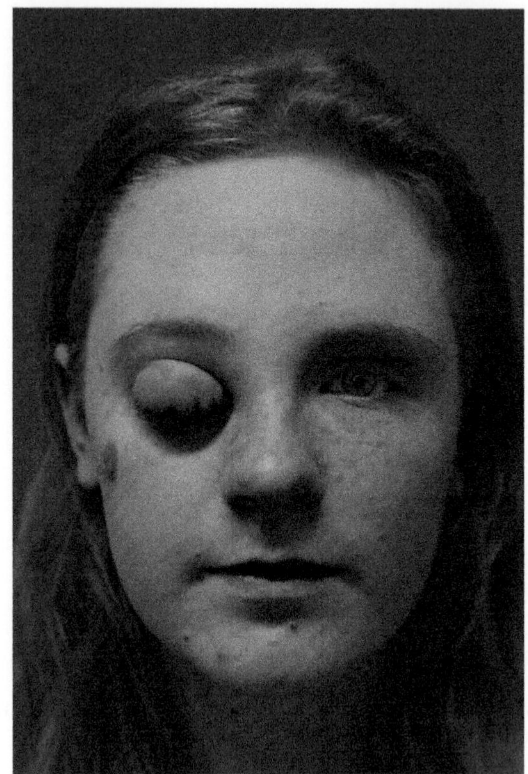

**Fig. 6.** A teenager with an orbital and upper eyelid LM. Her visual axis has been obstructed for many years and she has resultant amblyopia.

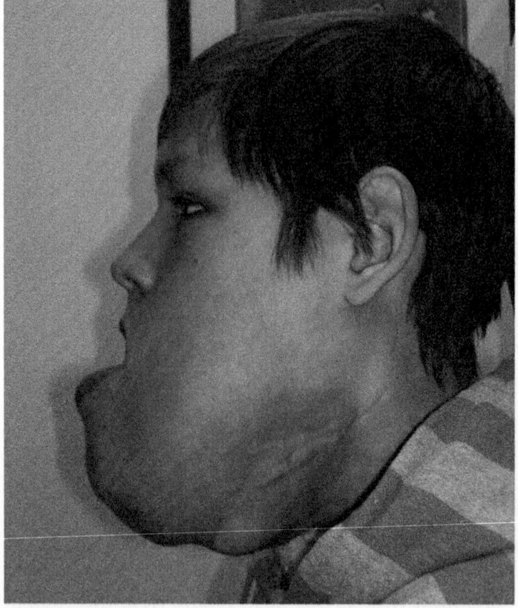

**Fig. 7.** A patient with an anterior open-bite deformity and class 3 malocclusion.

- Exacerbations/intralesional infections (15%)
- Airway issues (13%)
- Functional disability (12%)
- Bleeding (11%)
- Lymphorrhea (6%)

## DIAGNOSIS

The diagnosis is usually made on clinical presentation. In the absence of all the obvious features, MRI with and without contrast is needed. Lymph-filled macrocystic and/or microcystic lesions are the main diagnostic features. Hemorrhage into some of the lesions may result in a fluid-fluid level in 1 or more of the cysts. Because the lesion is made up of a large component of lymph, the lesion shows a high signal on T2-weighted images[18] (**Fig. 8**). Gadolinium enhancement is seen in the interstitial spaces between the cysts. Microcystic lesions show a hyperintense homogeneous T2 image. In some cases, a mixed lymphatic venous malformation may be present. These radiological features resemble both venous malformation and LM. In cases in which there has been bleeding into a cyst, a fluid-fluid level is seen.

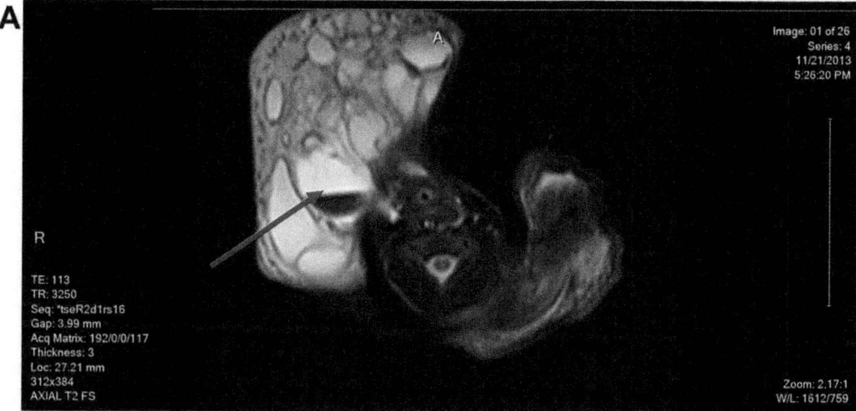


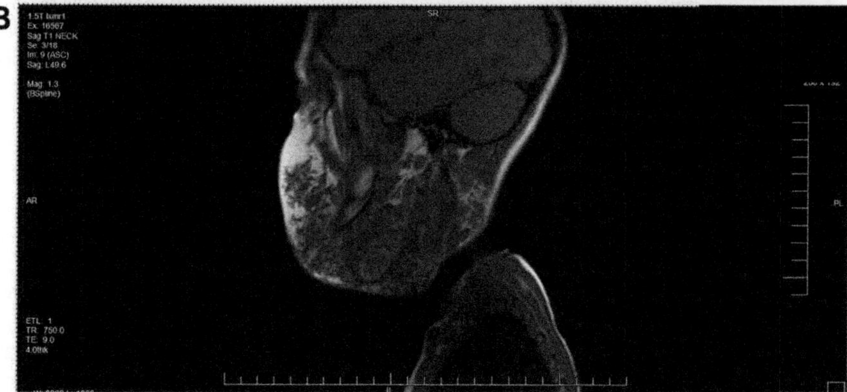


**Fig. 8.** (*A*) Axial T2-weighted MRI showing a macrocystic head and neck LM. Note the fluid-fluid level indicated by the arrow on this T2-weighted image. (*B*) Sagittal T2 MRI showing diffuse microcystic LM of the head and neck.

On ultrasonography imaging, a heterogeneous mix of cysts separated by echogenic septa is evident. Ultrasonography can also be helpful in identifying abnormal venous flow, which is common with mixed venous LMs (See Jared M. Steinklein and Deborah R. Shatzke's article, "Imaging of Vascular Lesions of the Head and Neck" for further details).

## TREATMENT

The treatment of LMs encompasses several modalities and is best undertaken by a multidisciplinary team. It is hoped that this will result in the most appropriate treatment. Treatment modalities include observation, surgery, sclerotherapy, and medical management. Management of the exacerbations as well as the various components of an LM is also considered.

### *General Considerations*

The risks and benefits of 3 modalities should be considered. They are sclerotherapy, surgery, and medical therapy. Each of these modalities can effectively treat an LM but may not be the treatment of choice for a particular lesion. In addition to this, Perkins and colleagues[28] advocate that, because a percentage of lesions in their series spontaneously shrunk, conservative management is appropriate in some cases. Given the tendency for lesions to exacerbate and remit, it is reasonable to wonder whether or not those lesions that had spontaneously regressed were in remission and would eventually exacerbate given enough time. However, because some lesions spontaneously regressed or were in remission for several years, conservative management is a reasonable approach in a select group of cases. These cases include patients in whom the lesion seems to have disappeared and in whom there are no other sequelae or complications. The work of Hassanein and colleagues[19] should also considered; they found that, in 85% of children with LMs, the lesions expanded and/or became symptomatic during childhood.

### *Sclerotherapy*

Sclerotherapy has been popularized as a primary modality for treating LMs. Although several agents have been used, the most commonly used are OK-432 (Picibanil) and bleomycin.[20] Smith and colleagues[13] showed that OK-432 was highly effective when used to treat macrocystic lesions; 94% had a complete or substantial response, whereas none of their patients with microcystic lesions responded. They also showed that, compared with aggregated surgical outcomes, OK-432 was 4 times more likely than surgery to result in a successful outcome and fewer complications. However, Balakrishnan and colleagues[21] showed no significant difference in efficacy between surgery and sclerotherapy. In a systematic review by Acevedo and colleagues[22] of patients treated with predominantly bleomycin and OK-432, 43% of patients had an excellent or complete response, whereas 45% had a good or fair response. Note that these rates of response do not apply to a single treatment but are the result of an aggregate of around 4 treatments.

Complication rates with bleomycin and OK-432 seem to be low.[23,24] Neither of these agents is neurotoxic and they are therefore safe when used adjacent to the facial nerve. Smith and colleagues[13] reported major complications in 3 of 30 patients treated with OK-432. These complications included airway obstruction, cellulitis, and proptosis.[23] Bleomycin is less likely to cause postoperative swelling and is therefore safe when used in the orbit. Precautions must be taken with skin adhesives and skin irritants because these can cause irreversible skin staining when used within 72 hours of bleomycin sclerotherapy. Electrocardiogram adhesives are therefore not removed for 72 hours and patients are told not to scratch themselves during this time.

### *Surgery*

Up until the advent of sclerotherapy, surgery formed the mainstay of treatment. High recurrence rates led to the search for alternative treatments as well as a better understanding of the nature of the disease. It is now known that macrocystic cervical lesions respond well to surgery and in most cases can be completely excised, whereas the likelihood of complete excision of a microcystic cervicofacial lesion is extremely low and therefore the risk of recurrence is high.[25,26]

A meta-analysis found that surgical recurrence rates are around 30%, whereas the morbidity is between 2% and 6%.[27,28] Note that, to compare the results of surgery with sclerotherapy is in essence to compare the results of a single round of surgery with the results of multiple (up to 5) rounds of sclerotherapy. Despite this, there does not seem to be an appreciable difference in recurrence rates between the two modalities.

### *Medical management*

**Sildenafil** After an initial encouraging report of a coincidental response in a patient and 2 subsequent patients, several studies were conducted, including a prospective cohort study.[29–32] However, the results of these studies have been mixed, with some showing improvement and some worsening. The use of sildenafil is currently still under investigation and, until further evidence warrants its use, the authors do not encourage its use in patients with LMs.

**Rapamycin (sirolimus)** Sirolimus is an mTOR inhibitor and is commonly used as an immunosuppressive drug in transplant patients.[33] The mTOR pathway forms the basis for cell growth and proliferation. It increases the expression of vascular endothelial growth factor, thereby playing a part in the regulation of angiogenesis and lymphangiogenesis. mTOR inhibitors block downstream protein synthesis and thereby have antitumoral as well as antiangiogenic activity.[34] Early reports using sirolimus for LMs have been encouraging.[6,35,36] More recently, Triana and colleagues[33] published a retrospective review of patients treated with sirolimus for vascular malformations. Eleven patients with LM were included in their series. All but 1 responded to treatment. Response was defined as shrinkage of the lesion and/or improvement of the symptoms. No patients had a complete response.

There are several issues that remain unresolved. Dosage of the drug has not been established. The duration of treatment is another issue. It seems that the duration of treatment is center specific.[33] Because many patients have been placed on "long-term sirolimus, the exact rebound rate is not known. The risk of lymphoma and skin cancer with long-term therapy in solid organ transplant patients is significant.[37] Will this also be a problem in children treated for LMs?

### *Combined treatment*

Because no single modality provides a satisfactory result, most patients should be treated with multiple modalities. Surgical resection as a primary treatment can adequately dispense with large macrocystic lesions as well as significantly debulk large microcystic lesions. Any remaining disease can be treated with sclerotherapy. Bleomycin is currently being used to treat residual microcystic disease with some success.[38] Several rounds of sclerotherapy may be necessary to treat any persistent disease. The authors prefer surgery as a primary modality in order to reduce the volume of disease. Initial medical treatment can reduce the volume of disease and it can then be surgically removed. Once again, any residuum can be treated with sclerotherapy. However, no published data evaluating multimodal therapy exist.

**Acute exacerbations** These are common in patients with active lesions and there is no uniformly accepted treatment. Exacerbations commonly commence after an upper respiratory infection (URI) or trauma to the lesion, but often there is no preceding URI or trauma. Acute swelling and inflammation herald the onset of such an event. Because the signs of an acute exacerbation resemble cellulitis, it is often assumed that this is caused by an acute bacterial infection and for this reason these patients are treated with an array of antibiotics, often to no avail. The exacerbation runs its course and this usually lasts 10 to 12 days. During these events, blood cultures are usually negative and there is often no direct evidence of a bacterial infection. Despite this, antibiotics have formed the mainstay of treatment. Adding corticosteroids to the regimen usually reverses the symptoms and shortens the course of the exacerbation.[39] Prednisone 1 to 2 mg/kg of body weight for 5 days and then a taper over a further 5 days is given.

**Vesicles/lymphorrhea** Vesicles of the oral cavity as well as cutaneous lesions should be treated. In the past, ablative modalities such as $CO_2$ laser ablation and coblation have been used.[20,40,41] Although these modalities have been able to provide relief, recurrence is common. More recently, local injections of bleomycin into the areas of involvement seem to be beneficial.[38] Although there has been no comparison of the modalities, it seems that bleomycin is at least as effective and possibly more so. A typical treatment consists of an intralesional injection of 1 or 2 mg/mL of bleomycin injected directly into the vesicles or into the mucosa or skin immediately deep to the affected area (**Fig. 9**). The authors prefer to avoid deep intramuscular injections of the tongue because this is likely to cause marked swelling.

After treatment, the area becomes indurated and swollen, and some purpura is common. Some patients experience pain. The mechanism for this is not understood. Pain usually lasts 5 to 6 days and then subsides. The acute changes usually subside in 10 to 14 days and the vesicles usually resolve. Any remaining disease can be treated with a second round of treatment 6 weeks later.

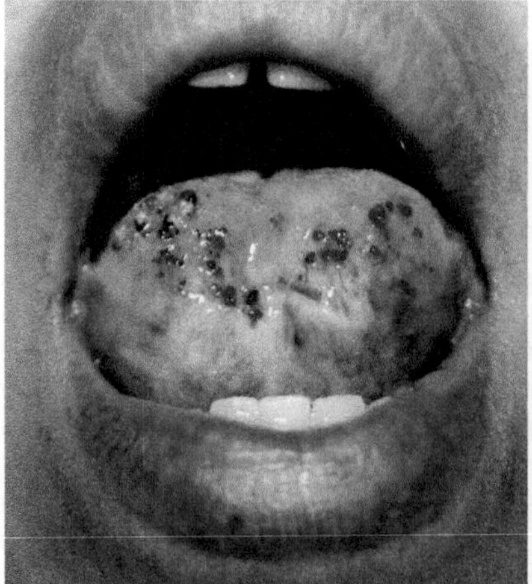

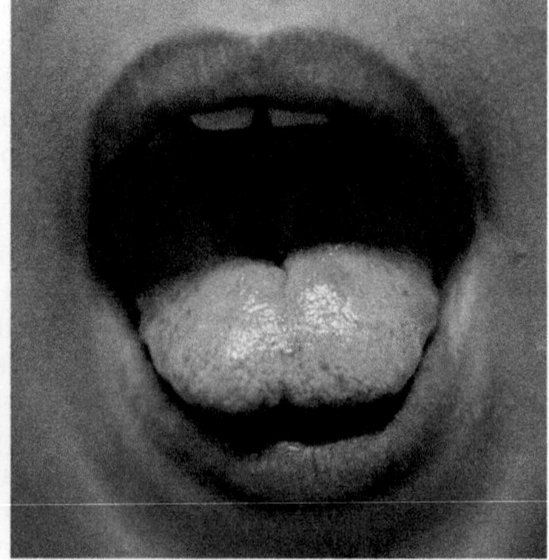

**Fig. 9.** A patient with extensive microcystic disease of her tongue and vesicles before (*left*) and after (*right*) treatment with bleomycin injections.

**Airway involvement** Once a tracheotomy has been performed, it is common to wait until the airway is large enough to compensate for the initial cause of the obstruction. This process may take many years and it is common for children to need a tracheotomy until the teenage years and sometimes even longer. For this reason, the authors have embarked on a more aggressive decannulation program. Each patient's airway is assessed and the site of obstruction is documented. Intralesional bleomycin injections with or without $CO_2$ laser ablation is performed periodically, usually every 3 months, in order to address the areas of obstruction[42] (**Fig. 10**). Bleomycin is administered via a 27-gauge butterfly needle. With the patient in direct suspension and under direct vision,

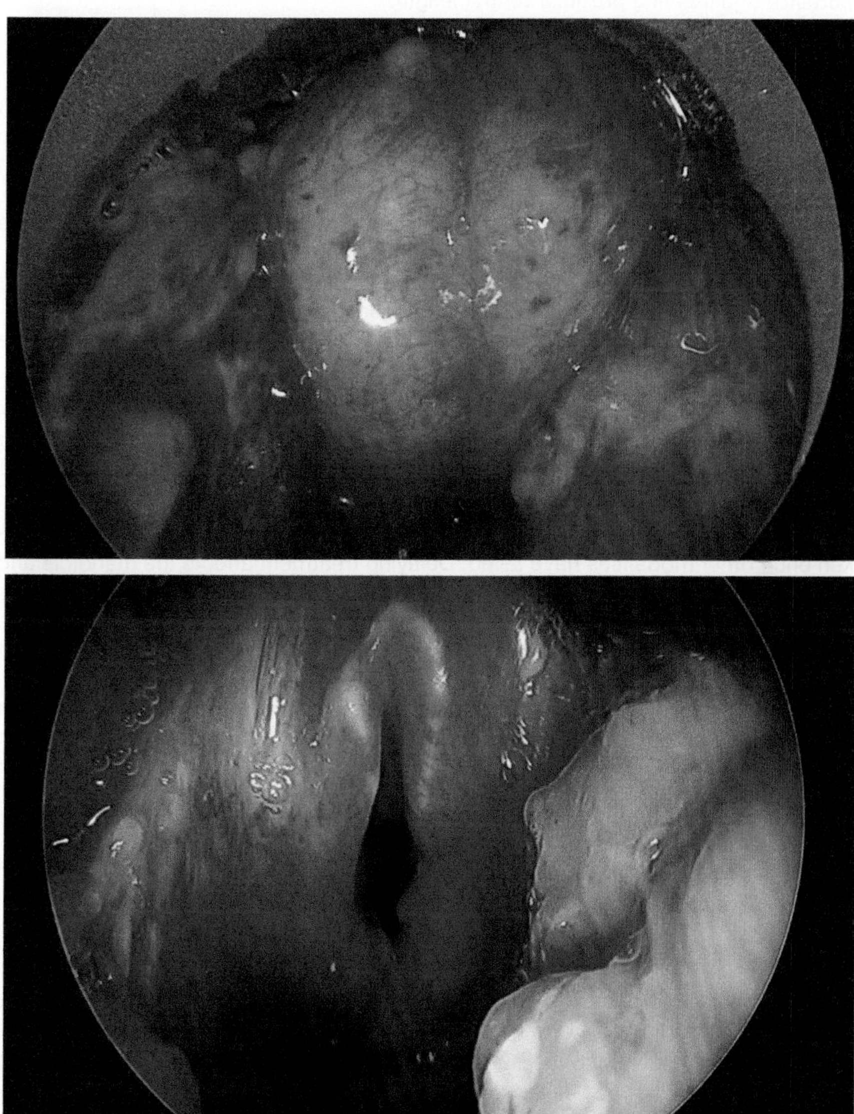

**Fig. 10.** A child with airway involvement before (*top*) and after (*bottom*) multiple treatments with transmucosal bleomycin injections.

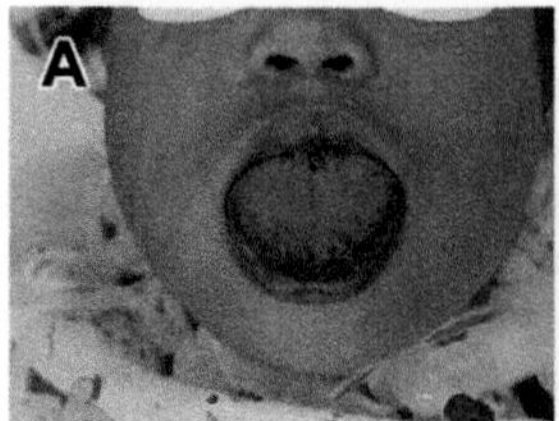

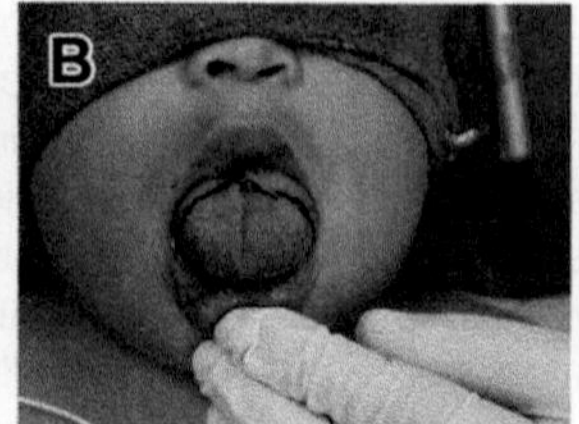

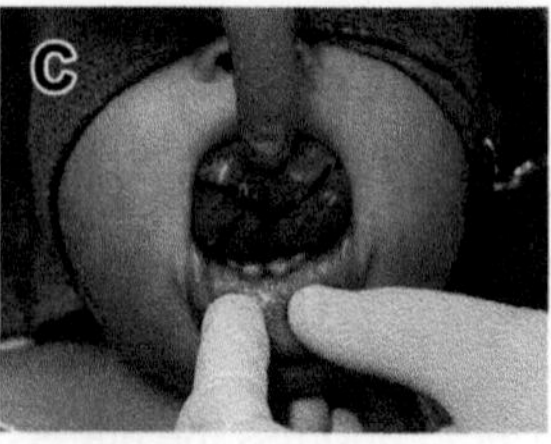


**Fig. 11.** Tongue wedge excision. (*A*) Young child with tongue LM, macroglossia and glossoptosis. (*B*) Dorsal markings for wedge excision. (*C*) Ventral markings for wedge excision. Note importance of perserving proximal ventral length.

the wings of the butterfly needle are trimmed. The syringe with bleomycin 3 mg or units per milliliter is attached to the butterfly and the apparatus is primed. The needle is then inserted into the area being treated with the aid of an alligator forceps and typically 0.1 to 0.2 mL are injected per supralaryngeal site. $CO_2$ laser ablation can also be used in conjunction with bleomycin. The laser is used with caution because of the risk of circumferential stenosis. Using these techniques, the authors have been able to decannulate many patients earlier than we would have had we not treated them aggressively.

More recently, medical management with sirolimus has been noted to improve airway obstruction.[35] Long-term medical management is usually necessary to accomplish this and the possibility of rebound after cessation of treatment should be considered.

**Glossoptosis/macroglossia** Long-standing glossoptosis in early childhood results in an open-bite deformity. Both speech intelligibility and mastication are compromised. Glossoptosis may be caused by macroglossia, floor of mouth involvement, or both. Medical management with sirolimus may be helpful. Intralesional bleomycin is also occasionally used. Surgical reduction of a massively enlarged tongue should be undertaken once other modalities have failed. Delaying treatment affects the mandible and dentition. A wedge resection of the excess should be done, keeping in mind that the tongue should be long enough to rest at the level of the teeth (**Fig. 11**). The apex of the wedge should be keyhole shaped so that the mucosal edges come together without redundancy.

Multimodal treatment, preferably in a major center where a multidisciplinary group is able to participate in management, provides significantly improved outcomes for patients.

## REFERENCES


1. de Serres LM, Sie KC, Richardson MA. Lymphatic malformations of the head and neck. A proposal for staging. Arch Otolaryngol Head Neck Surg 1995;121(5): 577–82.
2. Smith RJ. Lymphatic malformations. Lymphat Res Biol 2004;2(1):25–31.
3. Ethunandan M, Mellor TK. Haemangiomas and vascular malformations of the maxillofacial region–a review. Br J Oral Maxillofac Surg 2006;44(4):263–72.
4. Curran AJ, Malik N, McShane D, et al. Surgical management of lymphangiomas in adults. J Laryngol Otol 1996;110(6):586–9.
5. Kang GC, Song C. Forty-one cervicofacial vascular anomalies and their surgical management: retrospection and review. Ann Acad Med Singapore 2008;37: 165–79.

6. Hammill AM, Wentzel M, Gupta A, et al. Sirolimus for the treatment of complicated vascular anomalies in children. Pediatr Blood Cancer 2011;57(6):1018–24.
7. Mulliken J, Burrows PE, Fishman SJ, et al. Mulliken and Young's vascular anomalies: hemangiomas and malformations. New York: Oxford University Press; 2013.
8. Fonkalsrud EW. Lymphatic disorders. In: Grosfeld JL, O'Neil JA Jr, editors. Pediatric Surgery. 6th edition. Philadelpia: Elsevier; 2006. p. 2137–46.
9. Wiggs WJ Jr, Sismanis A. Cystic hygroma in the adult: two case reports. Otolaryngol Head Neck Surg 1994;110(2):239–41.
10. Surico D, Amadori R, D'Ajello P, et al. Antenatal diagnosis of fetal lymphangioma by ultrasonography. Eur J Obstet Gynecol Reprod Biol 2013;168(2):236.
11. Aslan A, Buyukkaya R, Tan S, et al. Efficacy of ultrasonography in lymphatic malformations: diagnosis, treatment and follow-up: a case report. Med Ultrason 2013;15(3):244–6.
12. Longstreet B, Balakrishnan K, Saltzman B, et al. Prognostic value of a simplified anatomically based nomenclature for fetal nuchal lymphatic anomalies. Otolaryngol Head Neck Surg 2015;152(2):342–7.
13. Smith MC, Zimmerman MB, Burke DK, et al. Efficacy and safety of OK-432 immunotherapy of lymphatic malformations. Laryngoscope 2009;119(1):107–15.
14. Eliasson JJ, Weiss I, Hogevold HE, et al. An 8-year population description from a national treatment centre on lymphatic malformations. J Plast Surg Hand Surg 2017;51(4):280–5.
15. O TM, Kwak R, Portnof JE, et al. Analysis of skeletal mandibular abnormalities associated with cervicofacial lymphatic malformations. Laryngoscope 2011; 121(1):91–101.
16. O TM, Rickert SM, Diallo AM, et al. Lymphatic malformations of the airway. Otolaryngol Head Neck Surg 2013;149(1):156–60.
17. Greene AK, Burrows PE, Smith L, et al. Periorbital lymphatic malformation: clinical course and management in 42 patients. Plast Reconstr Surg 2005;115(1):22–30.
18. Burrows PE, Laor T, Paltiel H, et al. Diagnostic imaging in the evaluation of vascular birthmarks. Dermatol Clin 1998;16(3):455–88.
19. Hassanein AH, Mulliken JB, Fishman SJ, et al. Lymphatic malformation: risk of progression during childhood and adolescence. J Craniofac Surg 2012;23(1): 149–52.
20. Morgan P, Keller R, Patel K. Evidence-based management of vascular malformations. Facial Plast Surg 2016;32(2):162–76.
21. Balakrishnan K, Bauman N, Chun RH, et al. Standardized outcome and reporting measures in pediatric head and neck lymphatic malformations. Otolaryngol Head Neck Surg 2015;152(5):948–53.
22. Acevedo JL, Shah RK, Brietzke SE. Nonsurgical therapies for lymphangiomas: a systematic review. Otolaryngol Head Neck Surg 2008;138(4):418–24.
23. Giguere CM, Bauman NM, Sato Y, et al. Treatment of lymphangiomas with OK-432 (Picibanil) sclerotherapy: a prospective multi-institutional trial. Arch Otolaryngol Head Neck Surg 2002;128(10):1137–44.
24. Mathur NN, Rana I, Bothra R, et al. Bleomycin sclerotherapy in congenital lymphatic and vascular malformations of head and neck. Int J Pediatr Otorhinolaryngol 2005;69(1):75–80.
25. Raveh E, de Jong AL, Taylor GP, et al. Prognostic factors in the treatment of lymphatic malformations. Arch Otolaryngol Head Neck Surg 1997;123(10): 1061–5.

26. Honig JF, Merten HA. Surgical removal of intra- and extraoral cavernous lymphangiomas using intraoperative-assisted intralesional fibrin glue injections. J Craniofac Surg 2000;11(1):42–5.
27. Elluru RG, Balakrishnan K, Padua HM. Lymphatic malformations: diagnosis and management. Semin Pediatr Surg 2014;23(4):178–85.
28. Perkins JA, Manning SC, Tempero RM, et al. Lymphatic malformations: review of current treatment. Otolaryngol Head Neck Surg 2010;142(6):795–803, 803.e1.
29. Swetman GL, Berk DR, Vasanawala SS, et al. Sildenafil for severe lymphatic malformations. N Engl J Med 2012;366(4):384–6.
30. Danial C, Tichy AL, Tariq U, et al. An open-label study to evaluate sildenafil for the treatment of lymphatic malformations. J Am Acad Dermatol 2014;70(6):1050–7.
31. Koshy JC, Eisemann BS, Agrawal N, et al. Sildenafil for microcystic lymphatic malformations of the head and neck: a prospective study. Int J Pediatr Otorhinolaryngol 2015;79(7):980–2.
32. Rankin H, Zwicker K, Trenor CC 3rd. Caution is recommended prior to sildenafil use in vascular anomalies. Pediatr Blood Cancer 2015;62(11):2015–7.
33. Triana P, Dore M, Cerezo VN, et al. Sirolimus in the treatment of vascular anomalies. Eur J Pediatr Surg 2017;27(1):86–90.
34. Hartford CM, Ratain MJ. Rapamycin: something old, something new, sometimes borrowed and now renewed. Clin Pharmacol Ther 2007;82(4):381–8.
35. Alemi AS, Rosbe KW, Chan DK, et al. Airway response to sirolimus therapy for the treatment of complex pediatric lymphatic malformations. Int J Pediatr Otorhinolaryngol 2015;79(12):2466–9.
36. Lackner H, Karastaneva A, Schwinger W, et al. Sirolimus for the treatment of children with various complicated vascular anomalies. Eur J Pediatr 2015;174(12): 1579–84.
37. Hortlund M, Arroyo Muhr LS, Storm H, et al. Cancer risks after solid organ transplantation and after long-term dialysis. Int J Cancer 2017;140(5):1091–101.
38. Cerrati EW, O TM, Binetter D, et al. Transmucosal bleomycin for tongue lymphatic malformations. Int J Otolaryngol Head Neck Surg 2015;4:81–5.
39. Kennedy TL, Whitaker M, Pellitteri P, et al. Cystic hygroma/lymphangioma: a rational approach to management. Laryngoscope 2001;111(11 Pt 1):1929–37.
40. Bloom DC, Perkins JA, Manning SC. Management of lymphatic malformations and macroglossia: results of a national treatment survey. Int J Pediatr Otorhinolaryngol 2009;73(8):1114–8.
41. Glade RS, Buckmiller LM. $CO_2$ laser resurfacing of intraoral lymphatic malformations: a 10-year experience. Int J Pediatr Otorhinolaryngol 2009;73(10):1358–61.
42. Oomen KP, Paramasivam S, Waner M, et al. Endoscopic transmucosal direct puncture sclerotherapy for management of airway vascular malformations. Laryngoscope 2016;126(1):205–11.

# Venous Malformations of the Head and Neck

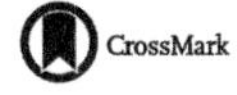

Emmanuel Seront, MD, PhD[a], Miikka Vikkula, MD, PhD[b,*], Laurence M. Boon, MD, PhD[b,c]

**KEYWORDS**

• Venous malformation • Head and neck • Vascular malformation

**KEY POINTS**

- Venous malformations (VMs) arise from deficits in the development of venous network, leading to dilated and dysfunctional venous channels that are deficient in smooth muscle cells.
- Clinical features of head and neck VMs are highly variable, ranging from small and asymptomatic varicosities to massive cervicofacial lesions.
- Several therapeutic approaches exist, including surgery; laser photocoagulation; sclerotherapy; and, more recently, systemic targeted drugs.

With an incidence of approximately 1 in 2,000 to 5,000, venous malformations (VMs) represent a vascular malformation frequently observed in specialized multidisciplinary centers.[1] They arise from deficits in the development of the venous network, leading to dilated and dysfunctional venous channels that are deficient in smooth muscle cells. These slow-flow venous sacs progressively expand with stagnation of venous blood. This results in growing lesions that do not spontaneously regress, and that ultimately infiltrate and compress normal adjacent tissues.[2,3]

More than 40% of VMs occur in the head and neck (H&N) region, representing, with infantile hemangiomas (IHs) and lymphatic malformations (LMs), the third most common vascular anomaly affecting this area.[4,5] Clinical features of H&N VMs are highly variable, ranging from small and asymptomatic varicosities to massive cervicofacial lesions. These VMs are not only disfiguring but also induce functional comorbidities with potential life-threatening complications. Several therapeutic approaches exist, including surgery; laser photocoagulation; sclerotherapy; and, more recently,

Disclosure: The authors have nothing they wish to disclose.

[a] Department of Medical Oncology, Institut Roi Albert II, Cliniques Universitaires Saint Luc, University of Louvain, Avenue Hippocrate 10, 1200 Brussels, Belgium; [b] Human Molecular Genetics, de Duve Institute, University of Louvain, Avenue Hippocrate 74, 1200 Brussels, Belgium; [c] Division of Plastic Surgery, Center for Vascular Anomalies, Cliniques Universitaires Saint Luc, University of Louvain, Avenue Hippocrate 10, 1200 Brussels, Belgium

* Corresponding author. Avenue Hippocrate 74, 5th Floor, PO Box B1.74.06, Avenue Hippocrate 74, 1200 Brussels, Belgium.

*E-mail address:* Miikka.Vikkula@uclouvain.be

Otolaryngol Clin N Am 51 (2018) 173–184
https://doi.org/10.1016/j.otc.2017.09.003

systemic targeted drugs. Even though superficial and small VMs are successfully treated by single-treatment modality, management of deep and infiltrative VMs represents a medical challenge and requires a multidisciplinary approach with individualized treatment modalities.

## NATURAL HISTORY AND SYMPTOMS

H&N VMs, as other VMs, are always present at birth but not always apparent. They grow with the child, slowly expand, and do not regress. The slow growth and deep location of some VMs can result in a late presentation during childhood, adolescence, or early adulthood. Environmental factors, such as traumatic injury, intervention, infection, or hormonal fluctuation (pregnancy or puberty) can exacerbate VM progression.[6–8]

More than 90% of VMs occur sporadically and consist of a unifocal lesion. Because VMs are able to arise in any location, tissue, or organ, H&N VMs can be well localized or extensive, superficial or deep (**Fig. 1**). They commonly involve buccal space, cheek, neck, eyelids, lips, parapharyngeal space, and submandibular triangle. Muscles of mastication, such as the temporal muscle, the masseter muscle, and the tongue muscles are also commonly affected. Other locations, such as pterygopalatine fossa and infratemporal fossa, may be affected, rendering the initial diagnosis difficult. Involvement of craniofacial skeleton can also occur, more commonly in the mandible and less commonly in maxilla, nasal, and cranial bones. Extensive H&N VMs diffusely spread along different tissue planes and ultimately involve adjacent structures, including skin, parotid gland, cervicofacial musculature, oral cavity, and respiratory and digestive tracts.[6,7,9]

Protrusion may be the only presenting symptom. Lesions typically present as a soft, compressible, and nonpulsatile mass with rapid refilling after compression. The overlying skin may appear normal or exhibit a bluish discoloration. Cutaneous involvement leads to a darker blue or purple discoloration. With time, calcified thrombi or phleboliths appear and are palpated within the venous mass.[10]

Symptoms are usually absent when the lesion is small or superficial; with expansion of the VM, symptoms appear, depending on the location and the mass effect on surrounding tissues and organs. Pain and swelling are observed in most patients. Sluggish flow progressively leads to increased blood stasis and alternated cycles of thrombosis and thrombolysis; that is, localized intravascular coagulopathy (LIC), which is responsible for chronic and recurrent pain. Physical activity, hormonal fluctuations (menstrual periods and puberty), extreme temperature, and Valsalva maneuver increase vein dilatation and exacerbate pain. Pain may also be more pronounced in the morning at awakening due to stasis and swelling. Acute pain should make suspect an acute venous thrombosis that leads to rapid enlargement of the malformation; this can sometimes be the first indication of a deep-seated H&N VM.[11,12]

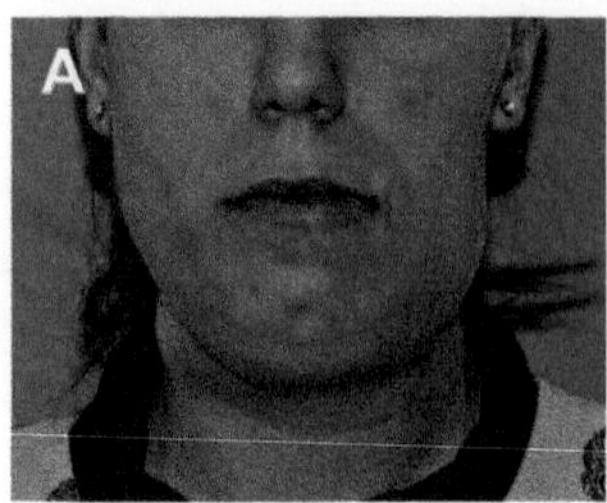

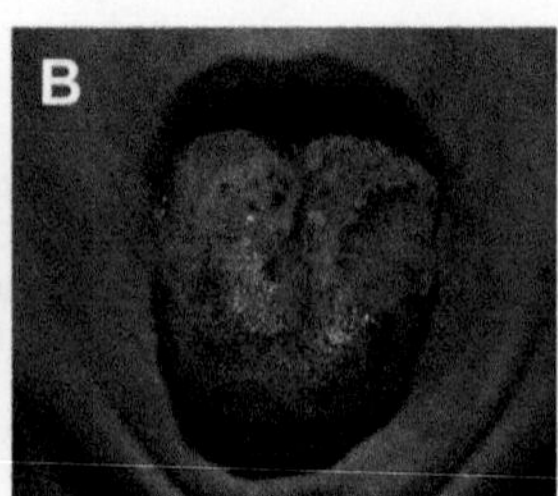

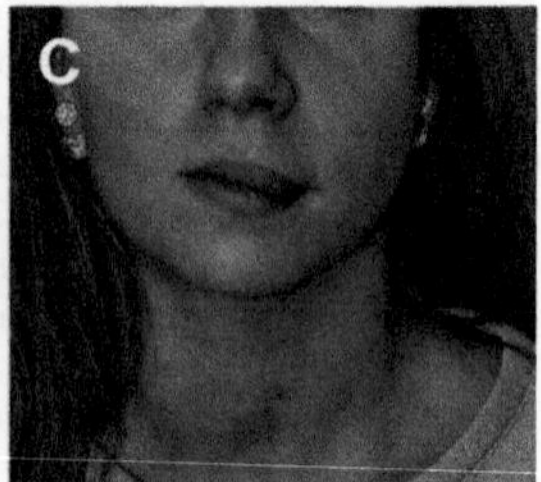


**Fig. 1.** Several aspects of facial VM. (*A*) Lower face involving the skin, mucosa, muscle and the tongue (*B*), causing facial asymmetry (*C*).

H&N VMs are often unilateral. Physical changes appear progressively and consist of deformities of the face and asymmetry. Orbital involvement (or involvement of the orbit) causes exophthalmia and proptosis, which is exacerbated when the patient is lying down. Oral lesions tend to cause dental malalignment due to a mass effect. Functional impairment is commonly observed and depends on the localization of the lesion; VMs in the buccal space and/or the tongue impedes speech, mastication, and/or swallowing. VMs in the parapharyngeal space, tongue, and soft palate are responsible for difficulties in swallowing and speech, as well as airway obstruction. Migraine is commonly seen in VMs located in the temporal muscle. Deep oropharyngeal lesions compress and deviate airways, causing snoring and sleep apnea. Laryngeal lesions can cause hoarseness, persistent coughing, stridor, and dyspnea. Involvement of the mucosal surfaces of the H&N also leads to other symptoms, such as ulceration or intermittent bleeding.[6,7,11]

A small proportion (less than 10%) of H&N VM patients present with multifocal lesions that are mostly inherited, yet sometimes occur sporadically. Glomuvenous malformation (GVM) is a rare venous anomaly that is inherited as an autosomal dominant trait. Although they are mostly located in the extremities, GVMs can also affect the H&N area. They always involve skin and subcutis, rarely involve mucosa, and extremely rarely extend more deeply into muscle. They are generally darker blue or purple, raised, and have a cobblestone-like appearance and slight hyperkeratosis. GVMs are painful to palpation. Cutaneomucosal VM (VMCM) is another inherited, multifocal VM (MVM) that involves cervicofacial area in 50% of cases. Lesions are small and superficial, easily compressible, and of various hues of blue. They often involve skin and oral mucosa and seldom invade muscle. They are often asymptomatic and not painful on compression. Some MVMs can also occur sporadically and do not differ clinically from VMCMs.[1] MVMs are also associated with the blue rubber bleb nevus syndrome (BRBN; or Bean) syndrome. This syndrome associates multiple VMs affecting the skin, soft tissue, and gastrointestinal tract. Skin lesions are often multiple, small, round, rubbery and located on the soles and palms, as well as in the H&N region. Gastrointestinal sessile lesions cause chronic bleeding and severe anemia.[13] Small cutaneous nodular MVMs occur in association with cerebral cavernous malformations (CCMs), typically in the H&N region.[14,15]

## DIAGNOSIS

### *Patient History and Clinical Examination*

A diagnosis of VM should be considered for a solitary lesion that presents as a light-to-dark-blue skin discoloration or a soft subcutaneous mass at birth. Further clues are slow growth during life that can be triggered by puberty, trauma, effort, or menstrual periods. They can be emptied by compression, which helps to distinguish them from LMs. There is no thrill or bruit, and the affected area is not warmer than a nonlesional site. Family history is useful to detect inherited forms. VMs are often associated with recurrent pain and tenderness, reflecting repeated thrombosis. Palpation of VMs frequently reveals phleboliths that are pathognomonic of VMs.[16,17]

### *Clinical Biology*

A coagulation abnormality known as LIC is present in about 50% of VMs, and is characterized by elevated D-dimer levels and normal-to-low fibrinogen levels. Patients with severe LIC (D-dimer level greater than twice the normal range with low fibrinogen level) are at high risk of decompensation into disseminated intravascular coagulopathy (DIC) in case of trauma or surgical procedure.[18]

### Imaging

Although superficial VMs are usually easily diagnosed by clinical examination, imaging is helpful for evaluation of the boundary and the organ infiltration, particularly in deep lesions. Ultrasound represents an excellent initial examination to confirm slow flow or absence of flow within the malformation. Generally, VMs appear hypoechogenic or heterogeneous and compressible (**Fig. 2**). Phleboliths appear as echogenic foci with associated acoustic shadowing; they are observed in about 20% of cases and are pathognomic of VM.[19]

Flexible endoscopy is often mandatory to evaluate the entire upper respiratory and digestive tracts. This endoscopic examination is also important to identify hidden VMs that are at risk of severe bleeding in case of intubation. The Trendelenburg position may help identify hidden laryngeal lesions in patients with atypical upper airway symptoms.

MRI is the optimal method to determine the extent of a VM and to evaluate the interaction with surrounding structures (**Fig. 3**).This is particularly useful for the recognition of adjacent neurovascular structures, particularly in the setting of preparation for surgery or sclerotherapy. VMs appear hyperintense on T2-weighted images, and hypointense and isointense on T1-weighted images, relative to muscle. The use of gadolinium contrast enables the differentiation of VM from LM and arteriovenous malformation. It should be noted that computed tomography is not effective in the imaging of venous lesions unless bony involvement is suspected.[20,21]

### Histopathology and Genetics

In the authors' current practice, biopsy is not usually needed to confirm the diagnosis. However, its place will be more and more important in clinical trials that evaluate systemic targeted therapies because the underlying causes of most VM-types have been identified.[22] More precisely, somatic mutations have been found in 2 genes, to date; 60% of VMs exhibit an activating mutation in the TEK gene, which encodes the TIE2 tyrosine kinase receptor present on endothelial cells,[23–25] and 20% of VMs exhibit a mutation in the PIK3CA gene, which leads to excessive activation of phosphoinositol 3 kinase (PI3K). These 2 mutations induce an excessive activation of intracellular signaling cascades and, importantly, the PI3K/AKT/mammalian target of rapamycin (mTOR) pathway, resulting in uncontrolled proliferation of endothelial cells and disrupted pericyte coverage.[22–28] A TEK mutation is also found in patients with VMCM (germline), MVM (mosaic), and BRBN (somatic), whereas inherited glomulin mutations associated with lesional glomulin second-hits are detected in GVMs.[29,30]

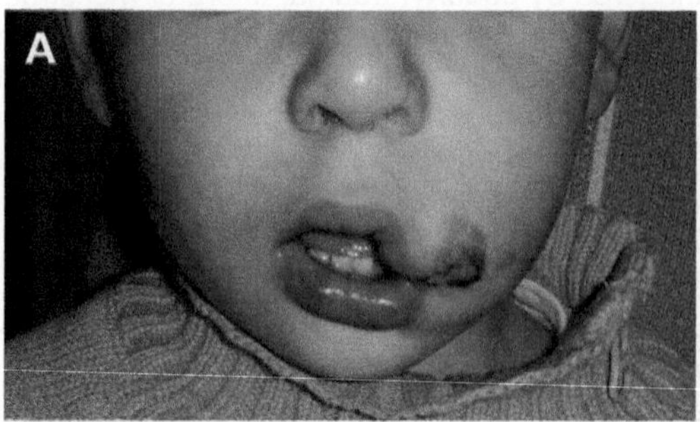


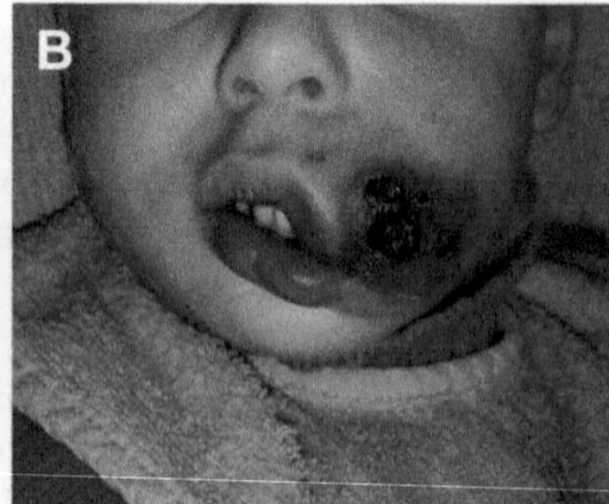


**Fig. 2.** Upper labial VM causing enlargement of the lip (*A*). Skin necrosis secondary to ethanol sclerotherapy (*B*).

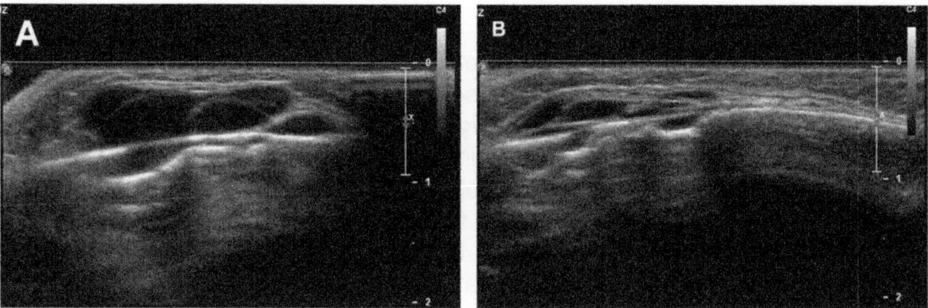


**Fig. 3.** Doppler ultrasound shows vascular spaces with thin membrane (*A*) that are compressible by the probe (*B*).

A germline mutation is seen in the CCM1, or KRIT1, gene in patients with nodular VMs of CCM.[14,15] Screening for these genetic alterations can thus help in differential diagnosis and are useful as predictive biomarkers for further targeted therapies, such as sirolimus.[28]

### *Differential Diagnosis*

Differential diagnosis includes IH and slow-flow vascular anomalies, such as LMs (**Fig. 4**). IH exhibits early rapid growth during the neonatal period, between 2 weeks and 2 months of life, and regresses spontaneously from 10 to 12 months onwards during several years. Doppler ultrasound is the best examination to differentiate a fast-flow IH from a slow-flow VM. D-dimer levels are normal in IH. It is not uncommon that patients have their malformation misdiagnosed as a hemangioma, resulting in a delay in treatment and inappropriate management.[31]

LMs typically appear as soft, noncompressible masses that can be discrete or diffuse with subsequent enlargement of the involved tissues. Unlike superficial VMs, changes in skin color are uncommon. However, in case of hemorrhage into the lymphatic cysts, LM is often difficult to distinguish from VM due to the blue coloration of the overlying skin.[32] Doppler ultrasound and/or MRI often allow the exact diagnosis.

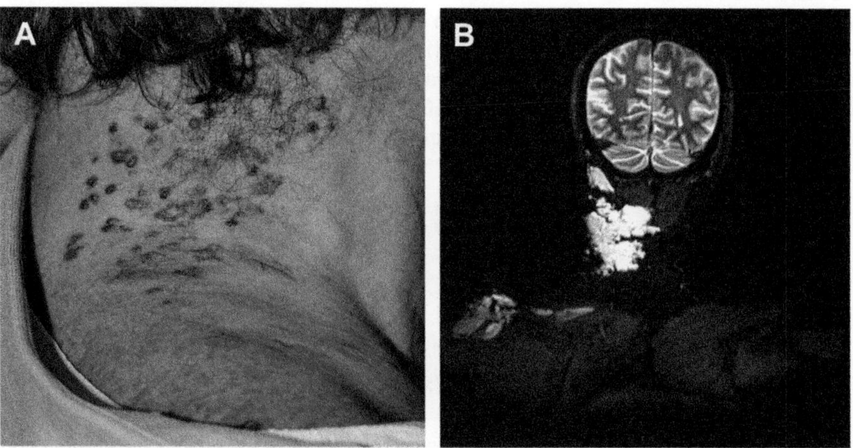


**Fig. 4.** Cervical VM (*A*). T2-weighted MRI image shows the extension of the lesion (*B*).

## MANAGEMENT

A multidisciplinary approach is essential for the appropriate management of all complex H&N VMs. Each patient should be discussed based on size, localization, depth, and symptomatology of his or her lesion (**Fig. 5**). Small and well-localized VMs are usually treated in a curative setting with a single modality: either surgical resection or sclerotherapy. In contrast, cure is rarely obtained for deep and extensive VMs infiltrating important anatomic structures. In these instances, the primary objective of treatment is to reduce the symptoms, prevent iatrogenic complications, and improve the quality of life. Therefore, active observation is often useful. Therapeutic modalities for VMs include conservative treatment, sclerotherapy, laser therapy, and surgery. Clinical trials are currently evaluating the efficacy of sirolimus as a targeted therapy.

## CONSERVATIVE MANAGEMENT

The aim of conservative management is to prevent complications from the progressive expansion of VMs and its associated intravascular coagulopathy. Elevation of the head during sleeping is important to decrease long periods of hydrostatic pressure that can lead to VM expansion. This helps decrease symptoms of airway obstruction, swelling, and pain that are experienced throughout the night and in the morning. When pain is associated with LIC (reflected by high D-dimer levels), low-molecular-weight heparin 100 antiXa IU/kg/day is introduced for 20 days, or longer if pain relapses. This may also be necessary to prevent intraoperative DIC in severe LIC. Some patients can benefit from low-dose aspirin and nonsteroidal anti-inflammatory medication in case of local thrombosis. Conservative management is applied for asymptomatic VM, as well as for large lesions being treated with other treatment modalities.[33]

## LASER

Laser therapy is a mainstay of management of mucosal and skin malformations. The light energy emitted by laser is selectively absorbed by intravascular proteins to heat, clot, and subsequently damage the vessel, resulting in occlusion and fibrosis. Neodymium-doped yttrium aluminum garnet (Nd:YAG) and potassium titanyl-phosphate lasers are used transcutaneously and transmucosally. Lasers can only penetrate 1 mm to 3 mm. Therefore, thicker VMs cannot be affected by intravascular laser.

Cutaneous VMs can be treated with Nd:YAG laser associated with a direct cooling system to decrease melatonin absorption and injury to the overlying skin. Airway lesions, such as distal pharyngeal, hypopharyngeal, laryngeal, and tracheal lesions, can be endoscopically managed with serial laser treatments using a flexible fiber delivery system. Surface noncontact Nd:YAG laser can be used to treat any mucosal lesion. Tracheal and laryngeal lesions are more sensitive, whereas larger lesions

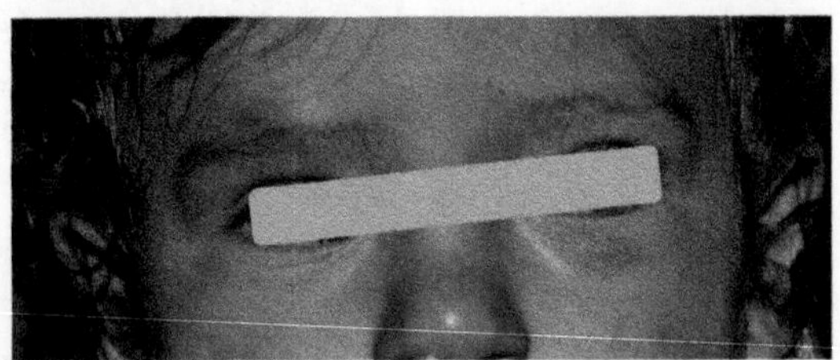

**Fig. 5.** IH of the lower eyelid that appeared a few days after birth. The lesion is not compressible on palpation.

require longer pulse duration. Mucosal VMs respond rapidly with an immediate shrinking. Serial laser treatments, performed with a minimum of a 3-month interval, are often required until satisfactory results are reached.[34]

Interstitial Nd:YAG laser can also be used for small and medium-size VMs with extensive communicating branches in deep layers. The Nd:YAG laser fiber is passed through a needle into a deep VM and is conducted radially in different directions. The duration of the laser exposure is determined by the lesion size. Results have been reported in the treatment of large tongue VM, deep parotid, neck, and masseteric muscle involvement; however, extensive data are still lacking. However, due to a high risk of facial nerve damage with interstitial laser in the parotid, this should be done only by experienced surgeons with facial nerve monitoring. Ultrasound guidance may be useful to avoid complications, such as neurovascular damage. After interstitial laser treatment, exudation, swelling, and fever can be severe, requiring a short course of intravenous corticosteroids, especially for lesions located in the oropharynx.[34–37]

## SCLEROTHERAPY

Sclerotherapy, the mainstay treatment of VMs, consists of the injection of an agent that obliterates the channels by causing damage to the endothelium with subsequent inflammation and fibrosis. This allows decreasing the volume of the malformation before surgical treatment or in case of technically unfeasible surgery. Multiple treatments are usually necessary. Sclerotherapy is usually done under general anesthesia with real-time fluoroscopic and ultrasonographic monitoring.[38–40]

The most commonly used agent used to be absolute ethanol, which has the most potent sclerosing property with a remission rate ranging between 75% and 96%.[38–41] However, its use has tremendously been reduced due to the frequent, severe complications associated with its use, such as blistering, skin necrosis, and nerve injury, which can occur in 12% to 30% of patients[42,43] (**Fig. 6**). Therefore, caution should be taken when ethanol injection is performed, for example, near the medial third of the parotid gland. Small doses with repeated procedures, rather than large injections with few procedures greatly reduce the chances of facial palsy. Other sclerosing agents, such as ethoxysclerol foam or bleomycin, are currently favored for this location.

Major localized swelling is another important side effect of ethanol sclerotherapy and compromises its use around the airway; these patients often remain intubated for 2 to 3 days postoperatively or need a prophylactic tracheotomy beforehand to avoid prolonged endotracheal postoperative intubation. Preoperative and postoperative injection of dexamethasone can ease tissue edema. The cumulative total dose of serial injections of ethanol in a single procedure should not exceed 1 mL/kg body weight of the patient.

Another severe complication of ethanol use is due its rapid flow into the pulmonary circulation, leading to pulmonary artery spasm, pulmonary hypertension, and pulmonary embolism. Renal failure, as well as cardiovascular collapse, has also been described. A balanced salt solution and sodium bicarbonate should be given intravenously to alkalinize urine to prevent acute renal failure.[44–47]

Currently, ethanol has been replaced by other sclerosing agents, including polidocanol (aka, lauromacrogol) foam, ethoxysclerol foam, sodium tetradecyl sulfate, and bleomycin. Although no randomized clinical trials exist, multiple reports suggest that these agents have a better tolerance but that they are also less effective than ethanol. Serious complications have been noticed with these agents, such as allergy, renal failure, transient ischemic attack, and stroke caused by emboli and bubbles.[48–54] After treatment with sclerosing agents, recurrence of the lesion is common.[55]

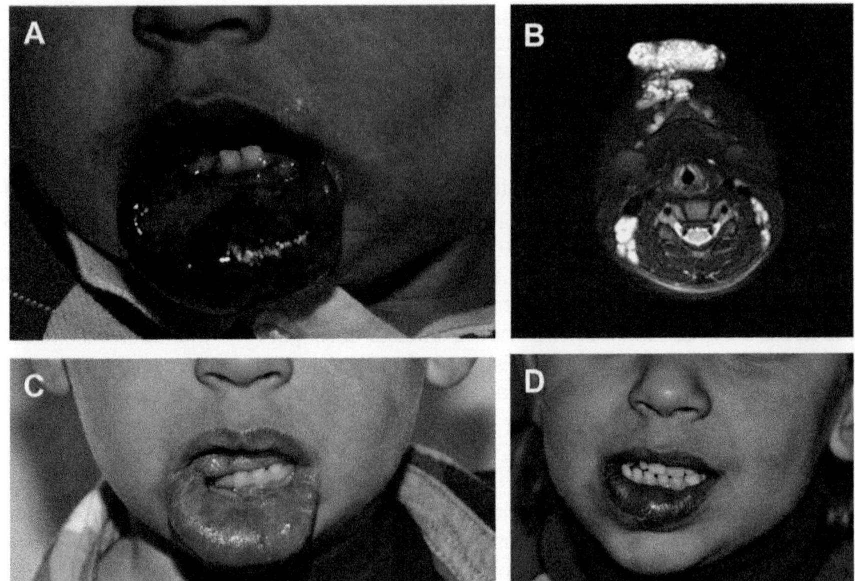


**Fig. 6.** VM of the lower lip (*A*). T2-weighted image confirms the diagnosis and determines its extension (*B*). Result after 3 sclerotherapy using bleomycin (*C*). One year postsurgical resection to restore the anatomy of the lip (*D*).

## SURGERY

Surgery remains a cornerstone treatment modality in H&N VM; however, its feasibility depends of the extent of the lesion, the venous drainage, and the relation with adjacent neurovascular structures. Small lesions (<2–4 cm), including mucosal and deep muscular VMs with minimal infiltration, are best managed with a wide local excision, resulting in nearly 100% cure rates. Submandibular VM and VM of the temporalis muscle are good candidates for excision because sclerotherapy in this localization can cause permanent nerve injury and recurrence.

In larger and infiltrative lesions, preoperative sclerotherapy is often recommended to decrease the volume of the VM and to induce local thrombosis, which will reduce blood loss during surgery and recurrence of the malformation. In these instances, surgery remains a challenge because VMs are rarely well-defined and intraoperative bleeding can make identification and preservation of important structures difficult. These lesions generally cannot be cured without compromising functional and cosmetic results. The appreciation that surgery is unfeasible is sometimes the key for management; strategy consists of controlling expansion of the malformation, alleviating pain, and maintaining a satisfactory aesthetic outcome. This requires multimodal therapy combining sclerotherapy to prevent excessive growth and surgery to remove large portions of the lesion while maintaining function and symmetry.[56]

## TARGETED THERAPY

Recently, sirolimus opened the era of targeted therapies for VM. The identification of activating mutations in the TIE2-PI3K-AKT-mTOR pathway led to the evaluation of the efficacy of sirolimus (aka, rapamycin). Sirolimus is an allosteric inhibitor of the 2 complexes that compose the mTOR protein, mTOR complex 1, and mTOR complex 2. In a preclinical study, sirolimus reduced the growth of VMs in TIE2 mutant murine models; inhibition of mTORC1 activity decreased the proliferation of endothelial cells and inhibition of mTORC2 inhibited the excessive activation of AKT, which is responsible of smooth muscle deficiency.[28]

Based on these results, a pilot study and a phase II clinical trial evaluated the efficacy of sirolimus (2 mg daily continuously) in 10 subjects with venous anomalies that were refractory to standard treatments.[28,57] All subjects rapidly experienced relief of pain, improved functional mobility, and increased self-perceived quality of life. Sirolimus had an on-off effect on bleeding and oozing. This efficacy was correlated with a decrease in D-dimer levels. Moreover, MRI images showed significant ($P<.05$) decrease in volume after 12 months on treatment.

Sirolimus was well-tolerated in these patients with minimal side effects, such as grade 1 and 2 mucositis, fatigue, cutaneous rash, and diarrhea, all easily manageable with symptomatic treatment. A prospective multicentric phase III trial is currently evaluating sirolimus in subjects (adult and children) with VM, including H&N VMs that are refractory to standard treatment (EudraCT 2015–001703–32 & NCT02638389). Sirolimus represents a promising agent for the treatment of these lesions because the radical treatment options, such as surgery and sclerotherapy, are not always feasible, and because the primary objective is to control disease and symptoms.

## DECISIONAL TREE

The therapeutic strategy in H&N VM depends on several factors, including the depth, the proximity of vital structures, and the presence of mucosal involvement. Airway obstruction always needs to be evaluated, especially when VM is located in the lower part of the face and/or in the neck. Identification of associated coagulation abnormalities is essential before any treatment to avoid excessive perioperative bleeding and to improve postoperative results.

Small and well-localized VMs can be successfully treated with surgical resection, laser therapy, or foam sclerotherapy. VMs involving the respiratory and digestive mucosa are best treated with Nd:YAG laser. Depending on the volume and extension, a multimodal therapeutic approach is often needed. Sclerotherapy, with ethoxysclerol foam or bleomycin, is usually the treatment of choice for extensive VMs. Surgery is usually programmed after sclerosing the lesion to reduce blood loss and long-term recurrence. Indications for sirolimus treatment still have to be defined, also in regard to surgery or sclerotherapy.

In conclusion, management of H&N VM needs a multidisciplinary approach that involves at least an interventional radiologist, an otorhinolaryngologist, a plastic and/or maxillofacial surgeon, and a hematologist, to choose the right treatment at the right moment. This is the way to improve the end result and to reduce possible iatrogenic complications.

## REFERENCES


1. Boon LM, Mulliken JB, Enjolras O, et al. Glomuvenous malformation (glomangioma) and venous malformation: distinct clinicopathologic and genetic entities. Arch Dermatol 2004;140:971–6.
2. Mulliken JB, Glowacki J. Hemangiomas and vascular malformations in infants and children: a classification based on endothelial characteristics. Plast Reconstr Surg 1982;69:412–20.

3. Wassef M, Blei F, Adams D, et al, ISSVA Board and Scientific Committee. Vascular anomalies classification: recommendations from the International Society for the Study of Vascular Anomalies. Pediatrics 2015;136:203–14.
4. Eifert S, Villavicencio JL, Kao TC, et al. Prevalence of deep venous anomalies in congenital vascular malformations of venous predominance. J Vasc Surg 2000; 31:462–71.
5. Richter GT, Braswell L. Management of venous malformations. Facial Plast Surg 2012;28:603–10.
6. Glade RS, Richter GT, James CA, et al. Diagnosis and management of pediatric cervicofacial venous malformations: retrospective review from a vascular anomalies center. Laryngoscope 2010;120:229–35.
7. Marler JJ, Mulliken JB. Current management of hemangiomas and vascular malformations. Clin Plast Surg 2005;32:99–116.
8. Duyka LJ, Fan CY, Coviello-Malle JM, et al. Progesterone receptors identified in vascular malformations of the head and neck. Otolaryngol Head Neck Surg 2009;141:491–5.
9. Hein KD, Mulliken JB, Kozakewich HP, et al. Venous malformations of skeletal muscle. Plast Reconstr Surg 2002;110:1625–35.
10. Legiehn GM, Heran MK. Venous malformations: classification, development, diagnosis, and interventional radiologic management. Radiol Clin North Am 2008;46(3):545–97.
11. Casanova D, Boon LM, Vikkula M. Venous malformations: clinical characteristics and differential diagnosis. Ann Chir Plast Esthet 2006;51(4–5):373–87.
12. Mavrikakis I, Heran MK, White V, et al. The role of thrombosis as a mechanism of exacerbation in venous and combined venous lymphatic vascular malformations of the orbit. Ophthalmology 2009;116:1216–24.
13. Bean WT, Charles C III. Vascular spiders and related lesions of the skin. Oxford: Blackwell Scientific Publications; 1959.
14. Revencu N, Vikkula M. Cerebral cavernous malformation: new molecular and clinical insights. J Med Genet 2006;43:716–21.
15. Sirvente J, Enjolras O, Wassef M, et al. Frequency and phenotypes of cutaneous vascular malformations in a consecutive series of 417 patients with familial cerebral cavernous malformations. J Eur Acad Dermatol Venereol 2009;23:1066–72.
16. Mulliken JB, Fishman SJ, Burrows PE. Vascular anomalies. Curr Probl Surg 2000; 37:517–84.
17. Elluru RG. Cutaneous vascular lesions. Facial Plast Surg Clin North Am 2013;21: 111–26.
18. Hermans C, Dessomme B, Lambert C, et al. Venous malformations and coagulopathy. Ann Chir Plast Esthet 2006;51:388–93.
19. Trop I, Dubois J, Guibaud L, et al. Soft-tissue venous malformations in pediatric and young adult patients: diagnosis with Doppler US. Radiology 1999;212(3): 841–5.
20. Dubois J, Soulez G, Oliva VL, et al. Soft-tissue venous malformations in adult patients: imaging and therapeutic issues. Radiographics 2001;21(6):1519–31.
21. Konez O, Burrows PE. Magnetic resonance of vascular anomalies. Magn Reson Imaging Clin N Am 2002;10(2):363–88, vii.
22. Vikkula M, Boon LM, Mulliken JB. Molecular genetics of vascular malformations. Matrix Biol 2001;20:327–35.
23. Limaye N, Wouters V, Uebelhoer M, et al. Somatic mutations in angiopoietin receptor gene TEK cause solitary and multiple sporadic venous malformations. Nat Genet 2009;41:118–24.

24. Soblet J, Limaye N, Uebelhoer M, et al. Variable somatic TIE2 mutations in half of sporadic venous malformations. Mol Syndromol 2013;4(4):179–83.
25. Vikkula M, Boon LM, Carraway KL 3rd, et al. Vascular dysmorphogenesis caused by an activating mutation in the receptor tyrosine kinase TIE2. Cell 1996;87(7): 1181–90.
26. Limaye N, Kangas J, Mendola A, et al. Somatic activating PIK3CA mutations cause venous malformation. Am J Hum Genet 2015;97:914–21.
27. Uebelhoer M, Nätynki M, Kangas J, et al. Venous malformation causative TIE2 mutations mediate an AKTdependent decrease in PDGFB. Hum Mol Genet 2013;22(17):3438–48.
28. Boscolo E, Limaye N, Huang L, et al. Rapamycin improves TIE2-mutated venous malformation in murine model and human subjects. J Clin Invest 2015;125: 3491–504.
29. Brouillard P, Boon LM, Mulliken JB, et al. Mutations in a novel factor, glomulin, are responsible for glomuvenous malformations ("glomangiomas"). Am J Hum Genet 2002;70(4):866–74.
30. Amyere M, Aerts V, Brouillard P, et al. Somatic uniparental isodisomy explains multifocality of glomuvenous malformations. Am J Hum Genet 2013;92(2): 188–96.
31. Drolet BA, Esterly NB, Frieden IJ. Hemangiomas in children. N Engl J Med 1999; 341:173–81.
32. Colbert SD, Seager L, Haider F, et al. Lymphatic malformations of the head and neck – current concepts in management. Br J Oral Maxillofac Surg 2013;51: 98–102.
33. Dompmartin A, Acher A, Thibon P, et al. Association of localized intravascular coagulopathy with venous malformations. Arch Dermatol 2008;144(7):873–7.
34. Eivazi B, Wiegand S, Teymoortash A, et al. Laser treatment of mucosal venous malformations of the upper aerodigestive tract in 50 patients. Lasers Med Sci 2010;25:571–6.
35. Clymer MA, Fortune DS, Reinisch L, et al. Interstitial Nd:YAG photocoagulation for vascular malformations and hemangiomas in childhood. Arch Otolaryngol Head Neck Surg 1998;124(4):431–6.
36. Chang CJ, Fisher DM, Chen YR. Intralesional photocoagulation of vascular anomalies of the tongue. Br J Plast Surg 1999;52(3):178–81.
37. Fisher DM, Chang CJ, Chua JJ. Potential complications of intralesional laser photocoagulation for extensive vascular malformations. Ann Plast Surg 2001; 47(3):252–6.
38. Berenguer B, Burrows PE, Zurakowski D, et al. Sclerotherapy of craniofacial venous malformations: complications and results. Plast Reconstr Surg 1999; 104(1):1–11.
39. Lee IH, Kim KH, Jeon P, et al. Ethanol sclerotherapy for the management of craniofacial venous malformations: the interim results. Korean J Radiol 2009;10: 269–76.
40. Uehara S, Osuga K, Yoneda A, et al. Intralesional sclerotherapy for subcutaneous venous malformations in children. Pediatr Surg Int 2009;25:709–13.
41. Orlando JL, Caldas JG, Campos HG, et al. Ethanol sclerotherapy of head and neck venous malformations. Einstein (Sao Paulo) 2014;12(2):181–6.
42. Fayad LM, Hazirolan T, Carrino JA, et al. Venous malformations: MR imaging features that predict skin burns after percutaneous alcohol embolization procedures. Skeletal Radiol 2008;37:895–901.

43. Lee KB, Kim DI, Oh SK, et al. Incidence of soft tissue injury and neuropathy after embolo/sclerotherapy for congenital vascular malformation. J Vasc Surg 2008;48: 1286–91.
44. Lee BB, Do YS, Byun HS, et al. Advanced management of venous malformation with ethanol sclerotherapy: mid-term results. J Vasc Surg 2003;37:533–8.
45. Burrows PE, Mason KP. Percutaneous treatment of low flow vascular malformations. J Vasc Interv Radiol 2004;15:431–45.
46. Mason KP, Michna E, Zurakowski D, et al. Serum ethanol levels in children and adults after ethanol embolization or sclerotherapy for vascular anomalies. Radiology 2000;217:127–32.
47. Hammer FD, Boon LM, Mathurin P, et al. Ethanol sclerotherapy of venous malformations: evaluation of systemic ethanol contamination. J Vasc Interv Radiol 2001; 12(5):595–600.
48. Chen WL, Huang ZQ, Zhang DM, et al. Percutaneous sclerotherapy of massive venous malformations of the face and neck using fibrin glue combined with OK-432 and pingyangmycin. Head Neck 2010;32(4):467–72.
49. Zheng JW, Yang XJ, Wang YA, et al. Intralesional injection of Pingyangmycin for vascular malformations in oral and maxillofacial regions: an evaluation of 297 consecutive patients. Oral Oncol 2009;45:872–6.
50. Mimura H, Fujiwara H, Hiraki T, et al. Polidocanol sclerotherapy for painful venous malformations: evaluation of safety and efficacy in pain relief. Eur Radiol 2009;19: 2474–80.
51. Stimpson P, Hewitt R, Barnacle A, et al. Sodium tetradecyl sulphate sclerotherapy for treating venous malformations of the oral and pharyngeal regions in children. Int J Pediatr Otorhinolaryngol 2012;76:569–73.
52. Bajpai H, Bajpai S. Comparative analysis of intralesional sclerotherapy with sodium tetradecyl sulfate versus bleomycin in the management of low flow craniofacial soft tissue vascular lesions. J Maxillofac Oral Surg 2012;11(1):13–20.
53. Forlee MV, Grouden M, Moore DJ, et al. Stroke after varicose vein foam injection sclerotherapy. J Vasc Surg 2006;43(1):162–4.
54. Marrocco-Trischitta MM, Guerrini P, Abeni D, et al. Reversible cardiac arrest after polidocanol sclerotherapy of peripheral venous malformation. Dermatol Surg 2002;28:153–5.
55. Dompmartin A, Blaizot X, Theron J, et al. Radioopaque ethylcellulose ethanol is a safe and efficient sclerosing agent for slow-flow vascular malformations. Eur Radiol 2011;21(12):2647–56.
56. Boon LM, Vanwijck R. Medical and surgical treatment of venous malformations. Ann Chir Plast Esthet 2006;51(4–5):403–11.
57. Hammer J, Seront E, Duez S, et al. Sirolimus treatment for extensive slow-flow vascular malformations: a monocentric prospective phase-II study. Ann Surg, in press.

# Arteriovenous Malformations of the Head and Neck

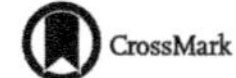

Tara L. Rosenberg, MD[a], James Y. Suen, MD[b], Gresham T. Richter, MD[c,*]

**KEYWORDS**

- Arteriovenous malformation • Extracranial • Vascular malformation • High-flow • Head and neck

**KEY POINTS**

- Arteriovenous malformations (AVMs) of the head and neck are vascular lesions (with potentially life-threatening symptoms) due to progressive and infiltrative disease without clear borders.
- AVMs are best characterized as either focal or diffuse disease but are staged by disease progression.
- Focal AVMs have good treatment outcomes, but diffuse lesions have high rates of recurrent disease requiring vigilant follow-up and repeat interventions.
- AVMs are diagnosed by a history of recalcitrant growth of a vascular lesion with examination findings of pulsations, warmth, superficial staining, telangiectasia, and dilated vessels.
- Diagnosis of AVM is supported by Doppler ultrasound, magnetic resonance angiography, computed tomography angiography, and traditional angiography.

## INTRODUCTION

Arteriovenous malformations (AVMs) of the head and neck are rare and complex vascular lesions thought to be present at birth and characterized by variable growth leading to disfiguring and life-threatening complications. Of all vascular malformations, AVMs can be the most dangerous and difficult to manage because of their high flow, bleeding risk, and infiltrative nature. Diagnosis is based on history, physical examination, and imaging characteristics. AVM histology reveals numerous

---

Disclosure: The authors have nothing they wish to disclose.

[a] Department of Otolaryngology–Head and Neck Surgery, Baylor College of Medicine, Texas Children's Hospital Vascular Anomalies Center, Houston, 6701 Fannin Street, Suite D.0640, Houston, TX 77030, USA; [b] Department of Otolaryngology–Head and Neck Surgery, University of Arkansas for Medical Sciences, 1 Children's Way, Slot 836, Little Rock, AR 72202, USA; [c] Department of Otolaryngology–Head and Neck Surgery, University of Arkansas for Medical Sciences, Arkansas Children's Hospital, 1 Children's Way, Slot 836, Little Rock, AR 72202, USA
* Corresponding author.
*E-mail address:* GTRichter@uams.edu

Otolaryngol Clin N Am 51 (2018) 185–195
https://doi.org/10.1016/j.otc.2017.09.005
0030-6665/18/
oto.theclinics.com

arteriovenous shunts and dilated capillary beds believed to lack autoregulation. The cause is attributed to somatic mutations and molecular mechanisms causing perivascular instability and vascular infiltration.[1–4] Progressive expansion of AVMs is attributed to vascular recruitment and collateralization, with the formation of a radiographic nidus.[5] Treatment of these lesions requires expert multimodal and multidisciplinary care. The recurrence rate of diffuse lesions is high, and cure is rarely achieved.[6,7] Focal lesions are more forgiving to treatment.[8]

## NATURAL HISTORY

AVMs are high-flow vascular malformations arising from direct and congenitally derived shunts between arteries and veins leading to vascular staining and soft tissue growth. Unlike infantile hemangiomas, AVMs never involute and are troubled by continued growth and destruction of superficial and deep local tissue. An older child or adult with an expanding, high-flow, vascular lesion should prompt suspicion of an AVM. Lack of vascular specification and poor perivascular regulation is thought to contribute to their continuous expansion. With a poor capillary network, important nutrients and oxygen fail to arrive at their intended soft tissue targets when AVM is present. The resultant release of inducible hypoxia and vascular growth factors with extracellular matrix degradation leads to further infiltration and disruption of adjacent normal tissue.[2,3,9] With persistent growth, AVMs can lead to significant bleeding and even heart failure.

AVMs may be classified as either a focal or diffuse disease (**Table 1**). A focal AVM is a single AVM with discrete borders and often firm to palpation with 1 to 2 arterial feeders found on ultrasound or arteriography. They are usually diagnosed early in life as a soft tissue mass with prominent vascularity. Focal AVM are frequently found in the tongue and lip.[7,8] Treatment outcomes for focal AVMs are very good because of the ability to manage the lesion and its single nidus directly. Surgical resection with or without preoperative embolization often leads to cure (**Fig. 1**).

Diffuse AVMs usually present in late childhood or in adulthood with a rapid phase of expansion that is often triggered during prepubescent or pubescent hormonal surges. Clinical evidence and histologic observation of hormone receptors on AVM samples suggest a hormonal influence.[10] These are commonly large lesions crossing multiple anatomic borders with skin to bone involvement and can be staged in this fashion.[7] Their boundaries are often difficult to ascertain radiographically and intraoperatively. Diffuse AVMs will recruit vessels, collateralize, and infiltrate adjacent normal tissue (**Fig. 2**). Thus, they are difficult to cure and are plagued with incomplete surgical excision or embolization.[7,11] Recurrent and staged treatment is, therefore, required to control the formation of collateral vessels. The management of diffuse AVMs requires vigilance because of their high recidivistic rates despite the therapeutic approach.[11,12] AVMs do not spontaneously regress. If left untreated, they will cause significant morbidity, social isolation, psychological distress, and possible mortality from ulceration, massive hemorrhage, and rarely high-output heart failure.

When diffuse AVMs are seen in childhood, they may present as a vascular blush of the skin but may be misdiagnosed or disregarded by the inexperienced eye. AVM of the skin may be differentiated from capillary malformations based on their increased warmth, mottled pattern, and sometimes pulsation. For unclear reasons, many AVMs do not present until adulthood. Some possible triggers are hormones and trauma. Forty-three percent of quiescent AVMs found in childhood progress before adolescence. All progress by adulthood. Diffuse lesions are more likely to progress early.[12] It is also unclear if these lesions were quiescent in childhood or if they are new malformations that formed during adulthood.[7,11,12]

**Table 1**
**Various classification systems for arteriovenous malformations**

| Focal vs Diffuse | | Schobinger | Suen-Richter |
|---|---|---|---|
| Focal | Diffuse | Stage I: Quiescence; cutaneous blush, warmth | T: Size of AVM<br>$T_1$: 1 cervicofacial subunit<br>$T_2$: 2 cervicofacial subunits<br>$T_3$: 3 cervicofacial subunits<br>$T_4$: bilateral/multifocal disease |
| Discrete borders with central nidus | Multiple or no discrete nidus | Stage II: Expansion; active growth, pulsations, bruit | D: Depth of AVM invasion<br>$D_1$: skin and/or subcutaneous involvement<br>$D_2$: subcutaneous and muscle involvement<br>$D_3$: subcutaneous, muscle, and cartilage or bone involvement<br>$D_4$: skull base or intracranial extension |
| Firm to palpation | Compressible with rapid rebound | Stage III: Destruction; same as stage II but symptomatic (pain, bleeding, disfigurement) | S: Schobinger stage modified: Kohout and colleagues[5]<br>$S_0$: quiescence<br>$S_1$: expansion (bruit, pulsation, rapid growth)<br>$S_2$: destruction (ulceration, bleeding, pain) |
| 1–2 arterial feeders | Multiple arterial feeders | Stage IV: Decompensation; same as stage III but with high-output cardiac failure | Stages<br>Stage I: $T_{1\text{-}2}D_1S_0$, $T_1D_1S_1$, $T_1D_2S_0$<br>Stage II: $T_1D_3S_0$, $T_2D_{1\text{-}2}S_{1\text{-}2}$, $T_2D_2S_0$<br>Stage III: $T_1D_3S_{1\text{-}2}$, $T_3D_{1\text{-}2}S_0$, $T_2D_3S_{0\text{-}2}$<br>Stage IV: $T_3D_3S_{0\text{-}2}$, any $D_4$, any $T_4$ |
| Good treatment outcomes | Higher risk of recurrence | — | — |

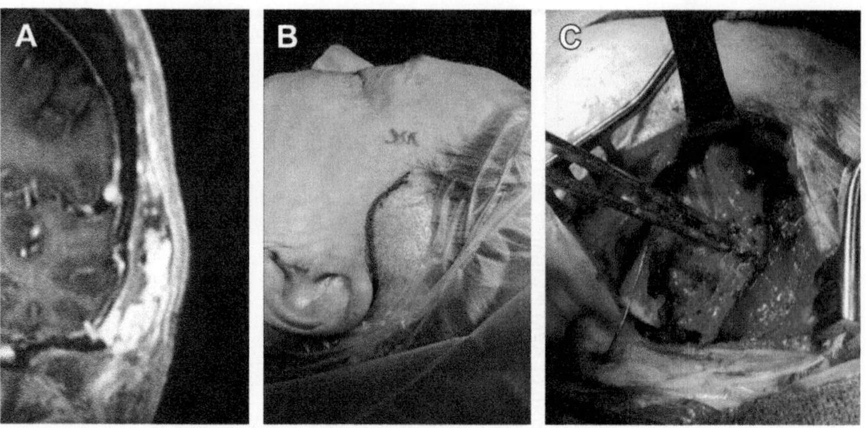


**Fig. 1.** Focal AVM of left temporalis muscle and associated soft tissue with MRI (*A*) and planned surgical resection after NCBA glue embolization (*B*) and intraoperative resection (*C*).

The Schobinger classification system is the most commonly used system for AVM clinical characterization and is outlined along with its associated features in **Table 1**. AVMs follow this natural course of progressive disease. Further modifications have been proposed to include the number of cervicofacial subunits involved and depth of invasion.[5,7]

## DIAGNOSIS

### *Clinical*

Clinical history is helpful in the diagnosis of AVMs. AVMs that present early in life frequently have a vascular blush or erythematous stain of the skin overlying the lesion in childhood, that later develops deeper soft tissue expansion. Because of the response to hormones, AVMs may grow rapidly when reaching puberty and often present during this age.[13] Common head and neck sites include the ear, oral cavity, lip, and midface. AVMs may also present very early in life with profuse bleeding. This point is particularly true during deciduous tooth disruption when the maxilla, mandible, or gingiva are involved.[5,14] AVMs that present later in life, usually after 40 years of age, may not have a prior history of a skin stain or lesion. Local trauma preceding

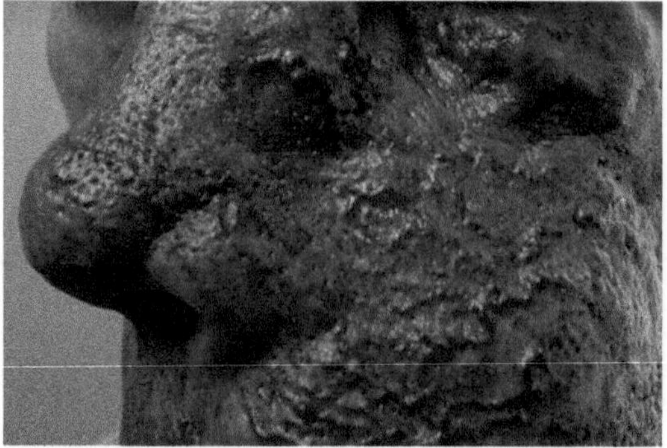

**Fig. 2.** Diffuse AVM of the left upper lip and cheek.

presentation may be garnered in the history. As AVMs grow, patients have pain, bleeding, and disfigurement caused by disease destruction of local tissue.[13] Patients also report feelings of throbbing or pulsing, pain with activity, or warmth in the area of the AVM.

The physical examination is also important for the diagnosis of AVMs. Early lesions demonstrate a vascular stain or blush of the overlying skin. Variable telangiectasias, ill-defined borders, and overgrowth help differentiate an AVM from capillary malformations. The deep portion of the AVM may not be clinically evident on the physical examination. However, thickening of the underlying tissue with pulsations and warmth compared with adjacent skin suggest its presence. Mucosal thickening with a red, vascular appearance indicates oral cavity involvement. Rarely do AVMs involve the airway. Advanced lesions are usually pulsatile and warm on palpation. They exhibit more noticeably dilated vessels superficially and may have ulceration and bleeding.[13]

### *Radiology*

After a thorough history and physical examination, imaging is imperative to confirm the diagnosis, determine the extent of disease (focal vs diffuse), and plan treatment. Ultrasound with color Doppler is initially helpful to differentiate AVM from other cutaneous lesions by demonstrating arteriovenous waveforms and high flow. MRI will determine the degree of soft tissue involvement and the magnitude of the lesion. T1- and T2-weighted imaging shows dilated, tortuous blood vessels with flow voids, indicating a high-flow lesion. Computed tomography (CT) is used mostly to identify bony involvement.[15] CT angiography (CTA) and magnetic resonance angiography (MRA) are also useful imaging studies. CTA is often preferred because of its reduced cost and shorter imaging time and because it characterizes adjacent normal soft tissue and bone better than MRA. CTA can also provide 3-dimensional reconstruction images to show primary arterial feeders of some AVMs.[13] Regardless, angiography remains the diagnostic gold standard and helps identify the central nidus and feeder arteries, information that can then be used for treatment planning and embolization (**Fig. 3**).[6,16]

## PATHOGENESIS

The pathogenesis of AVMs is still unclear, but emerging basic science is providing insight into this rare condition. AVMs are thought to be derived from congenital defects in vascular stabilization, differentiation, and endothelial cell function. Disturbances and mutations in Notch signaling and transforming growth factor-beta (TGF-beta)

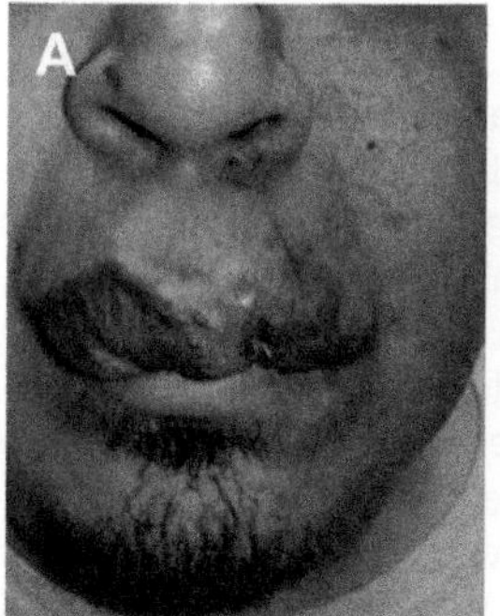


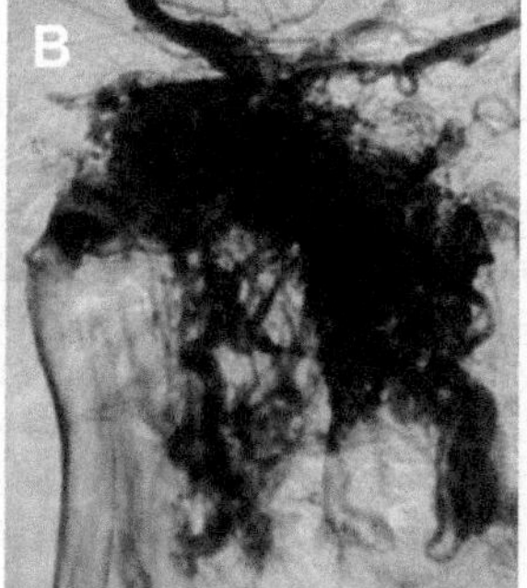


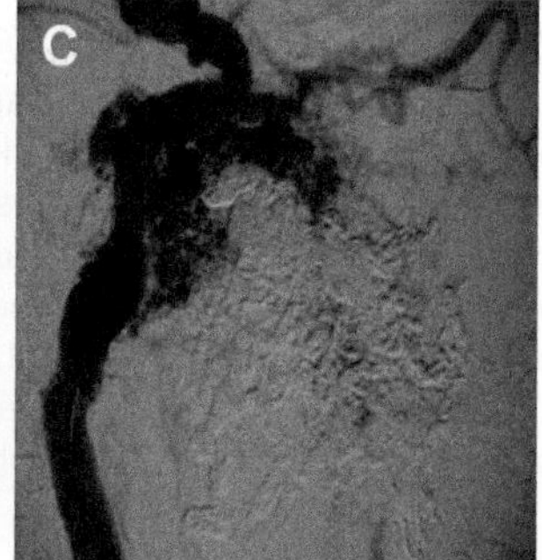


**Fig. 3.** Diffuse AVM of bilateral upper lip and cheek (*A*) with arteriogram before (*B*) and after (*C*) Onyx embolization.

pathways have been discovered in AVMs of the brain and hereditary hemorrhagic telangiectasia. Notch receptors (Notch 1, 3, and 4) and ligands (Dll, Jagged1) contribute to cell differentiation and specification of vessels into veins and arteries, whereas TGF-beta has a primary role in stabilization of vessels and their perivascular space. Variations in expression of TGF-beta, its downstream effectors, and receptors in AVMs suggest a role in their pathogenesis.[14] Similarly, increased expression of endothelial nitric oxide synthase (eNOS) and matrix metalloproteinase-9 in extracranial AVM implicate chronic hypoxia and the stimulation of angiogenesis with extracellular matrix degradation as a source of persistent vascular expansion and soft tissue destruction.[2] AVMs' expansion during prepubescence, puberty, or hormonal surges may be explained by the isolation of progesterone receptors within AVM tissue.[10,14]

Support of endothelial dysfunction comes from recent evidence of endothelial-derived somatic mutations of mitogen-activated protein kinase 1 in AVM.[1,3] Similarly, RAS p21 protein activator 1 (RASA1) is involved in vascular development. Mutations have been discovered in capillary malformation (CM)–AVM syndrome, which seems to have an autosomal dominant pattern of inheritance. These mutations are thought to be associated with a second-hit hypothesis, causing both alleles for *RASA1* to be abnormal. CM-AVM syndrome has phenotypic variability marked by cutaneous multifocal CMs with white halos and high-flow AVMs,[17] which may occur in the head and neck. There may also be a lymphatic malformation component in some patients.[18–20]

## MANAGEMENT

AVMs arise intertwined within healthy soft tissue and bone. The challenge is then to direct therapy to AVM vessels while preserving normal but involved tissue. Therapy shall be no worse than the disease for successful AVM outcomes. The traditional treatment of AVM includes multidisciplinary management with embolization and surgical excision, which are often used in combination. Focal AVMs, with 1 to 2 arterial feeders, respond well to either surgical resection or absolute ethanol embolization. In diffuse AVMs, early intervention with staged multimodal therapy reduces lesion size, controls growth, and maintains healthy soft tissue. Adjuvant therapy with laser and intralesional injections of small vessel cutaneous and subcutaneous disease also assists with the preservation of local tissue. Treatment should commence before aggressive disease infiltration. Because of the high recurrence rates of diffuse lesions, vigilant long-term follow-up with a multidisciplinary vascular anomalies team is imperative and treatment of local recurrence is necessary.[21] Identifying reliable pharmacotherapies for extracranial AVMs is still underway.[6,14,22]

### *Medical*

Currently, pharmacotherapy has a small role for evidence-based treatment in extracranial AVMs of the head and neck. Various medications have been tried (interferon, propranolol, thalidomide, and others),[23] but none has been identified as reliable options for AVM treatment.[6,11] Bevacizumab is a vascular endothelial growth factor antagonist, which is approved for use in the treatment of some cancers. Its intravenous use in the treatment of intranasal mucosal AVMs causing recurrent epistaxis in patients with hereditary hemorrhagic telangiectasia has been reportedly effective.[22,24] However, topical use of bevacizumab was recently shown ineffective for this same patient population.[25]

Chromosome 10 contains a tumor suppressor gene called *PTEN*. Mutation of this gene causes loss of function and has been associated with the development of vascular malformations. Sirolimus (rapamycin) is an inhibitor of mammalian target of rapamycin. It has been shown effective in treating hamartomas in patients with

*PTEN* mutations. In a recent study, sirolimus was shown effective in treating complex AVMs in patients with *PTEN* mutations, though additional research is needed.[22,26]

Matrix metalloproteinases (MMPs) are a family of molecules that have been found to have a role in angiogenesis and vascular remodeling. Particularly, MMP-9 has been associated with vascular instability and has been recently shown to be present in higher amounts in actively growing extracranial AVMs compared with normal tissue.[2,22] By decreasing MMP-9 activity using various MMP inhibitors, such as doxycycline, minocycline, or marimastat, the treatment of AVMs may be improved. However, they are not yet considered reliable treatment options for extracranial AVMs.[2,6,22] Medical therapy for extracranial AVMs is an area of needed research.

### *Endovascular*

One of the main treatment modalities for extracranial AVMs of the head and neck is embolization: the direct injection of agents caustic to the vascular endothelium under radiographic guidance and arteriography. Embolic agents include absolute ethanol, polyvinyl alcohol, n-butyl cyanoacrylate (NCBA) glue, onyx, and coils.[27] Embolization allows for temporary lesion control because of the selective embolization and destruction of the nidus. However, with embolization alone, recurrence rates are reportedly high (98%).[12,21] This recurrence is thought to be due to the incomplete destruction of the nidus that then recruits new vessels. Ideally, embolization is immediately followed by surgical excision; a solid embolic agent should be used in these conditions, such as onyx and NCBA. Embolization may also be used for large, diffuse, late-stage AVMs for palliation.[6,28] The potential risks of embolization include skin necrosis, ulceration and bleeding, nerve injury, and mucosal sloughing. When used for the embolization, onyx may stain the overlying skin with black discoloration.[14] Direct puncture sclerotherapy is another form of treatment of some AVMs with the goal to injure the vascular endothelium. Bleomycin, doxycycline, and other agents have been used in this treatment with some improvement, including interstitial injections of the soft tissue infiltrated by the disease.[28]

### *Surgery*

The surgical treatment of extracranial head and neck AVMs usually involves preoperative embolization, excision of diseased tissue, and reconstruction of the defect (**Fig. 4**).

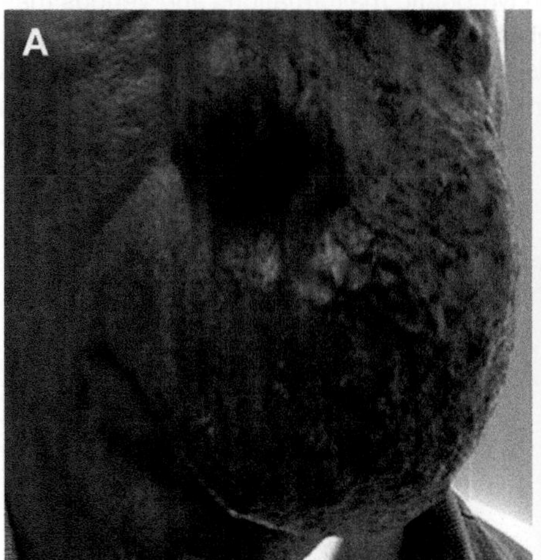


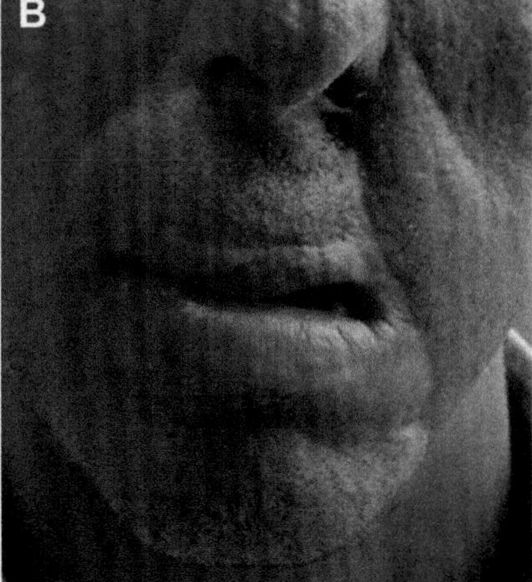


**Fig. 4.** Diffuse AVM of left face and upper lip before (*A*) and after (*B*) massive resection with preservation of local skin flap and reconstruction.

It may be difficult at times to determine the boundaries and the distinction between normal tissue from diseased. Therefore, over-resection and under-resection of diffuse AVMs may occur. Focal AVMs may be cured with surgical excision.[14,29] Diffuse AVMs, however, have high recurrence rates, about 90%.[21] For best treatment results, embolization is followed by complete surgical resection 6 to 48 hours later. Preoperative embolization allows for decreased intraoperative blood loss during excision and helps target the resection and identify the lesion boundaries.[14,30] Embolization with NCBA glue followed by immediate surgical excision has become the authors' preferred method of treatment. This treatment is staged for large lesions and depends on the amount of NCBA that can be used for one embolization. Repeat embolization and resection at 3-month intervals are performed to prevent vascular recruitment and collateralization. Onyx used for embolization of the malformation sparks when in contact with electrocautery during surgical excision. Nonstick bipolar cautery and absorbable gelatin sponge (Gelfoam) with thrombin may be helpful for intraoperative hemorrhage control. Preparation for intraoperative blood transfusions should be performed for large AVMs but is unlikely necessary if preoperative NCBA embolization is used.

### *Multimodal Adjuvant Therapy*

Preliminary data from the senior author's institution show improvement of cutaneous and mucosal disease control with laser therapy (**Fig. 5**). Laser therapy targets the small, superficial blood vessels of the malformation, including venules and veins. The highest flow components are not as responsive to laser. However, with hemoglobin and deoxyhemoglobin as chromophore targets, dual-laser therapy of superficial disease using the flash pump dye laser (595 nm) and GentleYAG (Nd:YAG) laser (1064 nm) can be effective to destroy small cutaneous components of AVM. Mucosal diseases is best targeted with the Nd:YAG laser. Laser therapy helps to selectively target infiltrated AVM while preserving and restoring normal soft tissue. It further helps to decrease lesion thickness and prevent superficial ulceration and bleeding.

Similarly, targeted interstitial therapy by injecting caustic agents to vascular endothelium can be effective to reduce tissue burden in superficial disease. This therapy offsets the need to resect skin and subcutaneous components that can affect reconstruction and postoperative cosmesis. Bleomycin and doxycycline are sclerotherapy agents with a known therapeutic effect on lymphatic malformations and venous malformations. Used in conjunction with embolization and surgery, interstitial injections can be of benefit to control residual disease. Staging these treatments in combination with laser therapy can help manage superficial and diffuse AVMs that would create an otherwise large defect if resected (**Fig. 6**). The intervals for treatment will gradually increase with disease control.

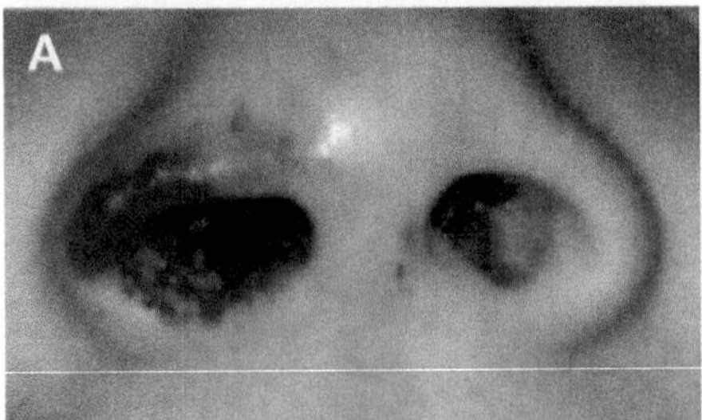


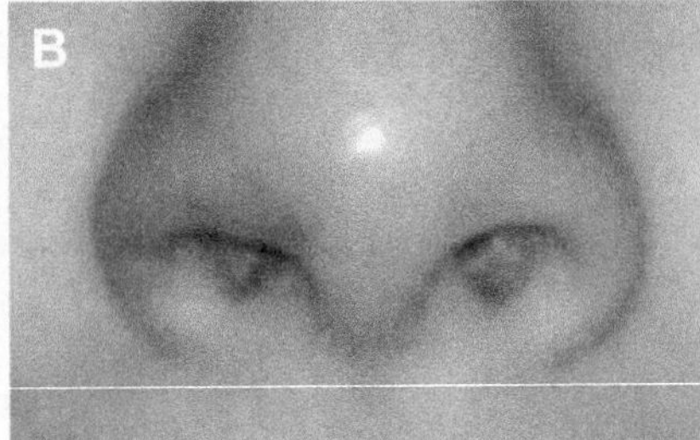


**Fig. 5.** Before (*A*) and after (*B*) GentleYAG (1064 nm) laser to nasal tip AVM. No other treatment performed at this location.

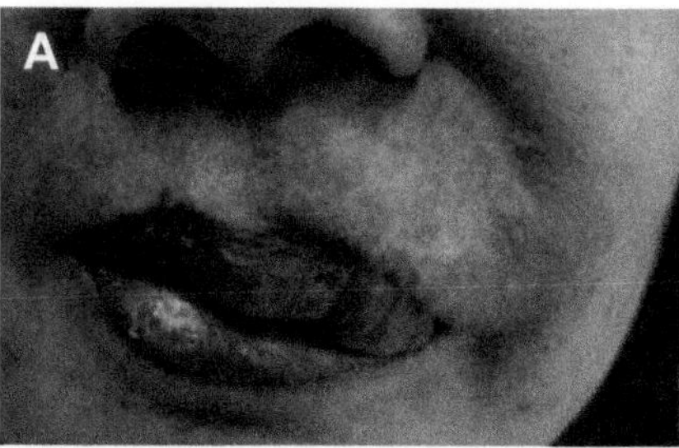


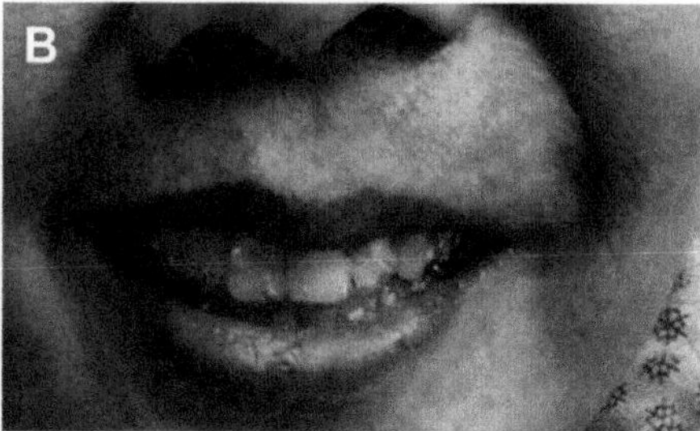


**Fig. 6.** Adult woman with diffuse upper lip AVM before (*A*) and after (*B*) multimodal and staged therapy every 3 months. Initial preoperative glue embolization and resection followed by repeated pulse dye and GentleYAG laser with subcutaneous and intramuscular bleomycin interstitial therapy. Note: Patient had multiple ethanol embolizations at outside institution before presenting with persistent disease.

## FOLLOW-UP

Patients with AVMs require vigilant follow-up for many years. The rate and risk of recurrence of diffuse disease warrants repeat visits with or without intervention to maintain control and confidence in disease eradication. Intermittent arteriography, MRA, or CTA is necessary; but intervals will depend on clinical signs and symptoms of recurrent disease. In asymptomatic but previously treated patients, angiography should be performed every couple of years, as quiescent or recurrent disease may not be fully apparent by examination. Superficial recurrent or recidivistic disease will be discoverable within 6 months as swelling, erythema, and vascular rebound.

## DISCUSSION

AVMs of the head and neck are fascinating lesions; despite their complexity, their management is possible. Diffuse AVMs are rarely cured but easily controlled with current treatment options. Despite this difficulty in successful treatment, there remains controversy with the timing of treatment commencement. Some physicians elect to postpone the treatment of known AVMs until they are symptomatic. However, delaying treatment allows the AVM to grow and infiltrate additional normal tissue, thus, making the treatment more difficult and outcome less successful. Because of this, many physicians (the authors included) advocate for early intervention to treat AVMs, even before symptoms arise. This early intervention may allow for improved lesion control. AVMs never spontaneously resolve. The best opportunity for treatment is early in the course of the disease before the AVM advances to later stages, when patients experience higher morbidity and treatment is more difficult and less successful.

There are reports in the literature of high success rates for head and neck AVMs by single-modality treatment, particularly embolization.[28,31] It is known that after embolization alone, collateralization, and new vessel recruitment can occur, allowing the lesion to expand and infiltrate adjacent normal tissue. The reported cure may be secondary to limited follow-up periods. Also, the term *cure* varies in the literature. Some use the term to indicate an asymptomatic state after embolization, not necessarily the absence of disease.

The management of head and neck AVMs requires multidisciplinary and multimodal care by appropriately trained physicians. Treatment requires repeated therapy for disease control. The overall goal of treating AVMs is to selectively manage the vessels involved. With this approach, management of head and neck AVMs is possible. Untreated lesions without expectation will cause significant morbidity in time. The rate of growth, however, may be unpredictable. Improving treatment outcomes and quality of life is imperative. Across the world, research is being conducted to help identify reliable medical options for treatment and, it is hoped, a cure.

## REFERENCES


1. Couto JA, Huang AY, Konczyk DJ, et al. Somatic MAP2K1 mutations are associated with extracranial arteriovenous malformation. Am J Hum Genet 2017;100(3): 546–54.
2. Wei T, Zhang H, Cetin N, et al. Elevated expression of matrix metalloproteinase-9 not matrix metalloproteinase-2 contributes to progression of extracranial arteriovenous malformation. Sci Rep 2016;6:24378.
3. Hou F, Dai Y, Dornhoffer JR, et al. Expression of endoglin (CD105) and endothelial nitric oxide synthase in head and neck arteriovenous malformations. JAMA Otolaryngol Head Neck Surg 2013;139(3):237–43.
4. Revencu N, Boon LM, Mulliken JB, et al. Parkes Weber syndrome, vein of Galen aneurysmal malformation, and other fast-flow vascular anomalies are caused by RASA1 mutations. Hum Mutat 2008;29(7):959–65.
5. Kohout MP, Hansen M, Pribaz JJ, et al. Arteriovenous malformations of the head and neck: natural history and management. Plast Reconstr Surg 1998;102(3): 643–54.
6. Hoff SR, Rastatter JC, Richter GT. Head and neck vascular lesions. Otolaryngol Clin North Am 2015;48(1):29–45.
7. Richter GT, Suen JY. Clinical course of arteriovenous malformations of the head and neck: a case series. Otolaryngol Head Neck Surg 2010;142(2):184–90.
8. Richter GT, Suen J, North PE, et al. Arteriovenous malformations of the tongue: a spectrum of disease. Laryngoscope 2007;117(2):328–35.
9. Lu L, Bischoff J, Mulliken JB, et al. Increased endothelial progenitor cells and vasculogenic factors in higher-staged arteriovenous malformations. Plast Reconstr Surg 2011;128(4):260e–9e.
10. Duyka LJ, Fan CY, Coviello-Malle JM, et al. Progesterone receptors identified in vascular malformations of the head and neck. Otolaryngol Head Neck Surg 2009;141(4):491–5.
11. Richter GT, Suen JY. Pediatric extracranial arteriovenous malformations. Curr Opin Otolaryngol Head Neck Surg 2011;19(6):455–61.
12. Liu AS, Mulliken JB, Zurakowski D, et al. Extracranial arteriovenous malformations: natural progression and recurrence after treatment. Plast Reconstr Surg 2010;125(4):1185–94.
13. Buckmiller LM, Richter GT, Suen JY. Diagnosis and management of hemangiomas and vascular malformations of the head and neck. Oral Dis 2010;16(5): 405–18.
14. Richter GT, Friedman AB. Hemangiomas and vascular malformations: current theory and management. Int J Pediatr 2012;2012:645678.
15. Griauzde J, Srinivasan A. Imaging of vascular lesions of the head and neck. Radiol Clin North Am 2015;53(1):197–213.
16. Lee BB, Baumgartner I, Berlien HP, et al. Consensus document of the International Union of Angiology (IUA)-2013. Current concept on the management of arterio-venous management. Int Angiol 2013;32(1):9–36.

17. Yadav P, De Castro DK, Waner M, et al. Vascular anomalies of the head and neck: a review of genetics. Semin Ophthalmol 2013;28(5–6):257–66.
18. Macmurdo CF, Wooderchak-Donahue W, Bayrak-Toydemir P, et al. RASA1 somatic mutation and variable expressivity in capillary malformation/arteriovenous malformation (CM/AVM) syndrome. Am J Med Genet A 2016;170(6):1450–4.
19. Larralde M, Abad ME, Luna PC, et al. Capillary malformation-arteriovenous malformation: a clinical review of 45 patients. Int J Dermatol 2014;53(4):458–61.
20. Revencu N, Boon LM, Mendola A, et al. RASA1 mutations and associated phenotypes in 68 families with capillary malformation-arteriovenous malformation. Hum Mutat 2013;34(12):1632–41.
21. Fearon JA. Discussion. Extracranial arteriovenous malformations: natural progression and recurrence after treatment. Plast Reconstr Surg 2010;125(4): 1195–6.
22. Blatt J, McLean TW, Castellino SM, et al. A review of contemporary options for medical management of hemangiomas, other vascular tumors, and vascular malformations. Pharmacol Ther 2013;139(3):327–33.
23. Colletti G, Dalmonte P, Moneghini L, et al. Adjuvant role of anti-angiogenic drugs in the management of head and neck arteriovenous malformations. Med Hypotheses 2015;85(3):298–302.
24. Dupuis-Girod S, Ginon I, Saurin JC, et al. Bevacizumab in patients with hereditary hemorrhagic telangiectasia and severe hepatic vascular malformations and high cardiac output. JAMA 2012;307(9):948–55.
25. Dupuis-Girod S, Ambrun A, Decullier E, et al. Effect of bevacizumab nasal spray on epistaxis duration in hereditary hemorrhagic telangectasia: a randomized clinical trial. JAMA 2016;316(9):934–42.
26. Adams DM, Trenor CC 3rd, Hammill AM, et al. Efficacy and safety of sirolimus in the treatment of complicated vascular anomalies. Pediatrics 2016;137(2): e20153257.
27. Vaidya S, Tozer KR, Chen J. An overview of embolic agents. Semin Intervent Radiol 2008;25(3):204–15.
28. Dmytriw AA, Ter Brugge KG, Krings T, et al. Endovascular treatment of head and neck arteriovenous malformations. Neuroradiology 2014;56(3):227–36.
29. Visser A, FitzJohn T, Tan ST. Surgical management of arteriovenous malformation. J Plast Reconstr Aesthet Surg 2011;64(3):283–91.
30. Goldenberg DC, Hiraki PY, Caldas JG, et al. Surgical treatment of extracranial arteriovenous malformations after multiple embolizations: outcomes in a series of 31 patients. Plast Reconstr Surg 2015;135(2):543–52.
31. Meila D, Grieb D, Greling B, et al. Endovascular treatment of head and neck arteriovenous malformations: long-term angiographic and quality of life results. J Neurointerv Surg 2017;9(9):860–6.

# Capillary Malformations (Portwine Stains) of the Head and Neck

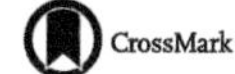

## Natural History, Investigations, Laser, and Surgical Management

Jeong Woo Lee, MD, PhD, Ho Yun Chung, MD, PhD*

**KEYWORDS**

- Capillary malformation • Port-wine stain • Natural history • Laser
- Surgical treatment

**KEY POINTS**

- Facial (capillary malformation) CM often occurs with a quasidermatomal distribution according to the sensory trigeminal nerve distribution.
- With time, CM darkens progressively, and soft tissue hypertrophy, bony hypertrophy, and/or nodule formation can develop.
- The mainstay and gold standard therapy for facial or aesthetically sensitive CM is still the pulsed dye laser (PDL) treatment.
- In patients with associated soft tissue/bony hypertrophy, surgical management is helpful in restoring the normal anatomy and in re-establishing a symmetric contour.

## CLINICAL FEATURES

Capillary malformations (CMs), also known as port-wine stains or nevus flammeus, are the most common type of congenital vascular malformations. They are present at birth and persist throughout life.[1–3] These lesions are initially flat and bright pink, red, or violaceous and typically affect the face (90%), followed by the neck, trunk, leg, arm, and hand.[4–6] They often seem to lighten significantly over the first few months of life. This is not indicative of spontaneous resolution, but it is probably caused by a drop in circulating blood hemoglobin concentration.[7] In contrast to other similar

Disclosure Statement: This research was supported by Basic Science Research Program through the National Research Foundation of Korea funded by the Ministry of Education (2014R1A1A4A01009584).

Department of Plastic and Reconstructive Surgery, Kyungpook National University School of Medicine, 130 Dongdeok-ro, Jung-gu, Daegu 41944, Republic of Korea
* Corresponding author.
*E-mail address:* hy-chung@knu.ac.kr

Otolaryngol Clin N Am 51 (2018) 197–211
https://doi.org/10.1016/j.otc.2017.09.004
oto.theclinics.com

birthmarks, most CMs become darker, thicker, and more nodular over time. This is particularly true of facial lesions.[8] The incidence rate is reported as 0.3% in newborns with an equal sex distribution, occurring spontaneously within the population.[9] In most affected individuals, CMs occur as a sporadic unifocal lesion and are not associated with any underlying abnormalities. However, CMs are sometimes associated with other underlying syndromes, such as Sturge-Weber syndrome; macrocephaly-CM syndrome; CM-arteriovenous malformation (AVM) syndrome; and overgrowth syndromes, such as Klippel-Trénaunay syndrome.[10,11]

The pathogenic mechanism of CM is still unknown. Shirley and colleagues[12] identified a somatic mutation in *GNAQ* with isolated CMs, disrupting vascular development. *GNAQ* encodes a guanine nucleotide-binding protein G(q) subunit alpha that mediates signals between G-protein-coupled receptors and downstream effectors. It has also been identified that the subclass of CMs associated with AVMs has an autosomal-dominant mutation in the *RASA1* gene, encoding Ras1, a GTPase-activating protein involved in cell growth, proliferation, and differentiation during angiogenesis.[13–16] Recently, Frigerio and colleagues[17] reported that novel somatic variants were found in *GNAQ* and *RASA1*.

Histologically, CMs are initially composed of a normal capillary network in the papillary dermis with no evidence of cellular proliferation; ectatic vessels with a small venular morphology in the papillary and occasionally reticular dermis become more evident over time.[2,18]

Facial CMs initially appear as a faint pink macule; however, some patients may develop soft tissue hypertrophy, bony hypertrophy, and/or nodule formation during adulthood.[5,6,19,20] Depending on the size and location, these changes can cause functional deficits in vision, speaking, or eating and significant psychological distress related to the resulting stigmatization or disfigurement.[19] The mucosa of the oral cavity, gingiva, tongue, larynx, nasal mucosa, soft tissue of the neck, and even the parotid gland have been demonstrated as possible sites of manifestation, leading to severe conditions, such as macrocheilia, painful cervical or parotid swelling, globus pharyngeus, dysphonia, dysphagia, gingival bleeding, epistaxis, and nasal and upper airway obstruction.[21]

Although multiple treatments have been reported, the mainstay and gold standard therapy for facial or aesthetically sensitive CMs is still the flashlamp-pumped pulsed dye laser (PDL) treatment.[22,23] However, laser therapy has a limited benefit for long-standing CMs with soft tissue hypertrophy, and a more satisfactory result is achieved after surgical intervention.[5,24]

Local complications of CMs include pyogenic granulomas and eczematous dermatitis occurring within the stain.[25–27] Pyogenic granulomas need to be excised or treated with electrodessication and curettage because they do not resolve spontaneously and are complicated by repeated bleeding and discomfort.

The differential diagnoses of CMs include other vascular lesions, including early infantile hemangioma, vascular stain associated with AVMs, and other vascular malformations. Doppler assessment may be helpful in differentiating between CMs and AVMs, based on a bruit and thrill associated with AVMs. Sometimes, it is difficult to distinguish between early CMs and infantile hemangiomas located on the face during infancy; the distribution (dermatomal in CM vs segmental in infantile hemangiomas) is a clue.[28] The endothelial cells of CMs do not stain for GLUT-1, a specific marker for infantile hemangiomas.

## NATURAL HISTORY

Facial CMs often occur with a quasidermatomal distribution according to the sensory trigeminal nerve distribution: V1, the ophthalmic region, including the forehead and upper eyelid; V2, the maxillary region; and V3, the mandibular region. Forty-five percent are restricted to one of the three regions, and those remaining include multiple dermatomes or those that cross the midline.[5,29] The mucous membranes are often contiguously involved. Although the cutaneous discoloration is usually evident at birth, it can be overlooked because of the stain being hidden by the erythema of the neonatal skin. With time, the faint, pink macules darken progressively to display the characteristic reddish-purple color, and soft tissue hypertrophy, bony hypertrophy, and/or nodule formation can develop.[30]

A retrospective chart review of patients with head and neck CM who presented to the Vascular Birthmark Institute of New York over a 7-year period (2004–2011) was conducted to classify the CMs based on location and to quantify the patients who had not received any treatment before the development of tissue hypertrophy and/or nodule formation.[19]

Of the 160 patients with CMs, 96 patients (60%) demonstrated disease progression to include either soft tissue/bony hypertrophy or nodule formation. Of these, 87 patients who had not received any previous treatment were enrolled, consisting of 36 men (41%) and 51 women (59%). Soft tissue hypertrophy began at an average age of 9 years (1–29 years). The V2 dermatome was the most commonly involved (28%), followed by a combined involvement of the V1 and V2 dermatomes (24%) (**Fig. 1**). With respect to anatomic distribution, upper lip hypertrophy was the most prominent (31%), followed by that of the cheek (14%), and nose (12%). Eight patients had gingival involvement, and five of them demonstrated gingival hypertrophy. Nodules, also known as cobblestones, were present in 38 of 87 (44%) patients with the average age of onset of 22 years (14–53 years). Eighty-two percent of patients with nodules also had soft tissue hypertrophy. Twelve patients (14%) presented with bony hypertrophy, which began at an average age of 15 years. Most involved the maxilla (**Fig. 2**), followed by the mandible, which can cause an occlusal cant (vertical maxillary overgrowth), increasing the incidence of dental show and malocclusion. All patients with bony hypertrophy also had anatomically related soft tissue hypertrophy.[19]

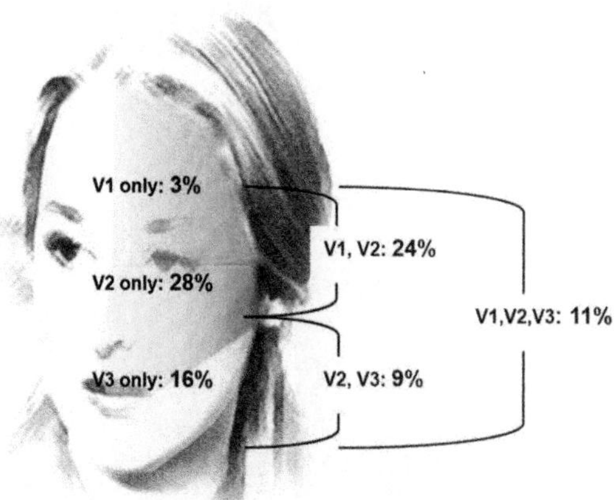


**Fig. 1.** Dermatome distribution of soft tissue hypertrophy. (*From* Lee JW, Chung HY, Cerrati EW, et al. The natural history of soft tissue hypertrophy, bony hypertrophy, and nodule formation in patients with untreated head and neck capillary malformations. Dermatol Surg 2015;41(11):1242; with permission.)

In 1980, Barsky and colleagues[2] reported the direct correlation between age and the increasing histologic changes in the dermis occupied by the vascular malformation. In 1984, Finley and colleagues[31] suggested that the nodule formation resulted from a localized vascular ectasia with their surrounding stroma. Mills and colleagues[4] reported that dermal thickening was found in 11% of patients and nodule formation in 10%, in their demographic study of 283 patients.

Another possible mechanism for nodule formation is the alteration in the neural regulation of cutaneous vascular flow. Because CMs lack proper innervation (high vessel-to-nerve ratio), continued blood flow, with decreased levels of autonomic nerves, could significantly shift blood flow regulation, leading to a progressive vascular ectasia.[32] As supported by this theory, Rydh and colleagues[33] reported that CMs show a deficit innervation with only occasional nerve fibers in connection to the ectatic vessels. Furthermore, they found that CMs lack not only sympathetic innervation but also sensory innervation.[34,35]

Klapman and Yao[36] reported that the onset of the thickening peaked in the 20- to 39-year age group. They also noted that the thickening continues to intensify as the patient ages with a greater tendency to develop nodules superimposed on the thickening. It was proposed that the increased incidence of facial thickening could be caused by the increased vascularity of the face or as an effect of sun exposure.

## CLINICAL MANAGEMENT

Multiple treatments for CMs have been reported, including excision, dermabrasion, external ionizing radiation, electrocautery, cryotherapy, use of sclerosing agents, photodynamic therapy (PDT), intense pulsed light (IPL), and laser therapy.[5,6,37,38] However, laser therapy is effective in approximately 70% of cases and has the lowest complication risk among these methods.[5,6,38] The flashlamp-pumped PDL and the neodymium-doped:yttrium-aluminum-garnet (Nd:YAG) laser are currently the criterion standard treatments for facial or aesthetically sensitive CMs.[6]

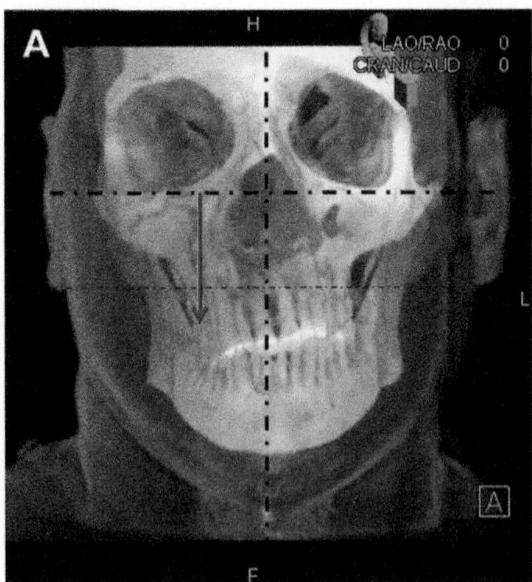


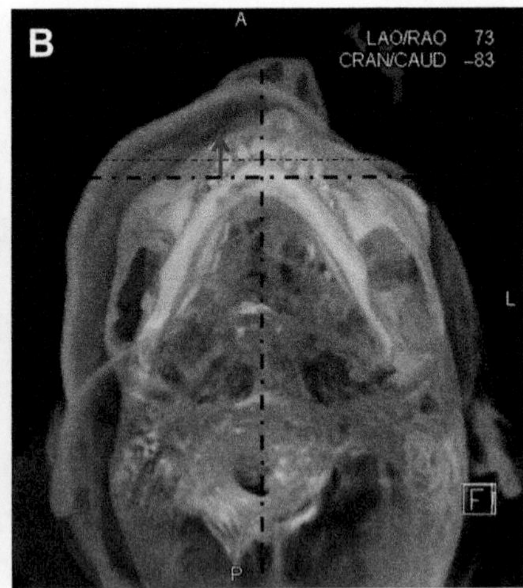


**Fig. 2.** Three-dimensional computed tomography findings of bony hypertrophy. Red arrows show skeletal hypertrophy with (*A*) elongation and (*B*) expansion of the maxilla. (*From* Lee JW, Chung HY, Cerrati EW, et al. The natural history of soft tissue hypertrophy, bony hypertrophy, and nodule formation in patients with untreated head and neck capillary malformations. Dermatol Surg 2015;41(11):1244; with permission.)

In patients with CMs, the decision on the treatment usually depends on the size and location of the lesion. The risks and benefits of each treatment and the natural history of CMs must be fully discussed with the patient and family.[39] Facial CMs can stigmatize a patient leading to stress and lowered self-esteem; thus, early laser therapy is recommended to lighten the stain before school age and to receive psychosocial benefits.[40–42] Currently, there is no prospective evidence that early intervention with PDL reduces the progression, such as darkening of the CMs, soft tissue hypertrophy, bony hypertrophy, and/or nodule formation of the involved structures over time.[43] However, in patients with associated soft tissue/bony hypertrophy, surgical management is helpful in restoring the normal anatomy and in re-establishing a symmetric contour.

### *Pulsed Dye Laser*

Until the early 1980s, there was no effective treatment available for CMs. Early lasers, such as the continuous-wave carbon dioxide and argon lasers, were nonselective and resulted in significant scarring.[44] The introduction of the concept of selective photothermolysis with the 577-nm PDL revolutionized CM treatment.[45] PDL emits a yellow light at wavelengths with a high absorption coefficient for oxyhemoglobin and deoxyhemoglobin.[46–49] In general, the laser wavelengths of 570 to 595 nm produce selective blood vessel damage to structures located in the superficial vascular plexus and to a depth of up to 2 mm. Most CMs have some degree of improvement after PDL treatment, because their superficial component is accessible to PDL.[50]

According to the principle of selective photothermolysis, hemoglobin-containing erythrocytes absorb photons on irradiation of the PDL, resulting in thermal denaturation of the blood (primary effect) and formation of thermal coagulum triggering thrombosis (secondary effect). It is suggested that these processes would induce an inflammatory reaction, and completely photocoagulated vasculature would be replaced by smaller diameter capillaries through angiogenesis and/or neovasculogenesis, which contain a lower blood volume. Incompletely photocoagulated vasculature may be remodeled into restructured vascular lumen. These underlying endovascular laser-tissue interactions and thrombosis lead to CM clearance.[51]

The most commonly used laser in clinical practice is the 595-nm PDL with a variable pulse width in combination with selective epidermal cooling by cryogen spray (**Fig. 3**).[46] Cryogen spray cooling during laser therapy has been used to selectively cool the most superficial layers of the skin and to provide sufficient epidermal protection, while minimally affecting deeply located targets.[52,53] To minimize complications after laser treatment, such as dyspigmentation, scarring, and rarely, infection, patients should be advised to use sunblock and avoid sun exposure to minimize dyspigmentation, barrier emollients to protect the skin from bacterial infections, and oral acyclovir to prevent more disseminated infections in patients with known herpes simplex infection.[54–56]

PDL treatments almost completely lighten the stain in approximately 20% of cases, with 50% of patients achieving approximately 70% improvement.[57] The remaining patients, especially those who have large CMs involving the V2 dermatome and soft tissue hypertrophy, tend to respond less to PDL. Many other laser modalities have been studied to treat the resistant and hypertrophic CMs refractory to PDL, because the deeper dermal capillaries may be inaccessible to PDL, which only penetrates up to 2 mm of the skin.

To manage this, longer wavelength systems (which penetrate deeper areas because of decreased optical scattering and epidermal melanin absorption), such as 755-nm alexandrite, 810-nm diode, and 1064-nm Nd:YAG laser, have been developed. However, these wavelengths have lesser hemoglobin absorption; thus, higher laser

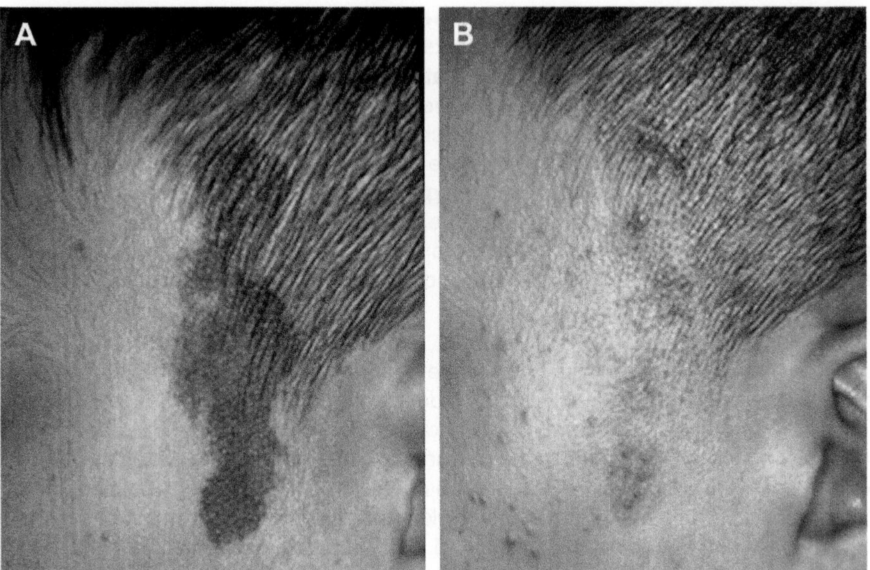


**Fig. 3.** Capillary malformation of the left cheek. Before (*A*) and after (*B*) five pulsed dye laser treatments.

fluences are required to achieve adequate capillary heating, increasing the risk of epidermal and dermal side effects.[57]

### *Long-Pulsed Neodymium-Doped:Yttrium-Aluminum-Garnet Laser*

In patients with CMs refractory to PDL, nodularity and darkening can persist despite repeated treatments, because the deeper and larger vessels are not ablated by PDL. The long-pulsed Nd:YAG laser has a wavelength of 1064 nm and penetrates more deeply than the PDL.

Because of the depth of penetration and increased risk of scarring with long-pulsed Nd:YAG laser, the treatment should be reserved for patients with CMs refractory to PDL and used with caution.[58,59]

### *Combined Pulsed Dye Laser and Neodymium-Doped:Yttrium-Aluminum-Garnet Laser Systems*

There are some studies showing that a single type of laser cannot properly treat all CMs because of the great heterogeneity of phenotypic presentation as color, depth, and site of the lesion.[60] A new combined PDL and Nd:YAG laser system delivers sequential pulses of 595 nm (PDL) followed by 1064 nm (Nd:YAG laser).[57] The initial 595-nm pulse induces methemoglobin formation, which has a significant absorption peak at approximately 1064 nm. Thus, the absorption rate of the following 1064-nm pulse after an interval of 50 to 2000 milliseconds can be increased.[57] This combined laser system results in a deeper coagulation effect within the treated capillaries than a single type of laser and it can treat CMs safely and effectively.[61,62]

### *Alexandrite Laser*

According to the principle of selective photothermolysis, the deeper vessels in the resistant and hypertrophic CMs can be treated with a more deeply penetrating laser that has the selective absorption for deoxyhemoglobin and oxyhemoglobin.[63] From this perspective, the alexandrite laser, which emits an infrared light (wavelength, 755 nm), has been used effectively in treating resistant or hypertrophic CMs. Although the absorption coefficient of the 1064-nm laser is greater for oxyhemoglobin than deoxyhemoglobin, the 755-nm alexandrite laser has a higher absorption coefficient for deoxyhemoglobin than oxyhemoglobin. Because the venous vessels contain 30% deoxyhemoglobin and 70% oxyhemoglobin and the arterial vessels contain almost purely oxyhemoglobin, the preferential targeting of deoxyhemoglobin by the 755-nm alexandrite laser provides at least a theoretic advantage over the 1064-nm Nd:YAG laser when treating the primarily venous vessels of the CMs, where the flow is stagnant and accumulation of deoxyhemoglobin is greater. However, this deeply penetrating laser should be used carefully to avoid deep dermal burns that can cause scarring.[50]

### *Intense Pulsed Light*

IPL is used as an alternative to laser systems for the treatment of CMs. In contrast to lasers, the IPL systems emit noncoherent light with variable pulse durations and variable wavelength bands. Thus, the IPL system may have a broader range of absorption coefficients and thermal relaxation times, and they may be matched to a broader range of CMs, compared with laser systems.[64] Several reports show that patients with CMs and PDL-resistant CMs showed a good response to IPL with fewer complications, such as bleeding, dyspigmentation, and scarring.[65–68] Recently, Faurschou and colleagues[69] reported that a higher proportion of patients obtained good or excellent clearance rates on using the PDL (75%) compared with IPL (30%) in a randomized controlled trial. Additional research studies on the safety and efficacy of IPL in the management of CMs are needed.

### *Photodynamic Therapy*

PDT, which was started as an antitumor therapy, is a new modality that involves either topical or an intracirculatory exposure to an exogenous chromophore in the dilated capillaries of CMs. The most widely used chromophores are the porphyrin precursors, such as hematoporphyrin and benzoporphyrin (administered intravenously) and aminolevulinic acid (administered topically).[46] These drugs are highly concentrated inside vessels with CMs and their diffusion to normal tissue is negligible. After the administration of the chromophores, a photosensitizer is excited using a laser, thereby producing cytotoxic-activated oxygen species including singlet oxygen, which destroy the malformed vessels, while inflicting little damage to normal tissue.[70] Evans and colleagues[71] reported that there was no significant difference in clearance between the patients with CM treated with topical aminolevulinic acid followed by PDL and with PDL alone. Recently, several large reports from China have shown that using systemic photosensitizers followed by exposure to the copper vapor laser, which emits two wavelengths of light at 510.6 and 578.2 nm, is effective in treating CMs.[72–74] Additional studies are needed to demonstrate the safety and efficacy of PDT in the management of CMs.

### *Antiangiogenic Therapy*

The steadily emerging antiangiogenic therapy for the management of CMs involves the concomitant use of PDL and topical agents, such as imiquimod and rapamycin, to inhibit angiogenesis or neovascularization.[46] Angiogenesis is a normal process in growth and wound healing, but it is also a contributing factor in a wide range of disease processes. Based on these findings, many researchers investigated whether the topical application of these agents after laser exposure could inhibit the reperfusion of the photocoagulated blood vessels. Imiquimod is a topically administered immune response modulator for treating various skin diseases, such as external genital warts, superficial basal cell carcinoma, and actinic keratosis.[75–78] It is also known as an inhibitor of pathologic neovascularization and has been used successfully to treat vascular proliferative lesions, such as infantile hemangiomas, pyogenic granulomas, Kaposi sarcoma, and hemangiosarcomas.[79] Rapamycin is a specific inhibitor of "mammalian target of rapamycin" and it was approved by the Food and Drug Administration for use as an immunosuppressive agent to prevent allograft rejection after organ transplantation and for coating coronary stents to prevent restenosis.[80,81] Recently, the inhibition of mammalian target of rapamycin–mediated functions has led to the speculation that it is involved in the downregulation of hypoxia-inducible factor synthesis, which in turn regulates vascular endothelial growth factor expression.[76,77] Additional studies are needed to demonstrate safety and efficacy of antiangiogenic therapy in the management of CMs.

### *Surgical Management Using a Staged Zonal Approach*

In patients with long-standing CMs with soft tissue hypertrophy, laser therapy has limited benefit, and a more satisfactory result is achieved after surgical approaches

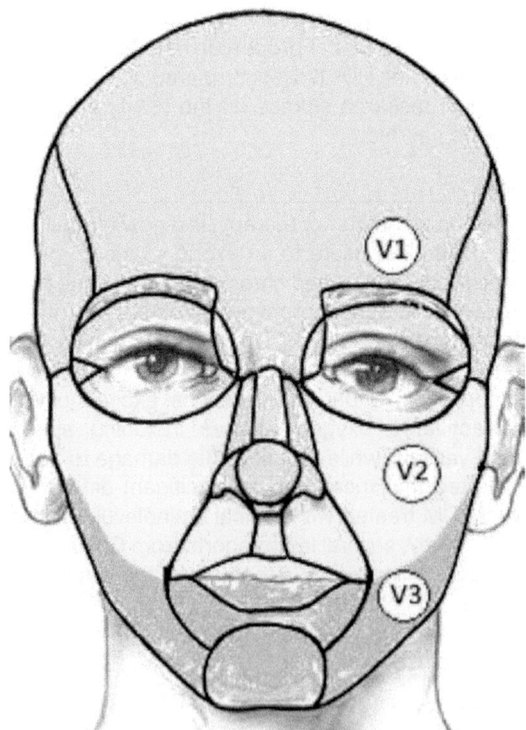


**Fig. 4.** The face is divided into six major aesthetic units: the forehead, eye/eyebrow, nose, lips, chin, and cheek. Each of these is further subdivided into additional anatomic subunits as demonstrated. The facial dermatomes have also been colored and labeled. (*From* Cerrati EW, O TM, Binetter D, et al. Surgical treatment of head and neck port-wine stains by means of a staged zonal approach. Plast Reconstr Surg 2014;134(5):1004; with permission.)

and managements.[5,24] Soft tissue hypertrophy secondary to a growth signal abnormality begins at an average age of 9 years; many of these patients also experience negative psychosocial effects.[2,19,30] Although there is no absolute age for initial surgical interventions, soft tissue reduction is performed at any age to re-establish symmetry.

Cerrati and colleagues[82] proposed the surgical management of head and neck CMs using a staged zonal approach, based on the facial horizontal thirds, relaxed skin tension lines, and aesthetic facial subunits (**Figs. 4** and **5**).[83–85] If the CMs involved two adjacent dermatomes or horizontal thirds, a combined or extended approach could be used for the resection. However, if the CMs spanned more than two dermatomes or involved multiple adjacent facial subunits, the excision was staged (**Fig. 6**). When a planned excision was not located near a facial subunit border, either an elliptical excision was placed in the direction of the relaxed skin tension line or a local rotational or advancement flap was used.

Once the lesion was removed, the flap was redraped toward the boundaries of the subunits, and any redundant or involved tissue was excised using a parallel incision

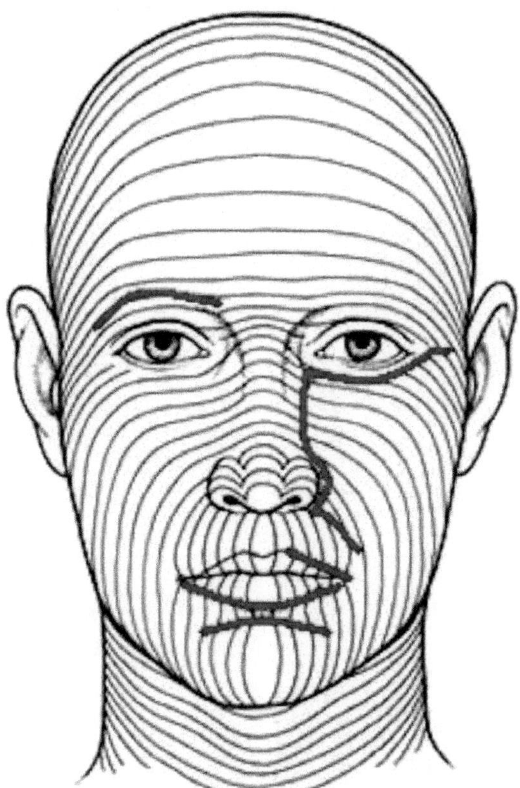

**Fig. 5.** The relaxed skin tension lines run perpendicular to the underlying muscular contraction. By creating an incision along one of these lines, a narrow and strong scar line results with an excellent cosmesis. Our most common approach is the combination of the marked incisions. (*From* Cerrati EW, O TM, Binetter D, et al. Surgical treatment of head and neck port-wine stains by means of a staged zonal approach. Plast Reconstr Surg 2014;134(5):1006; with permission.)

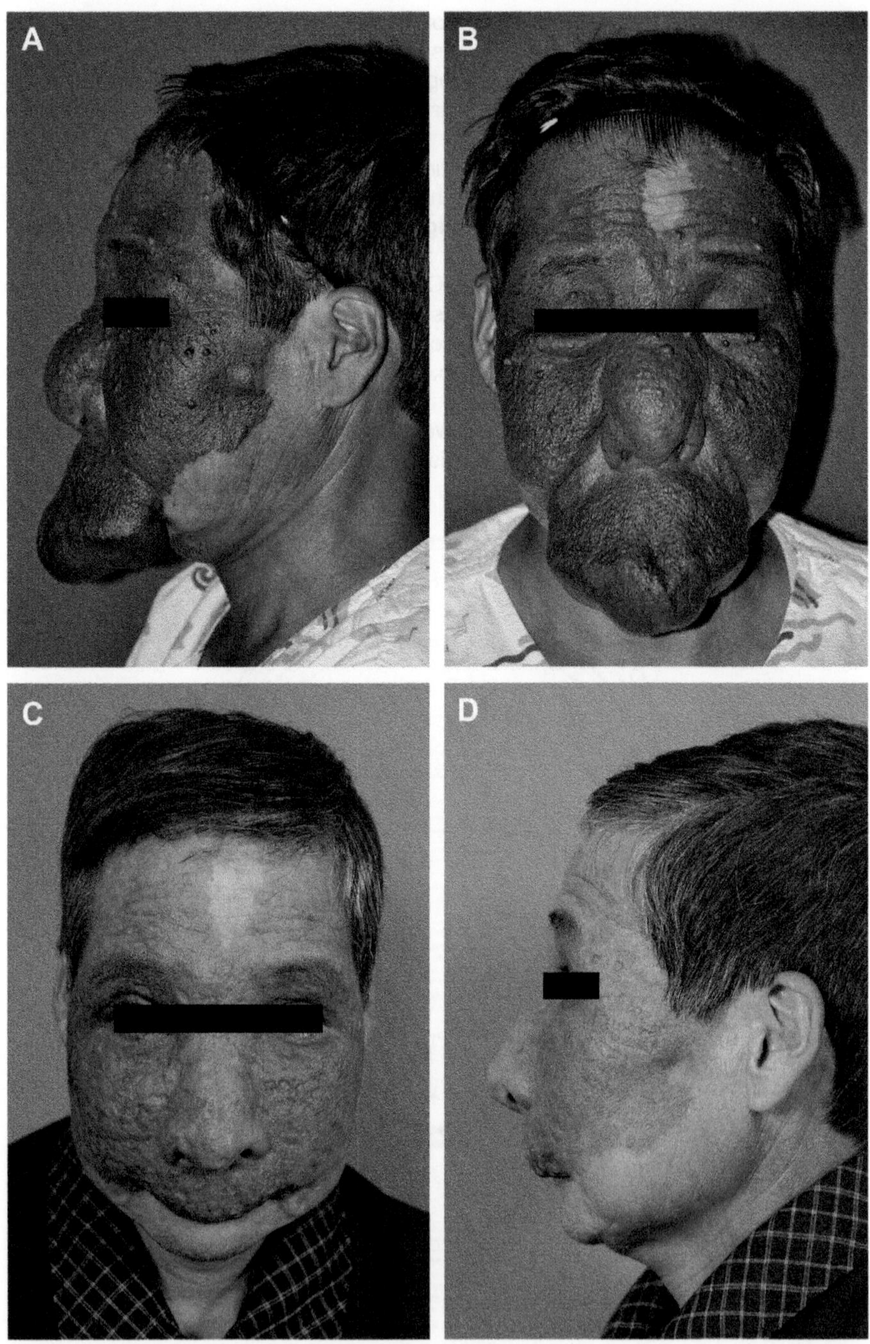


**Fig. 6.** (*A, B*) Preoperative photograph demonstrates a V1/V2 capillary malformation crossing the midline. The soft tissue hypertrophy progressed and resulted in a serious disfigurement. These changes caused functional deficits in vision, speaking, and eating. (*C, D*) After four times of excisions based on the facial aesthetic subunits and following multiple pulsed dye laser treatments, the gross facial contouring was restored, and the patient's quality of life improved.

created next to the initial incision. Each of these procedures can and usually does involve a staged approach to avoid overresection. The associated soft tissue hypertrophy and nodularity are never uniform in height and density, making the prediction of how the skin flap will heal once it has been redraped over the surgical bed extremely difficult. As the duration of the operation increases, the degree of edema also increases, resulting in tissue distortion and difficulty for the surgeon to assess accurately the aesthetic subunits. Furthermore, preoperative and/or postoperative laser treatments can reduce the amount of tissue that needs to be removed.

The appearance of the resulting scar is dependent on the amount of tension placed on the incision. Although the initial scar can appear hypochromic when surrounded by an area of the involved skin, this resolves over time as the scar matures and the surrounding skin is treated with laser therapy. Bleeding is only present when the skin incision is created through CMs located primarily in the superficial dermis; this is easily controlled because CMs are low-flow vascular malformations consisting of small-diameter vessels. Facial nerve monitoring is rarely used during operations, because the lesion is located in a more superficial layer than the facial nerves.

The goals of surgical treatment of CMs include not only to remove as much of the lesion as necessary to re-establish a symmetric contour but also to improve the patients' quality of life. Any remaining lesions are treated with either repeated excision or PDL at a later date.

## REFERENCES

1. Johnson WC. Pathology of cutaneous vascular tumors. Int J Dermatol 1976;15(4): 239–70.
2. Barsky SH, Rosen S, Geer DE, et al. The nature and evolution of port wine stains: a computer-assisted study. J Invest Dermatol 1980;74(3):154–7.
3. Enzinger FM, Wiess SW. Soft tissue tumors. 2nd edition. St Louis (MO): Mosby; 1988. p. 521–2.
4. Mills CM, Lanigan SW, Hughes J, et al. Demographic study of port wine stain patients attending a laser clinic: family history, prevalence of naevus anaemicus and results of prior treatment. Clin Exp Dermatol 1997;22(4):166–8.
5. Renfro L, Geronemus RG. Anatomical differences of port-wine stains in response to treatment with the pulsed dye laser. Arch Dermatol 1993;129(2):182–8.
6. Orten SS, Waner M, Flock S, et al. Port-wine stains. An assessment of 5 years of treatment. Arch Otolaryngol Head Neck Surg 1996;122(11):1174–9.
7. Cordoro KM, Speetzen LS, Koerper MA, et al. Physiologic changes in vascular birthmarks during early infancy: mechanisms and clinical implications. J Am Acad Dermatol 2009;60(4):669–75.
8. Brouillard P, Vikkula M. Genetic causes of vascular malformations. Hum Mol Genet 2007;16(Spec No. 2):R140–9.
9. Jacobs AH, Walton RG. The incidence of birthmarks in the neonate. Pediatrics 1976;58(2):218–22.
10. Wright DR, Frieden IJ, Orlow SJ, et al. The misnomer "macrocephaly-cutis marmorata telangiectatica congenita syndrome": report of 12 new cases and support for revising the name to macrocephaly-capillary malformations. Arch Dermatol 2009;145(3):287–93.
11. Gonzalez ME, Burk CJ, Barbouth DS, et al. Macrocephaly-capillary malformation: a report of three cases and review of the literature. Pediatr Dermatol 2009;26(3): 342–6.

12. Shirley MD, Tang H, Gallione CJ, et al. Sturge-Weber syndrome and port-wine stains caused by somatic mutation in GNAQ. N Engl J Med 2013;368(21):1971–9.
13. Boon LM, Ballieux F, Vikkula M. Pathogenesis of vascular anomalies. Clin Plast Surg 2011;38(1):7–19.
14. Yadav P, De Castro DK, Waner M, et al. Vascular anomalies of the head and neck: a review of genetics. Semin Ophthalmol 2013;28(5–6):257–66.
15. Behr GG, Liberman L, Compton J, et al. CM-AVM syndrome in a neonate: case report and treatment with a novel flow reduction strategy. Vasc Cell 2012;4(1):19.
16. Eerola I, Boon LM, Mulliken JB, et al. Capillary malformation-arteriovenous malformation, a new clinical and genetic disorder caused by RASA1 mutations. Am J Hum Genet 2003;73(6):1240–9.
17. Frigerio A, Wright K, Wooderchak-Donahue W, et al. Genetic variants associated with port-wine stains. PLoS One 2015;10(7):e0133158.
18. Mulliken JB, Young AE. Vascular birthmarks: hemangiomas and malformations. Philadelphia: WB Saunders; 1988.
19. Lee JW, Chung HY, Cerrati EW, et al. The natural history of soft tissue hypertrophy, bony hypertrophy, and nodule formation in patients with untreated head and neck capillary malformations. Dermatol Surg 2015;41(11):1241–5.
20. Koster PH, Bossuyt PM, van der Horst CM, et al. Characterization of portwine stain disfigurement. Plast Reconstr Surg 1998;102(4):1210–6.
21. Eivazi B, Roessler M, Pfützner W, et al. Port-wine stains are more than skin-deep! Expanding the spectrum of extracutaneous manifestations of nevi flammei of the head and neck. Eur J Dermatol 2012;22(2):246–51.
22. Goldman MP, Fitzpatrick RE. Laser treatment of cutaneous vascular lesions. In: Goldman MP, Fitzpatrick RE, editors. Cutaneous laser surgery: the art and science of selective photothermolysis. 2nd edition. St Louis (MO): Mosby-Year Book; 1999. p. 37–74.
23. Sivarajan V, Maclaren WM, Mackay IR. The effect of varying pulse duration, wavelength, spot size, and fluence on the response of previously treated capillary vascular malformations to pulsed-dye laser treatment. Ann Plast Surg 2006; 57(1):25–32.
24. Tierney EP, Hanke CW. Alexandrite laser for the treatment of port wine stains refractory to pulsed dye laser. Dermatol Surg 2011;37(9):1268–78.
25. Swerlick RA, Cooper PH. Pyogenic granuloma (lobular capillary hemangioma) within port-wine stains. J Am Acad Dermatol 1983;8(5):627–30.
26. Rajan N, Natarajan S. Impetiginized eczema arising within a port-wine stain of the arm. J Eur Acad Dermatol Venereol 2006;20(8):1009–10.
27. Fonder MA, Mamelak AJ, Kazin RA, et al. Port-wine-stain-associated dermatitis: implications for cutaneous vascular laser therapy. Pediatr Dermatol 2007;24(4): 376–9.
28. Haggstrom AN, Lammer EJ, Schneider RA, et al. Patterns of infantile hemangiomas: new clues to hemangioma pathogenesis and embryonic facial development. Pediatrics 2006;117(3):698–703.
29. Enjolras O, Riche MC, Merland JJ. Facial port-wine stains and Sturge-Weber syndrome. Pediatrics 1985;76(1):48–51.
30. Chang CJ, Yu JS, Nelson JS. Confocal microscopy study of neurovascular distribution in facial port wine stains (capillary malformation). J Formos Med Assoc 2008;107(7):559–66.
31. Finley JL, Noe JM, Arndt KA, et al. Port-wine stains. Morphologic variations and developmental lesions. Arch Dermatol 1984;120(11):1453–5.

32. Smoller BR, Rosen S. Port-wine stains. A disease of altered neural modulation of blood vessels? Arch Dermatol 1986;122(2):177–9.
33. Rydh M, Malm M, Jernbeck J, et al. Ectatic blood vessels in port-wine stains lack innervation: possible role in pathogenesis. Plast Reconstr Surg 1991;87(3): 419–22.
34. Nilsson J, von Euler AM, Dalsgaard CJ. Stimulation of connective tissue cell growth by substance P and substance K. Nature 1985;315(6014):61–3.
35. Haegerstrand A, Dalsgaard CJ, Jonzon B, et al. Calcitonin gene-related peptide stimulates proliferation of human endothelial cells. Proc Natl Acad Sci U S A 1990;87(9):3299–303.
36. Klapman MH, Yao JF. Thickening and nodules in port-wine stains. J Am Acad Dermatol 2001;44(2):300–2.
37. Gao K, Huang Z, Yuan KH, et al. Side-by-side comparison of photodynamic therapy and pulsed-dye laser treatment of port-wine stain birthmarks. Br J Dermatol 2013;168(5):1040–6.
38. Xiao Q, Li Q, Yuan KH, et al. Photodynamic therapy of port-wine stains: long-term efficacy and complication in Chinese patients. J Dermatol 2011;38(12):1146–52.
39. Maguiness SM, Liang MG. Management of capillary malformations. Clin Plast Surg 2011;38(1):65–73.
40. Minkis K, Geronemus RG, Hale EK. Port wine stain progression: a potential consequence of delayed and inadequate treatment? Lasers Surg Med 2009; 41(6):423–6.
41. Chapas AM, Eickhorst K, Geronemus RG. Efficacy of early treatment of facial port wine stains in newborns: a review of 49 cases. Lasers Surg Med 2007;39(7): 563–8.
42. Troilius A, Wrangsjö B, Ljunggren B. Potential psychological benefits from early treatment of port-wine stains in children. Br J Dermatol 1998;139(1):59–65.
43. van der Horst CM, Koster PH, de Borgie CA, et al. Effect of the timing of treatment of port-wine stains with the flash-lamp-pumped pulsed-dye laser. N Engl J Med 1998;338(15):1028–33.
44. Olbricht SM, Stern RS, Tang SV, et al. Complications of cutaneous laser surgery. A survey. Arch Dermatol 1987;123(3):345–9.
45. Anderson RR, Parrish JA. Selective photothermolysis: precise microsurgery by selective absorption of pulsed radiation. Science 1983;220(4596):524–7.
46. Cordisco MR. An update on lasers in children. Curr Opin Pediatr 2009;21(4): 499–504.
47. Lam SM, Williams EF 3rd. Practical considerations in the treatment of capillary vascular malformations, or port wine stains. Facial Plast Surg 2004;20(1):71–6.
48. Tan E, Vinciullo C. Pulsed dye laser treatment of port-wine stains: a review of patients treated in Western Australia. Med J Aust 1996;164(6):333–6.
49. Wimmershoff MB, Wenig M, Hohenleutner U, et al. Treatment of port-wine stains with the flash lamp pumped dye laser. 5 years of clinical experience. Hautarzt 2001;52(11):1011–5.
50. Izikson L, Anderson RR. Treatment endpoints for resistant port wine stains with a 755 nm laser. J Cosmet Laser Ther 2009;11(1):52–5.
51. Heger M, Beek JF, Moldovan NI, et al. Towards optimization of selective photothermolysis: prothrombotic pharmaceutical agents as potential adjuvants in laser treatment of port wine stains. A theoretical study. Thromb Haemost 2005;93(2): 242–56.

52. Nelson JS, Milner TE, Anvari B, et al. Dynamic epidermal cooling during pulsed laser treatment of port-wine stain. A new methodology with preliminary clinical evaluation. Arch Dermatol 1995;131(6):695–700.
53. Chang CJ, Nelson JS. Cryogen spray cooling and higher fluence pulsed dye laser treatment improve port-wine stain clearance while minimizing epidermal damage. Dermatol Surg 1999;25(10):767–72.
54. Owens WW 3rd, Lang PG. Herpes simplex infection and colonization with *Pseudomonas aeruginosa* complicating pulsed-dye laser treatment. Arch Dermatol 2004;140(6):760–1.
55. Strauss RM, Sheehan-Dare R. Local molluscum contagiosum infection as a side-effect of pulsed-dye laser treatment. Br J Dermatol 2004;150(5):1047–9.
56. Chen T, Frieden IJ. Development of extensive flat warts after pulsed dye laser treatment of a port-wine stain. Dermatol Surg 2007;33(6):734–5.
57. Jasim ZF, Handley JM. Treatment of pulsed dye laser-resistant port wine stain birthmarks. J Am Acad Dermatol 2007;57(4):677–82.
58. Yang MU, Yaroslavsky AN, Farinelli WA, et al. Long-pulsed neodymium:yttrium-aluminum-garnet laser treatment for port-wine stains. J Am Acad Dermatol 2005;52(3 Pt 1):480–90.
59. Kono T, Frederick Groff W, Chan HH, et al. Long-pulsed neodymium:yttrium-aluminum-garnet laser treatment for hypertrophic port-wine stains on the lips. J Cosmet Laser Ther 2009;11(1):11–3.
60. Al-Dhalimi MA, Al-Janabi MH. Split lesion randomized comparative study between long pulsed Nd:YAG laser 532 and 1,064 nm in treatment of facial port-wine stain. Lasers Surg Med 2016;48(9):852–8.
61. Borges da Costa J, Boixeda P, Moreno C, et al. Treatment of resistant port-wine stains with a pulsed dual wavelength 595 and 1064 nm laser: a histochemical evaluation of the vessel wall destruction and selectivity. Photomed Laser Surg 2009;27(4):599–605.
62. Alster TS, Tanzi EL. Combined 595-nm and 1,064-nm laser irradiation of recalcitrant and hypertrophic port-wine stains in children and adults. Dermatol Surg 2009;35(6):914–8.
63. Izikson L, Nelson JS, Anderson RR. Treatment of hypertrophic and resistant port wine stains with a 755 nm laser: a case series of 20 patients. Lasers Surg Med 2009;41(6):427–32.
64. Bjerring P, Christiansen K, Troilius A. Intense pulsed light source for the treatment of dye laser resistant port-wine stains. J Cosmet Laser Ther 2003;5(1):7–13.
65. Ho WS, Ying SY, Chan PC, et al. Treatment of port wine stains with intense pulsed light: a prospective study. Dermatol Surg 2004;30(6):887–90.
66. Reynolds N, Exley J, Hills S, et al. The role of the Lumina intense pulsed light system in the treatment of port wine stains-a case controlled study. Br J Plast Surg 2005;58(7):968–80.
67. Raulin C, Schroeter CA, Weiss RA, et al. Treatment of port-wine stains with a noncoherent pulsed light source: a retrospective study. Arch Dermatol 1999; 135(6):679–83.
68. Ozdemir M, Engin B, Mevlitoğlu I. Treatment of facial port-wine stains with intense pulsed light: a prospective study. J Cosmet Dermatol 2008;7(2):127–31.
69. Faurschou A, Togsverd-Bo K, Zachariae C, et al. Pulsed dye laser vs. intense pulsed light for port-wine stains: a randomized side-by-side trial with blinded response evaluation. Br J Dermatol 2009;160(2):359–64.
70. Wang X, Tian C, Duan X, et al. A medical manipulator system with lasers in photodynamic therapy of port wine stains. Biomed Res Int 2014;2014:384646.

71. Evans AV, Robson A, Barlow RJ, et al. Treatment of port wine stains with photodynamic therapy, using pulsed dye laser as a light source, compared with pulsed dye laser alone: a pilot study. Lasers Surg Med 2005;36(4):266–9.
72. Yuan KH, Li Q, Yu WL, et al. Comparison of photodynamic therapy and pulsed dye laser in patients with port wine stain birthmarks: a retrospective analysis. Photodiagnosis Photodyn Ther 2008;5(1):50–7.
73. Yuan KH, Li Q, Yu WL, et al. Photodynamic therapy in treatment of port wine stain birthmarks-recent progress. Photodiagnosis Photodyn Ther 2009;6(3–4):189–94.
74. Gu Y, Huang NY, Liang J, et al. Clinical study of 1949 cases of port wine stains treated with vascular photodynamic therapy (Gu's PDT). Ann Dermatol Venereol 2007;134(3 Pt 1):241–4.
75. Chang CJ, Hsiao YC, Mihm MC Jr, et al. Pilot study examining the combined use of pulsed dye laser and topical imiquimod versus laser alone for treatment of port wine stain birthmarks. Lasers Surg Med 2008;40(9):605–10.
76. Kimel S, Svaasand LO, Kelly KM, et al. Synergistic photodynamic and photothermal treatment of port-wine stain? Lasers Surg Med 2004;34(2):80–2.
77. Phung TL, Oble DA, Jia W, et al. Can the wound healing response of human skin be modulated after laser treatment and the effects of exposure extended? Implications on the combined use of the pulsed dye laser and a topical angiogenesis inhibitor for treatment of port wine stain birthmarks. Lasers Surg Med 2008;40(1):1–5.
78. Wagstaff AJ, Perry CM. Topical imiquimod: a review of its use in the management of anogenital warts, actinic keratoses, basal cell carcinoma and other skin lesions. Drugs 2007;67(15):2187–210.
79. Tremaine AM, Armstrong J, Huang YC, et al. Enhanced port-wine stain lightening achieved with combined treatment of selective photothermolysis and imiquimod. J Am Acad Dermatol 2012;66(4):634–41.
80. Saunders RN, Metcalfe MS, Nicholson ML. Rapamycin in transplantation: a review of the evidence. Kidney Int 2001;59(1):3–16.
81. Morice MC, Serruys PW, Sousa JE, et al. A randomized comparison of a sirolimus-eluting stent with a standard stent for coronary revascularization. N Engl J Med 2002;346(23):1773–80.
82. Cerrati EW, O TM, Binetter D, et al. Surgical treatment of head and neck port-wine stains by means of a staged zonal approach. Plast Reconstr Surg 2014;134(5):1003–12.
83. Burget GC, Menick FJ. The subunit principle in nasal reconstruction. Plast Reconstr Surg 1985;76(2):239–47.
84. Calhoun KH. Reconstruction of small- and medium-sized defects of the lower lip. Am J Otolaryngol 1992;13(1):16–22.
85. Hicks DL, Watson D. Soft tissue reconstruction of the forehead and temple. Facial Plast Surg Clin North Am 2005;13(2):243–51, vi.

# The Management of Vascular Malformations of the Airway

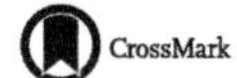

## Natural History, Investigations, Medical, Surgical and Radiological Management

Tristan Klosterman, MD[a], Teresa M. O, MD, MArch[b,*]

**KEYWORDS**

- Airway • Congenital • Vascular lesion • Lymphatic malformation
- Venous malformation • Arteriovenous malformation

**KEY POINTS**

- Airway vascular malformations affect all areas of the airway and each have a characteristic appearance and distribution.
- Airway lymphatic malformations involve the supraglottis and above; venous malformations may be transglottic, whereas arteriovenous malformations occur in vascular "choke zones" and are often found in the base of tongue or parapharyngeal spaces.
- Problems with speaking, swallowing, oral competence, glossoptosis, and sleep apnea often coexistent and require simultaneous management.
- Sclerotherapy with bleomycin is a safe and effective agent in both venous and lymphatic airway disease.
- Posttherapy inflammation should be anticipated with proper consideration to airway protection.

## UPPER AIRWAY CONGENITAL VASCULAR LESIONS

Congenital vascular malformations of the upper airway present unique problems for the patient and the medical team and often require a multidisciplinary approach.[1,2] The upper airway is defined anatomically from its anterior superior boundary of the

Disclosure Statement: The authors have nothing they wish to disclose.
[a] Vascular Birthmark Institute of New York, Head and Neck Institute, Lenox Hill Hospital, 150 East 77th Street, New York, NY 10075, USA; [b] Department of Otolaryngology–Head and Neck Surgery, Vascular Birthmark Institute of New York, Facial Nerve Center, Manhattan Eye, Ear and Throat Hospital, 210 East 64th Street, 7 Floor, New York, NY 10065, USA
* Corresponding author.
*E-mail address:* to@vbiny.org

Otolaryngol Clin N Am 51 (2018) 213–223
https://doi.org/10.1016/j.otc.2017.09.013
oto.theclinics.com
0030-6665/18/

lips to the carina of the trachea. This definition covers a large and varied topography including the oral cavity, oropharynx, larynx, glottis, and trachea.

Morbidity includes difficulty with mastication, airway obstruction, speech intelligibility, oral incompetence, sialorrhea, and dysphagia. These concerns necessitate special consideration, with focused evaluation and treatment modalities, which may differ from other locations. Recent studies have shown a high propensity of obstructive sleep apnea in this population with 47% to 85% affected.[1,3,4]

Vascular tumors and malformations may be present in the airway. The most common vascular tumor involving the airway is infantile hemangioma (IH), (see David H. Darrow's article, "Management of Infantile Hemangiomas of the Airway," in this issue). Vascular malformations are defined by their vessel type and may be lymphatic, venous, capillary (port wine stains), or arteriovenous. Each type is discussed with a focus on specific presentation and management.

## AIRWAY VASCULAR MALFORMATIONS

Similar to the classification of airway IHs into focal and segmental lesions, airway vascular malformations may also be classified according to their distribution (focal or diffuse).[5] All patients with extensive head and neck cutaneous lesions have a high risk of airway involvement and thus should be evaluated by an otolaryngologist. The treatment is often multidisciplinary. Unlike airway IHs, which proliferate and involute, vascular malformations of the airway persist and enlarge over time.

## LYMPHATIC MALFORMATIONS

Patients with lymphatic malformations (LMs) of the head and neck have up to a 73% rate of upper airway involvement.[6] The oral cavity, tongue, oropharynx, base of tongue, and supraglottis are all commonly involved (**Fig. 1**). Lymphatic malformations of the airway may extend from the lips to the supraglottis. To date, we have never seen involvement of the true vocal folds, subglottis, or trachea.[6] Patients with massive bilateral cervicofacial disease will require a tracheostomy in up to 30% of cases. Lesions may be microcystic (<1–2 cm cysts), macrocystic, or mixed. More commonly, in diffuse disease, they are mixed.

### *Presentation*

Upper airway LMs most commonly involve the tongue.[6] These lesions are characterized by mucosal colored or hemorrhagic vesicles on the tongue surface. They have been described as frog's eggs–type vesicles. Patients may also present with tongue swelling, bleeding, pain, halitosis, difficulty eating spicy or acidic foods, speech intelligibility, sleep-disordered breathing, and, in some cases, airway compromise. Tongue base enlargement is an important finding and is often associated with an Ω-shaped edematous epiglottis. Involvement of the floor of mouth, tongue, or tongue base can also result in glossoptosis, which may be characterized by floor-of-mouth involvement, macroglossia, or both. Differentiation of the root cause of glossoptosis is important in the choice of treatment.

A hallmark of LMs is exacerbations and remissions. An exacerbation is characterized by acute swelling and pain with or without the presence of hemorrhagic vesicles. The swelling may resolve fully or may not fully recede after each event. Trauma and hormonal changes also lead to growth and enlargement.[6]

Severe disease with macroglossia is usually detected during prenatal ultrasound fetal screening. In extreme cases, an EXIT procedure (Ex-utero Intrapartum Tracheostomy) may be planned to control the airway at delivery.[6–10]

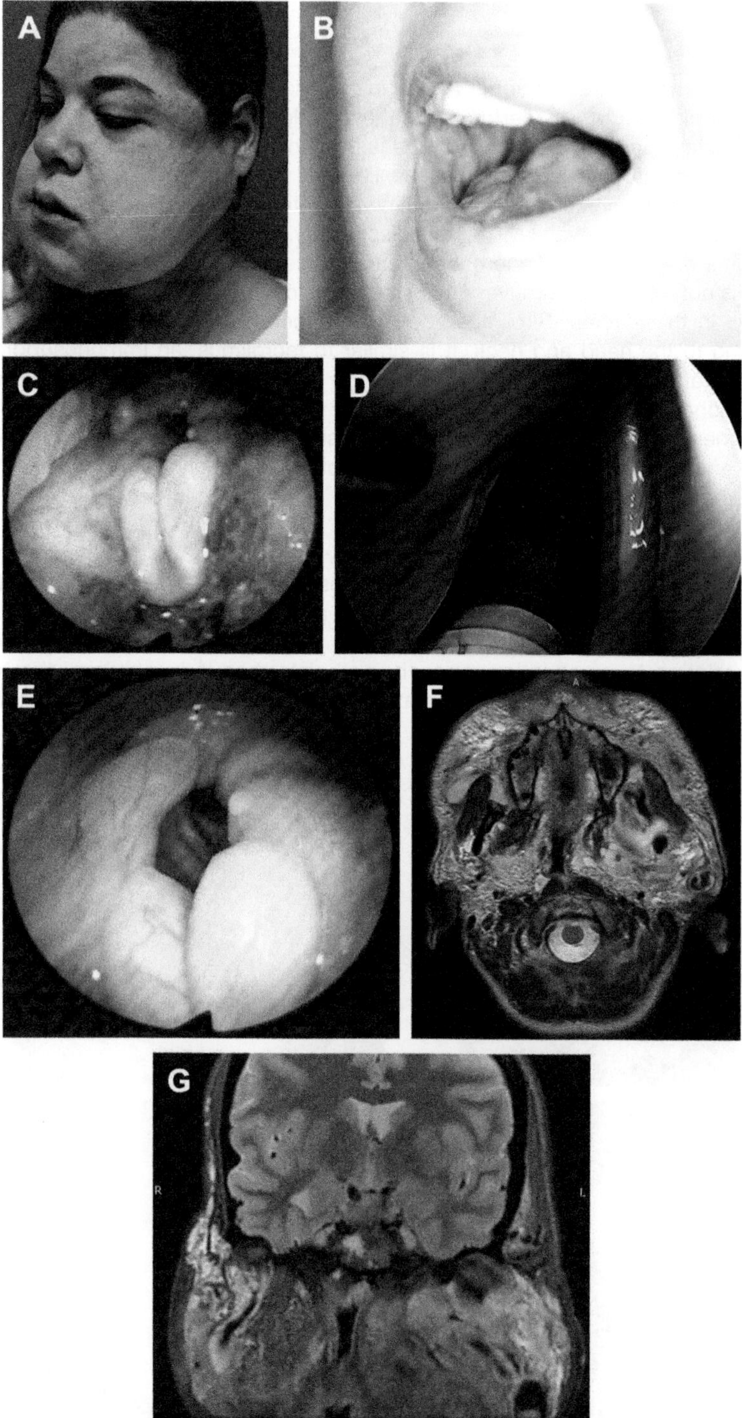


**Fig. 1.** (*A–C*) Extensive cervicofacial LM with oral and laryngoscopy view. Note base of tongue LM hypertrophy with Ω-shaped edematous epiglottis and supraglottic involvement. (*D, E*) The true vocal folds and trachea are free of disease. (*F, G*) T2-weighted MRI, axial and coronal views of the same patient.

## Management

Because of the high risk of upper airway involvement in cervicofacial LMs, an airway survey should be routinely performed in these patients. An office fiberoptic laryngoscopy is initially performed if airway disease is suspected. MR imaging is important in assessing the anatomic extent of disease. Bilateral involvement is an important finding and is associated with a higher risk of airway obstruction.[11]

The treatment of airway LMs is multidisciplinary. Medical treatment can temporize symptoms during acute exacerbations and induce remission of lymphangitis. However, it is not ultimately curative. The use of corticosteroids and antibiotics are highly effective in these roles. Sirolimus has recently been used in extensive airway LM extending to the head and neck. It is similar to tacrolimus, an immunosuppressant used in graft rejection; however, it works on the mammalian target of rapamycin and the phosphoinositide-3-kinase pathway, which has been associated with the pathogenesis of vascular malformations. Data show effectiveness in shrinking disease burden and relieving some of the symptoms of LMs, but long-term side effects and control remain to be seen.[12,13]

Diffuse LMs involving multiple anatomic areas require a staged multimodal approach. Depending on the degree of airway obstruction, a tracheostomy may be necessary during the treatment period, because surgical or interventional radiology procedures may temporarily increase swelling and obstruction.

Macroglossia is difficult to manage and has additional considerations outside the airway relating to mastication, speech, and sialorrhea.[14] In children, the tongue affects the growth of the palate, maxilla, and mandible (**Fig. 2**). Macroglossia,

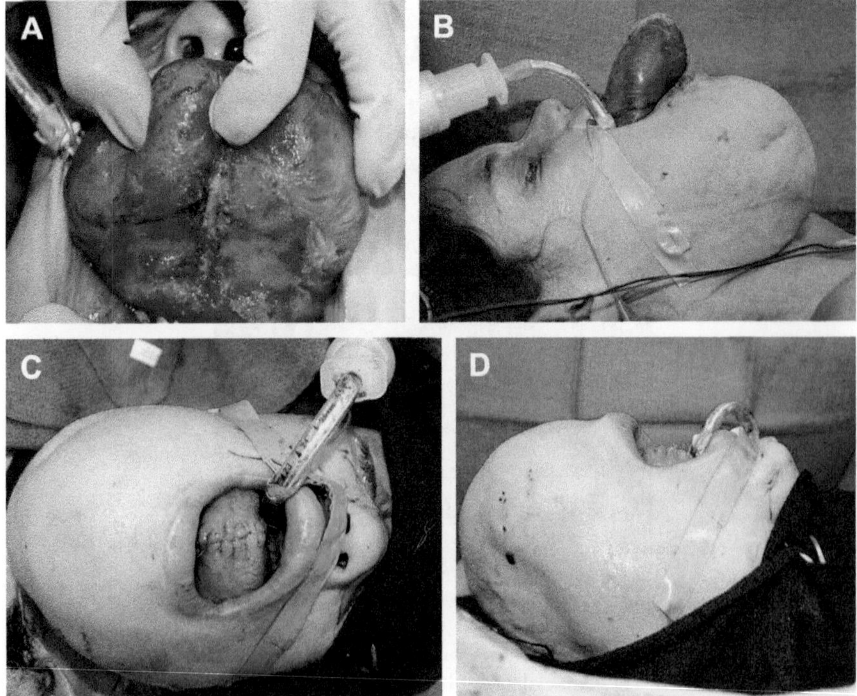


**Fig. 2.** Extensive cervicofacial LM involvement with macroglossia. (*A,B*) Before and (*C,D*) Immediately after surgical excision.

glossoptosis, and floor-of-mouth disease exerts a mass effect on the developing mandible and dentition leading to malocclusion and other dental complications. For these reasons, the first goal is to reduce the size of the tongue. Many surgical interventions have been described for debulking with the simple wedge and keyhole incisions being the most commonly preferred.[14] The height and width of the tongue can be addressed in stages in advanced cases if necessary. Floor-of-mouth involvement may be excised. Direct transmucosal sclerotherapy may also be used as a primary or adjunctive therapy for mucosal and subcutaneous disease.

Interventional procedures, such as direct puncture transmucosal bleomycin sclerotherapy with direct laryngoscopy, are effective and cause minimal edema and scarring (**Fig. 3**).[15] This therapy is effective for all mucosal lesions including the lip, tongue, and upper airway.[12,16,17] The medication may be used in its pure form and injected as the needle is withdrawn. Fluoroscopic or ultrasound guidance may be used for small retropharyngeal or lateral pharyngeal lesions not clinically visible. Bleomycin is a chemotherapeutic agent that inhibits DNA synthesis. Its sclerosant effect may be caused by vascular fibrosis via endothelial cell differentiation to myofibroblast and inhibition of endothelial cell migration and capillary tube formation.[18] Risks are rare given the small dosages used; however, they include hyperpigmentation, interstitial pneumonia, and pulmonary fibrosis.[17,18] The pulmonary risks are dose related. It is effective in both macrocystic and microcystic lesions and it is believed to spread via lymphatic channels.

$CO_2$ ablative laser can be effective if used judiciously in superficial mucosal lesions (**Fig. 4**).[19,20] However, stenosis is a known complication that should be considered when determining the aggressiveness of treatment. In bilateral disease, ablation of one side at a time is recommended to reduce the risk of airway compromise.

High-dose corticosteroids should be considered postoperatively after any intervention including surgery or sclerotherapy. In surgical cases, intralesional steroid injections are useful 4 to 6 weeks after intervention to quell the common and extensive fibrotic reaction typical of healing LM. With staged multidisciplinary therapy, decannulation is possible.

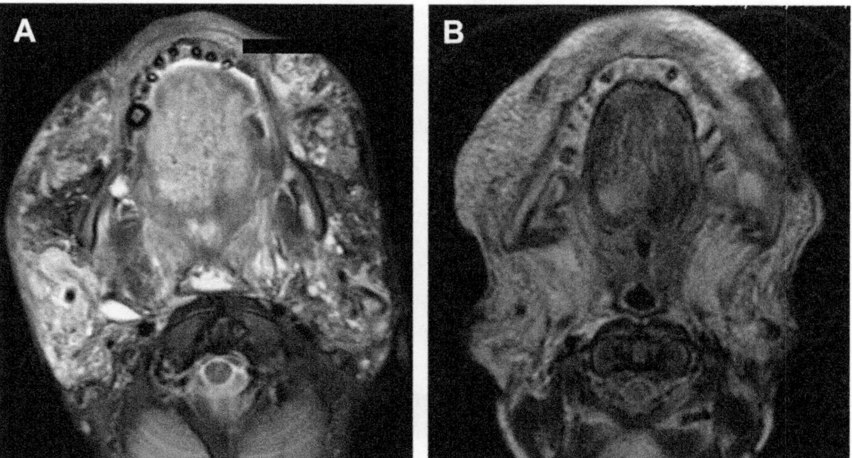


**Fig. 3.** (*A*) Before and (*B*) after direct puncture sclerotherapy.

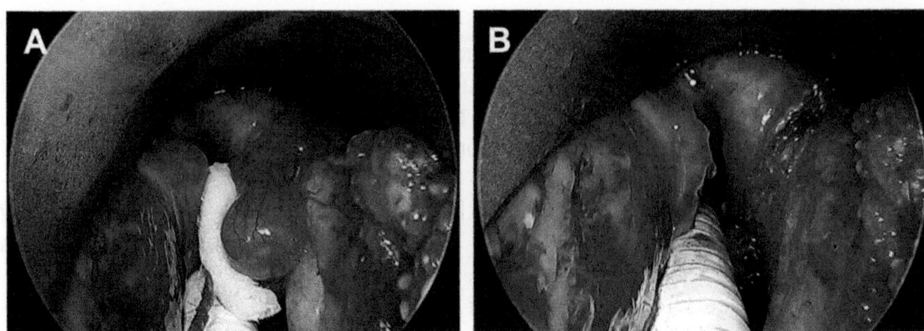


**Fig. 4.** (*A*) Before and, (*B*) After CO2 laser ablation.

## AIRWAY VENOUS MALFORMATIONS

### *Presentation*

In contrast to other vascular lesions of the head and neck, venous malformations (VMs) are compressible, and expand with Valsalva or in the dependent position (**Fig. 5**). Mucosal or cutaneous lesions present as a bluish mass. Phleboliths may be present and can be palpated as small firm stonelike masses. Clinical presentation depends on the site and extent of the lesion. Oral cavity or tongue lesions will be clinically obvious. In advanced stages, patients may experience oral cavity bleeding with minor trauma. Airway VMs may involve all areas of the upper airway: lip, tongue, oral cavity, palate, pharynx, and larynx. They may also present at a later stage in life with dysphagia and dysphonia. Extensive laryngeal lesions will present with orthopnea, obstructive sleep apnea, and, later, frank upper airway obstruction when recumbent.[1,3,4]

Airway VMs may be focal, multifocal, or diffuse (**Fig. 6**). Multifocal disease involves all areas of the upper aerodigestive tract. When the larynx is affected, the disease may

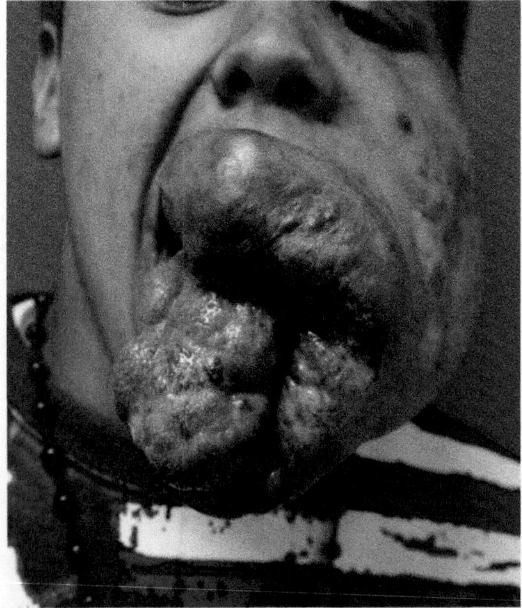

**Fig. 5.** Extensive facial, oral, and airway involvement of VM. Note enlarged lips and macroglossia and glossoptosis. Patient sleeps in an upright position.

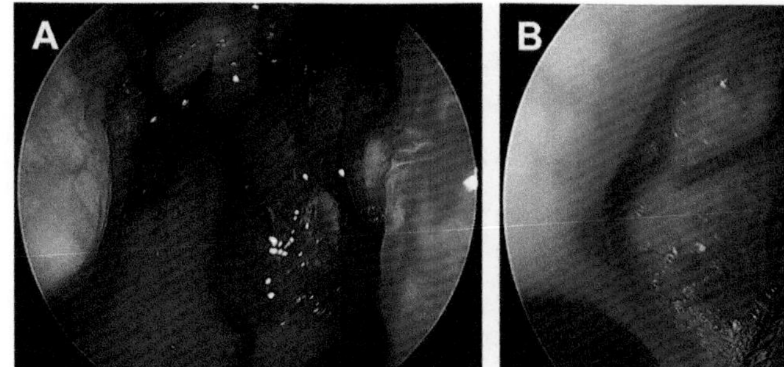

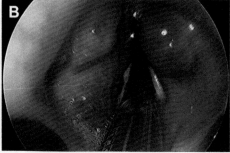

**Fig. 6.** (*A*) Airway VM in the supraglottis with Ω-shaped epiglottis. (*B*) Laryngeal involvement near the anterior commissure and false vocal cords.

be transglottic involving the supraglottis, glottis, and subglottis. Facial cutaneous disease is an important marker of airway disease, with up to 70% affected (poster presentation, ISSVA 2012[21]).

MRI is a crucial study to fully evaluate the extent and anatomic distribution of VMs. These lesions exhibit high signal intensity on T2-weighted images, and the presence of phleboliths is usually seen in the form of tubular flow voids.[19] Ultrasound scans can be helpful, and lesions will appear hypoechoic, heterogeneous, and compressible. Monophasic low velocity flow is also characteristic.

### *Management*

Because of the high incidence of concurrent airway disease in patients with head and neck cutaneous lesions, all patients with head and neck cutaneous VMs require flexible fiberoptic airway evaluation in the office. Several factors determine the type of intervention including the extent of the disease, its depth, and the concern for airway obstruction.

Superficial disease can often be treated with a Neodymium-doped:yttrium aluminum, garnet (Nd:YAG) laser. This treatment is a mainstay for mucosal lesions. The laser is used in the noncontact mode, 1 to 3 mm away from the lesion, and light is delivered through a 600-μm optical quartz fiber in a nonoverlapping "snowstorm pattern" (**Fig. 7**). Using this method can prevent necrosis because of its extended depth (1 cm) and width of penetration.[19] Multimodal therapy of surgery, laser, or sclerotherapy is an option for smaller focal lesions.

Large compound lesions with superficial components can be first treated with laser therapy to induce a submucosal fibrotic plane in anticipation of surgical excision. Special care should be taken with extensive mucosal VM because of increased risk of flap necrosis, bleeding, and poor healing with either surgery or sclerotherapy. Surgery or sclerotherapy should be delayed approximately 4 to 6 weeks after any initial laser treatment.

As with other malformations, laryngeal disease requires direct rigid laryngoscopy with microscopy. Nd:YAG light is delivered via a quartz fiber. Direct transmucosal puncture sclerotherapy is also a frequently performed modality and can be very effective. Sclerotherapy agent choice depends on the safety of the airway. If there is no tracheostomy, bleomycin is the agent of choice because of the minimal risk of posttherapy swelling. Bleomycin has been used safely in several cases and can be introduced through an endoscopic transmucosal approach.[15] Foamed bleomycin has also been used with improved success in a recent study versus ethanol.[18] If the airway is secure, a variety of different agents can be used and will depend on the

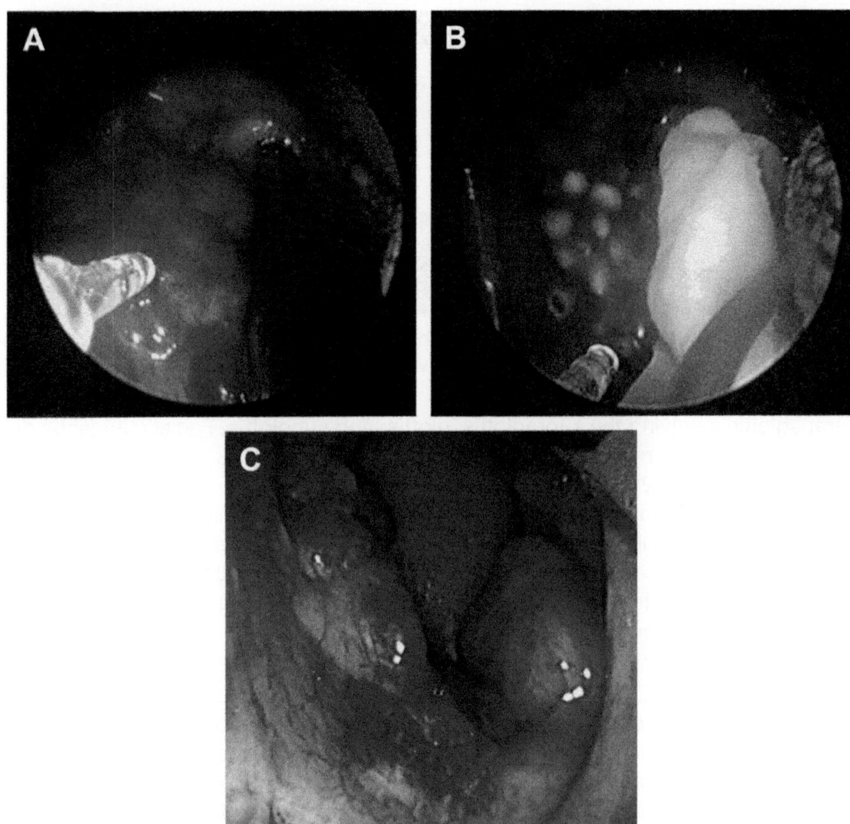


**Fig. 7.** (*A, B*) VM treated with Nd:YAG laser in a "snowstorm" pattern. (*C*) Image of postoperative image 6 months later after 1 treatment.

expertise of the interventional radiologist. In cases of extensive bilateral disease, unilateral treatment may be prudent to reduce the chance of airway compromise; however, a temporary tracheostomy should be considered during the treatment period.

## AIRWAY CAPILLARY MALFORMATIONS/PORT WINE STAINS

### *Presentation*

Airway capillary malformations often affect the oral cavity and oropharynx. Specifically, the lips, buccal mucosa, floor of mouth, tongue, soft and hard palate, gingiva, oropharynx (tonsil), and lateral pharyngeal wall are commonly involved. Soft tissue hypertrophy often occurs in cutaneous and mucosal disease, especially in long-standing cases. These patients are usually disfigured by lip hypertrophy and experience sleep apnea caused by increased airway tissue mass and reduced elasticity (**Fig. 8**).

### *Management*

Pulsed dye laser treatment is the gold standard treatment of cutaneous port wine stains. Photodynamic therapy is also effective, but at this stage is still experimental.[22] However, soft tissue hypertrophy can only be eliminated through surgical excision. Presurgical evaluation includes fiberoptic endoscopy in the upright and supine

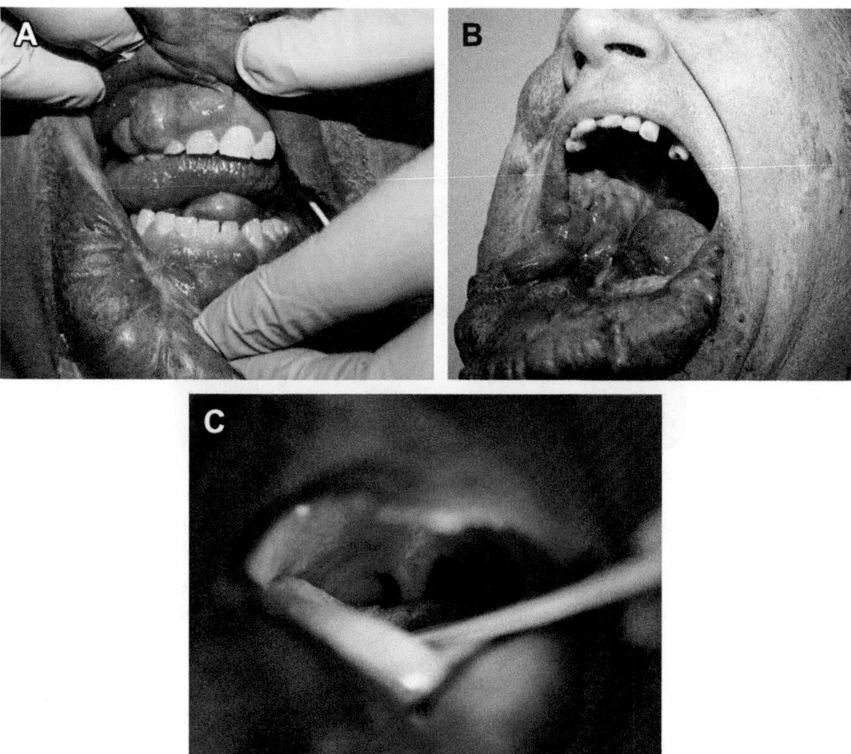


**Fig. 8.** Oral port wine stain involvement in 2 patients. (*A*) Note soft tissue hypertrophy of lips, gingiva, floor of mouth, and tongue. Patient also has right nasal soft tissue hypertrophy of nasal mucosa, inferior turbinate hypertrophy, and obstruction (*B*). Soft tissue hypertrophy of right face, bilateral lower lip, buccal mucosa, tongue, and floor of mouth. (*C*) Staining of soft palate from the patient in B in segmental pattern. Both patients have sleep apnea.

positions. The Muller maneuver can help determine the degree of pharyngeal collapse and guide intervention strategies. In patients with significant disease, care should be taken during intubation, as obstruction can occur owing to redundant pharyngeal tissue. It is best to intubate these patients awake using a video laryngoscope or fiberoptic scope. Standard obstructive sleep apnea surgery methods including tonsillectomy and uvulopalatopharyngoplasty are commonly used. Ipsilateral tongue or tongue base reduction and floor of mouth resection may also be necessary. Gingival hypertrophy is treated with $CO_2$ ablative procedures.

## AIRWAY ARTERIOVENOUS MALFORMATIONS

Laryngeal arteriovenous malformations (AVMs) are extremely rare but when present typically result in progressive upper airway obstruction. The underlying condition is thought to be related to vascular choke zones or areas between 2 main arteries, which are relatively limited in the larynx and glottis.[23,24] AVMs of the tongue are seen more frequently and can involve both the anterior and posterior segments. Infrequently, lesions have been seen arising from the supraglottis.[25] Adjacent AVMs of the tongue or parapharyngeal space can compress the airway or hemorrhage requiring intervention. Intravascular embolization with or without surgery is the treatment of choice in these cases (**Fig. 9**).

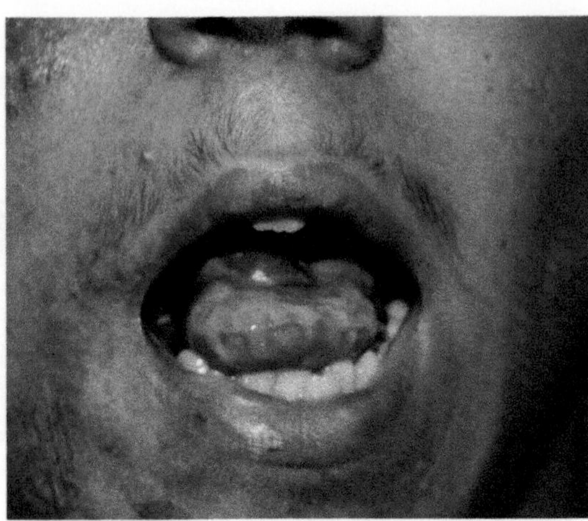

**Fig. 9.** Tongue and oral AVM in a young adult.

Surgical excision with or without preoperative embolization is recommended in select lesions.

Gingival hypertrophy is sometimes seen and usually indicates the presence of adjacent bony involvement, which is almost always treated with embolization.

## REFERENCES

1. Clarke C, Lee EI, Edmonds J Jr. Vascular anomalies and airway concerns. Semin Plast Surg 2014;28(2):104–10.
2. Waner M, Suen J. Treatment for the management of hemangiomas. Hemangiomas and vascular malformations of the head and neck. New York: Wiley-Liss; 1999. p. 234–9.
3. Durr ML, Meyer AK, Kezirian EJ, et al. Sleep-disordered breathing in pediatric head and neck vascular malformations. Laryngoscope 2017;127(9):2159–64.
4. Jolink F, van Steenwijk RP, van der Horst CM. Consider obstructive sleep apnea in patients with oropharyngeal vascular malformations. J Craniomaxillofac Surg 2015;43(10):1937–41.
5. O TM, Alexander RE, Lando T, et al. Segmental hemangiomas of the upper airway. Laryngoscope 2009;119(11):2242–7.
6. O TM, Rickert SM, Diallo AM, et al. Lymphatic malformations of the airway. Otolaryngol Head Neck Surg 2013;149:156–60.
7. Mychaliska GB, Bealer JF, Graf JL, et al. Operating on placental support: the ex utero intrapartum treatment procedure. J Pediatr Surg 1997;32(2):227–30 [discussion: 230–1].
8. Stefini S, Bazzana T, Smussi C, et al. EXIT (Ex utero Intrapartum Treatment) in lymphatic malformations of the head and neck: discussion of three cases and proposal of an EXIT-TTP (Team Time Procedure) list. Int J Pediatr Otorhinolaryngol 2012;76(1):20–7.
9. Otteson TD, Hackam DJ, Mandell DL. The ex utero intrapartum treatment (EXIT) procedure: new challenges. Arch Otolaryngol Head Neck Surg 2006;132(6):686–9.
10. Schwartz MZ, Silver H, Schulman S. Maintenance of the placental circulation to evaluate and treat an infant with massive head and neck hemangioma. J Pediatr Surg 1993;28(4):520–2.

11. De Serres LM, Sie KC, Richardson MA. Lymphatic malformations of the head and neck. A proposal for staging. Arch Otolaryngol Head Neck Surg 1995;121(5):577–82.
12. Alemi AS, Rosbe KW, Chan DK, et al. Airway response to sirolimus therapy for the treatment of complex pediatric lymphatic malformations. Int J Pediatr Otorhinolaryngol 2015;79(12):2466–9.
13. Lackner H, Karastaneva A, Schwinger W, et al. Sirolimus for the treatment of children with various complicated vascular anomalies. Eur J Pediatr 2015;174(12):1579–84.
14. Klosterman T, Tatum SA. Current surgical management of macroglossia. Curr Opin Otolaryngol Head Neck Surg 2015;23(4):302–8.
15. Oomen KP, Paramasivam S, Waner M, et al. Endoscopic transmucosal direct puncture sclerotherapy for management of airway vascular malformations. Laryngoscope 2016;126(1):205–11.
16. Bagrodia N, Defnet AM, Kandel JJ. Management of lymphatic malformations in children. Curr Opin Pediatr 2015;27(3):356–63.
17. Defnet AM, Bagrodia N, Hernandez SL, et al. Pediatric lymphatic malformations: evolving understanding and therapeutic options. Pediatr Surg Int 2016;32(5):425–33.
18. Azene E, Mitchell S, Radvany M, et al. Foamed bleomycin sclerosis of airway venous malformations: the role of interspecialty collaboration. Laryngoscope 2016;126(12):2726–32.
19. Waner M, Suen J. The treatment of vascular malformations. Hemangiomas and vascular malformations of the head and neck. New York: Wiley-LIss; 1999.
20. Glade RS, Buckmiller LM. CO laser resurfacing of intraoral lymphatic malformations: a 10-year experience. Int J Pediatr Otorhinolaryngol 2009;73(10):1358–61.
21. Venous Malformations of the Upper Aerodigestive Tract. O TM, Chung HY, Waner M. Poster presentation. International Society for the Study of Vascular Anomalies (ISSVA). June 16–19, Malmo, Sweden.
22. Brightman LA, Geronemus RG, Reddy KK. Laser treatment of port-wine stains. Clin Cosmet Investig Dermatol 2015;12(8):27–33 [review].
23. Houseman ND, Taylor GI, Pan WR. The angiosomes of the head and neck: anatomic study and clinical applications. Plast Reconstr Surg 2000;105(7):2287–313.
24. Mitchell EL, Taylor GI, Houseman ND, et al. The angiosome concept applied to arteriovenous malformations of the head and neck. Plast Reconstr Surg 2001;107(3):633–46.
25. Griffin AS, Gunasena R, Schaefer NR, et al. An unusual cause of dysphagia: a large expectorated arteriovenous malformation. Ochsner J 2015;15(2):203–5.

# Orthognathic Considerations of Vascular Malformations

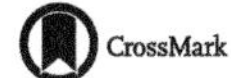

Luis Delgado, DMD[a], Avanti Verma, MD[b], Teresa M. O, MD, MArch[c], Stuart Super, DMD[a,*]

**KEYWORDS**

• Orthognathic • Skeletal abnormalities • Vascular malformations • Malocclusion • Open bite

**KEY POINTS**

- Vascular malformations affect the craniofacial skeleton in several ways, depending on the type of lesion and its location.
- Vascular malformations may remodel the mandible causing bony hypertrophy or thinning or expansion.
- Orthognathic abnormalities are addressed after the soft tissues are adequately debulked.

Congenital vascular lesions affect the craniofacial skeleton in several ways depending on the type of lesion and its location. Infantile hemangiomas (IHs), the most common congenital vascular lesions, rarely affect adjacent osseous structures.[1] Vascular malformations, on the other hand, may have either a direct or indirect effect on the adjacent bony skeleton.[2,3] All types of vascular malformations (lymphatic [LM, capillary [CM], venous [VM], or arteriovenous [AVM]) may present with bony changes[4,5] and cause functional and aesthetic concerns. Especially with regard to the lower third of the face, patients present with facial asymmetry, dental caries, and malocclusion, which contribute further to oral incompetence, speech intelligibility, and psychosocial concerns. Cervicofacial LMs, for example, are associated with characteristic structural abnormalities such as winging of the mandibular rami, widening of the gonial angles, and increased lower facial and mandibular anterior dentoalveolar height.[2] With

Disclosure: The authors have nothing they wish to disclose.
[a] Department of Oral and Maxillofacial Surgery, Lenox Hill Hospital, New York, NY, USA; [b] Department of Otolaryngology–Head and Neck Surgery, Vascular Birthmark Institute of New York, Manhattan Eye, Ear, and Throat Hospital, New York, NY, USA; [c] Department of Otolaryngology–Head and Neck Surgery, Vascular Birthmark Institute of New York, Facial Nerve Center, Manhattan Eye, Ear and Throat Hospital, 210 East 64th Street, 7 Floor, New York, NY 10065, USA
* Corresponding author. 30 East 60th Street Suite 1401, New York, NY 10022.
*E-mail address:* drstuartsuper@yahoo.com

Otolaryngol Clin N Am 51 (2018) 225–235
https://doi.org/10.1016/j.otc.2017.09.016
0030-6665/18/

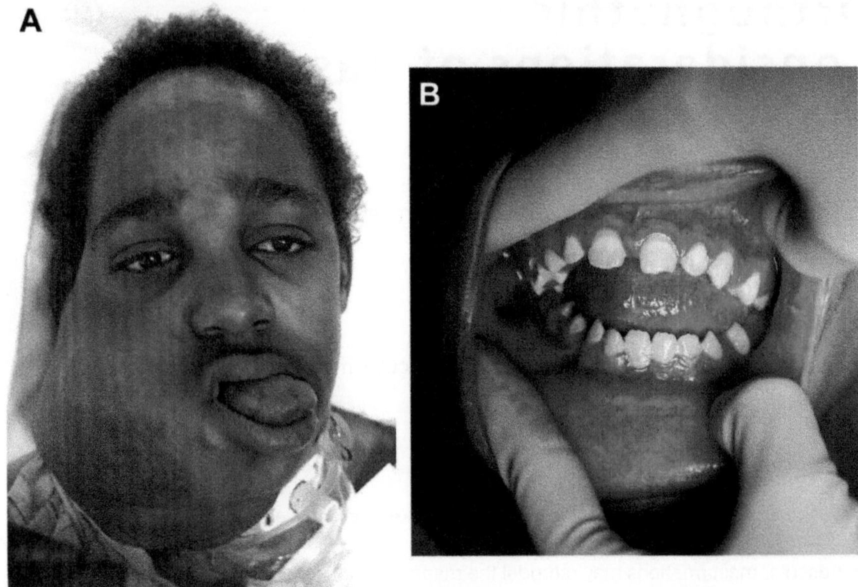


**Fig. 1.** 17-year-old patient with right cervicofacial venous malformation involving the premandible, oral cavity (tongue, floor of mouth), oropharynx and larynx. (*A*) Note macroglossia and open bite deformity. Patient also required a tracheotomy for advancing airway disease prior to treatment. (*B*) After tongue reduction.

regard to occlusion and mandibular displacement, there can be anterior displacement of the condyle in addition to class III occlusion and an anterior open bite deformity. These same findings are also seen in venous malformation (**Figs. 1–3**). Patients with untreated capillary malformations (CMs) may develop soft tissue hypertrophy, bony hypertrophy, and nodule formation in the distribution of the lesion[6] (**Fig. 4**). The maxilla and zygoma were noted to be hypertrophied in a case series of patients with Sturge-Weber syndrome in addition to facial soft tissue hypertrophy.[7] One patient had class II

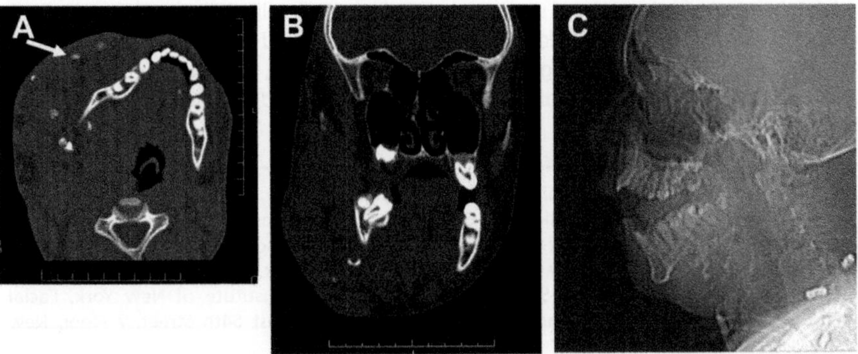


**Fig. 2.** (*A*) Axial CT image from patient in **Fig. 1** shows anterior displacement of the right mandibular body and ramus with bulky right premandibular, parotid, and parapharyngeal space disease. Radio-opaque lesions denote phleboliths (*arrow*). Airway is shifted to the left. (*B*) Coronal CT. Abnormal eruption of path of right molar medially into oral cavity. (*C*) Sagittal scout film shows anterior open bite deformity.

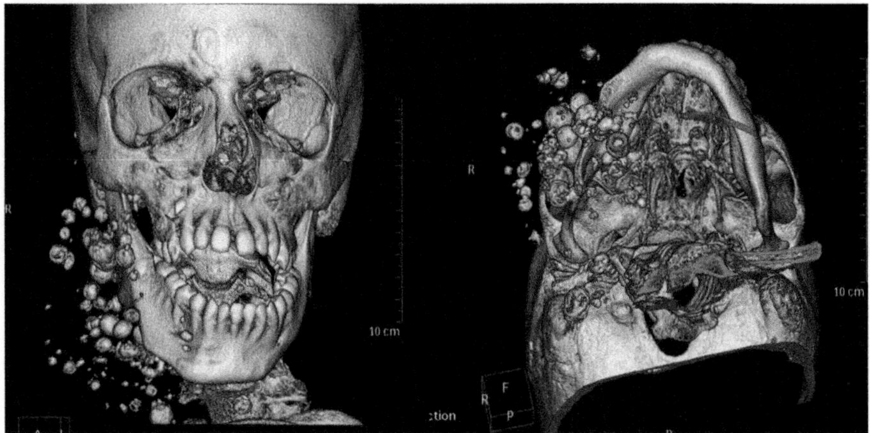


**Fig. 3.** Same patient with 3-dimensional CT showing skeletal abnormality with open bite and VM represented by phleboliths.

malocclusion caused by regional osseous overgrowth, while another had an anterior open bite deformity.

The etiology of osseous changes remains unclear at this time. One theory is that there is direct bony infiltration by the vascular malformation. For example, prior studies showed abnormal lymphatic channels in specimens of hypertrophied bone in patients with LM.[8] CMs caused by primary venous dysplasia can lead to focal venous hypertension, which may cause hypertrophy of adjacent bone.[7] Another possibility is the mass effect of adjacent soft tissues on skeletal growth. This is especially common with large LMs. The presence of a large mass of vascular malformation can mold bony growth, resulting in a misshapen facial skeleton. Lastly, with respect to CMs, the soft tissue overgrowth seen in some patients appears to be caused by a growth signal abnormality, which is present within the bony structures of the affected dermatome.

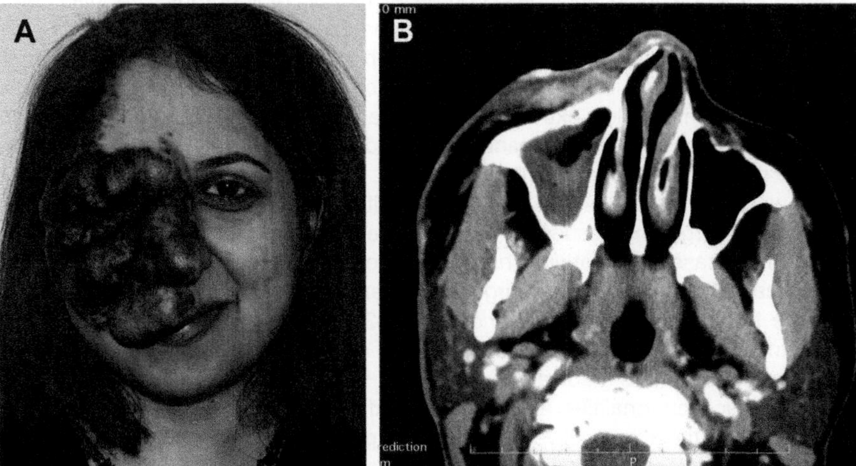


**Fig. 4.** (*A*) Right V1, V2 capillary malformation with extensive soft tissue hypertrophy. (*B*) Axial CT showing right maxillary bone hypertrophy with overlying soft tissue hypertrophy.

Although less than 1% of bony tumors are intraosseous vascular malformations,[1] direct bone involvement also causes orthognathic concerns. Patients often present with dental problems such as pain, tooth loss, and bleeding. As the vascular malformation infiltrates the alveolar bone, there is a loss of periodontal support, and finally exfoliation of the related dentition. Intraosseous vascular malformations are difficult to initially diagnose due to a varied radiographic appearance and may be confused with other lesions.[9,10] It is for this reason that patients may undergo a biopsy or tooth extraction for dental complaints, resulting in life-threatening bleeding in an outpatient setting.[11,12] Both a computed tomography (CT) scan and an MRI are necessary to evaluate the bone lesion. Venous malformations and arteriovenous malformations are associated with osteolytic changes. In some cases, the bone may be expanded, causing a contour deformity. Adjacent soft tissues may also be involved.

Depending on the type of vascular malformation and its location, treatment can include embolization, sclerotherapy, surgical resection, or a combination of these treatments. Intraosseous lesions may be addressed with embolization or with a resection, which may require reconstruction with a bone graft or osteomyocutaneous free flap.[13] Orthognathic abnormalities are typically corrected with surgery secondarily after the soft tissues have been treated.

## TREATMENT OF ORTHOGNATHIC ABNORMALITIES

Patients with malocclusion and widening or elongation of facial proportions require orthodontics and orthognathic surgery. Typically, this involves patients with lymphatic or venous malformation. The authors advocate for a multidisciplinary, multimodal approach to the treatment of skeletal abnormalities, including physicians from otolaryngology-head and neck surgery, oral and maxillofacial surgery, pediatric dentistry, and orthodontia.

In the past, the timing of orthognathic surgery was delayed until the adolescent years to accommodate eruption of the permanent teeth and because of concerns of damaging growth centers in the craniofacial skeleton (maxilla and mandible). The authors and others have previously argued the benefit of early intervention, with risk of some recidivism given the high social and functional cost of an open bite deformity.[2,14] Also of note is that the mandibular growth center is located at the condyle and not the ramus or body.

Preoperative planning includes complete dental radiographs, cephalometric studies, CT, and 3-dimensional medical and stereolithic modeling.

Presurgical orthodontics are a crucial first step to align the teeth. Next, the type of ostetomies will depend on the presentation. For example, a lone class III may be approached via intraoral or extraoral bilateral sagittal split osteotomies. If the difference is great, a combination of maneuvers to advance the maxilla and withdraw the mandible may be necessary.

Here, we present a case series of 3 patients with large-volume cervicofacial LM and associated orthognathic issues to demonstrate the principles of management for these difficult cases. All patients had macroglossia and were treated with tongue and cervical soft tissue reduction surgeries. Patients ranged in age from 11 to 17 years and were treated over a 2-year period (2014–2015). They presented unique challenges. In all 3 cases, medical modeling was obtained in order to preoperatively plan osteotomies on the medical model.

Orthognathic abnormalities are addressed after the soft tissues are adequately debulked. If not, the abnormal vector of skeletal growth will progress. Also, soft tissue overgrowth may mask any obvious bony changes. In some cases, further soft tissue reduction is performed at the time of orthognathic surgery. Two patients (11 years old) received presurgical orthodontic correction to align their teeth. A classic Le Fort

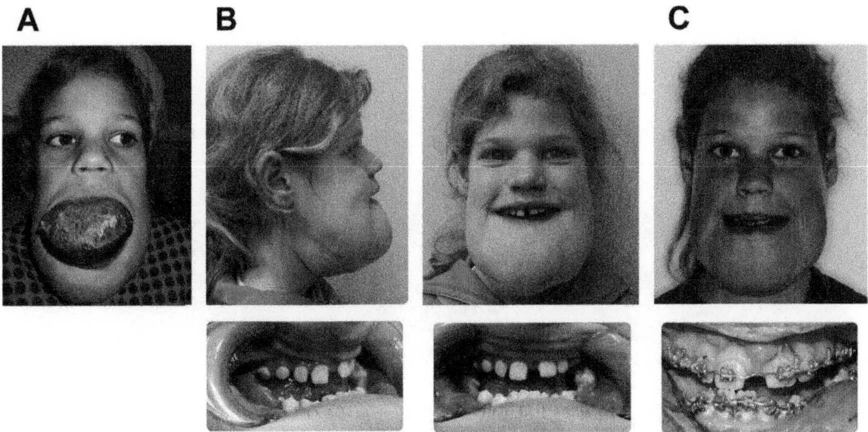


**Fig. 5.** Patient 1. 11-year-old girl with large cervicofacial LM with macroglossia, glossoptosis, open bite deformity, and class III malocclusion. (*A*) Before tongue reduction. (*B*) After tongue reduction showing class III open bite deformity. (*C*) After orthognathic procedure, patient undergoing elastic therapy. She will need further soft tissue surgery.

I osteotomy procedure via an intraoral approach was performed in all 3 patients. One patient required a nonvascularized bone graft for an inlay procedure to mobilize the maxilla anteroinferiorly. The procedures used overall were vertical ramus osteotomy (VRO), gonial angle osteotomy (GAO), or bilateral sagittal split osteomy (BSSO).

The first patient (Patient 1) is an 11-year-old girl who has had multiple premandibular and cervical excisions with dentofacial deformity and class III malocclusion. Airway evaluation showed a class I Mallampati scale and patent airway. She received preoperative orthodontics. Radiographic images and CT of the head and neck were obtained. Medical models and stereolithic models were then fabricated and used to plan the osteotomies.

A prophylactic tracheotomy was placed. Pre-existing cervical incisions were used to excise soft tissue LM and to access the mandible. A Le Fort I osteotomy was performed to advance the maxilla 4 to 5 mm (mm), and the mandible was recessed by 7 mm using bilateral vertical ramus osteotomies. Titanium (2.0 KLS martin) bone plates and 7.0 mm screws were placed through a Risdon approach. Dental elastics were used postoperatively, and orthodontics were continued. Once the swelling resolved, the tracheotomy was removed (**Figs. 5–8**).

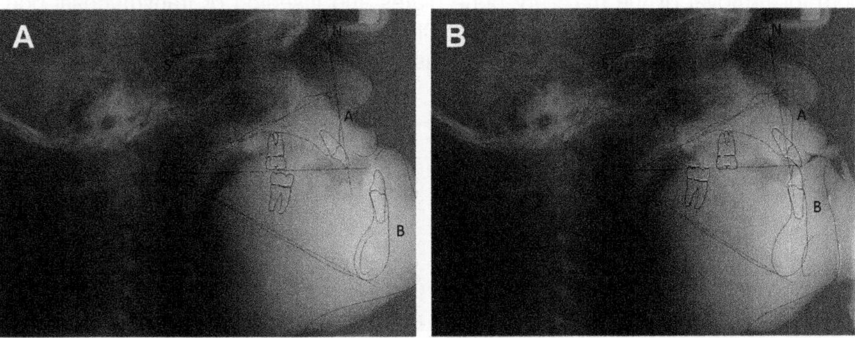


**Fig. 6.** Patient 1. (*A*) Cephalometric planning (patient 1) shows significant underbite or class III malocclusion. (*B*) Planned correction of malocclusion.

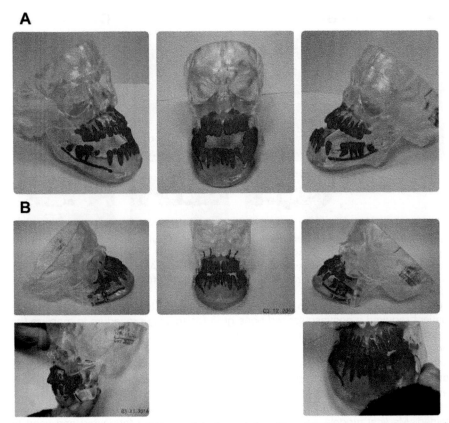

**Fig. 7.** Patient 1 - (*A*) Stereolithic models show deformities. (*B*) Planning osteotomies and plate placement.

The second patient (Patient 2) is an 11-year-old girl with anterior open bite deformity and malocclusion. She also received presurgical orthodontics. The patient had an existing tracheotomy secondary to base of tongue obstruction. A Le Fort I osteotomy was performed to position the mandible into a more anatomic and functionally acceptable position. Complete dental occlusion was not obtained secondary to dental decay and hypoplasia. One month postoperatively, the patient returned to the operating room for removal of the maxillary bone plates and insertion of transmucosal bone screws into the mandibular symphysis. Class III heavy elastics were placed, and distraction osteogenesis of the maxilla was used to correct the bite over a 4-week

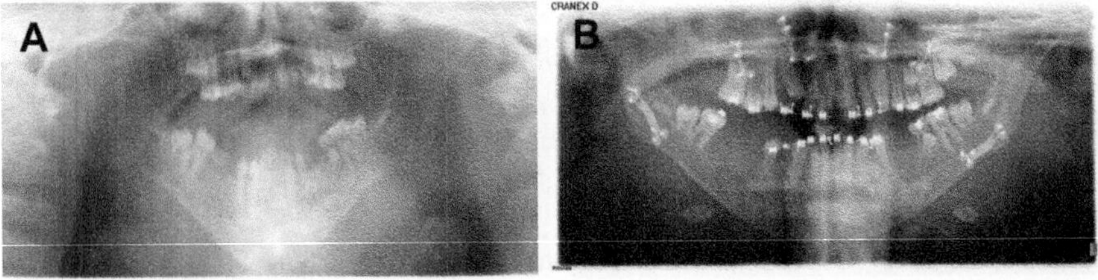


**Fig. 8.** Patient 1. (*A*) Preoperative panoramic radiograph. (*B*) Postoperatively with continued orthodontic treatment.

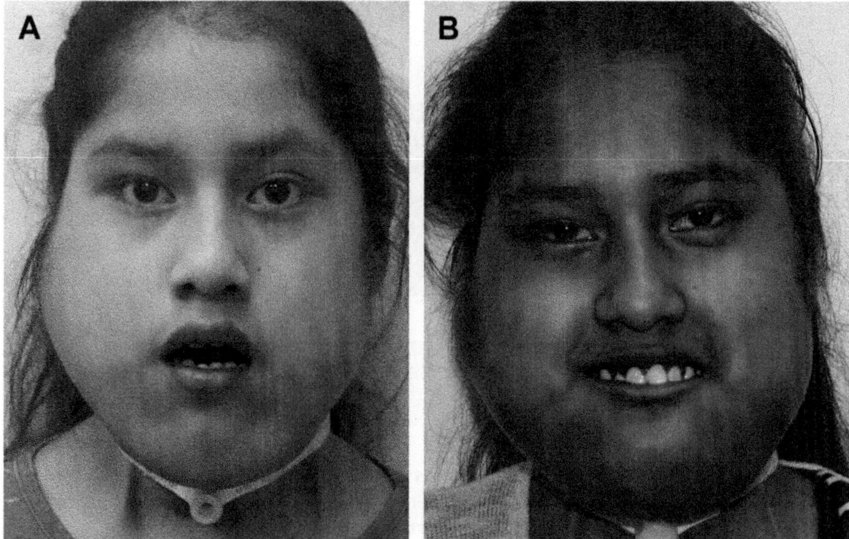

**Fig. 9.** Patient 2. (*A*) 11-year-old girl with cervicofacial LM and open bite deformity. (*B*) After orthognathic and dental restorative treatment. She requires further soft tissue debulking overlying bilateral mandible and sclerotherapy to the airway.

period. Elastics were used for a further 8 weeks to stabilize the dental occlusion. The patient returned for bony reduction of the menton with a bone rasp and bilateral osteotomies of the gonial angles and medial rotation of the splayed gonial angles (**Figs. 9–11**).

The third patient (Patient 3) is a 17-year-old boy with skeletal dentofacial deformity and class III malocclusion with anterior open bite deformity. The plan involved advancement and downward clockwise rotation of the maxilla with bone graft and setback and counterclockwise rotation of the mandible. A Le Fort I osteotomy with an interpositional nonvascularized anterior iliac crest bone graft was performed. Bilateral sagittal split osteotomy with intraoral and transcutaneous approaches was also

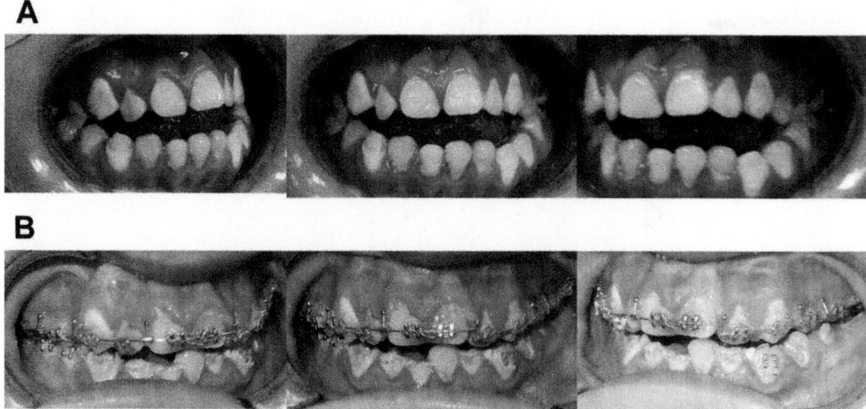

**Fig. 10.** Patient 2. (*A*) Open bite deformity. Note dental caries and evidence of prior restorative treatment. (*B*) After orthognathic surgery, with orthodontics. Underlying poor dental health is revealed.

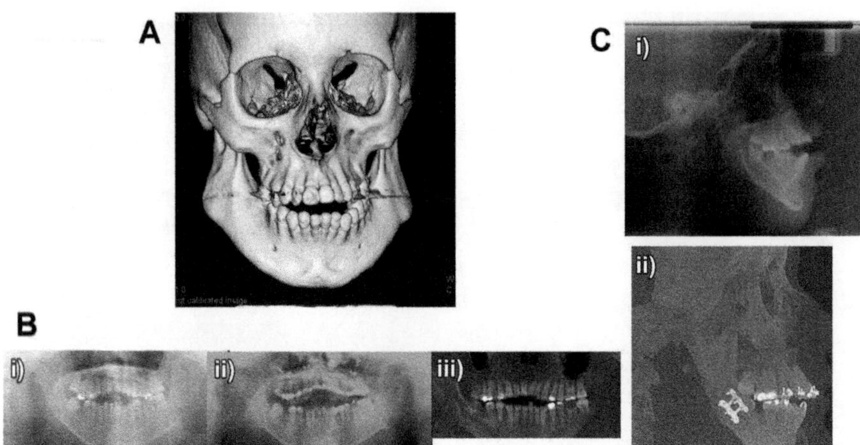


**Fig. 11.** Patient 2 - (*A*) 3dimensional CT shows outward winging of mandibular rami and open bite. (*B*) Panoramic radiographs i) preoperatively, ii) after LeFort I osteotomy, iii) after removal of maxillary plates, orthodontic adjustment. (*C*) Lateral radiographs. i) preoperatively, ii) after treatment with ongoing dental restoration.

performed. He also received tongue and soft tissue reduction surgery. His intraoperative course was complicated by a 2 L blood loss requiring multiple transfusions. He was then discharged after 5 days. The patient was nonadherent with postoperative elastic therapy and had some evidence of relapse after 3 months (**Figs. 12–15**).

In this small series, class III malocclusion was corrected in 3 patients. One patient partially relapsed after a short time secondary to nonadherence to

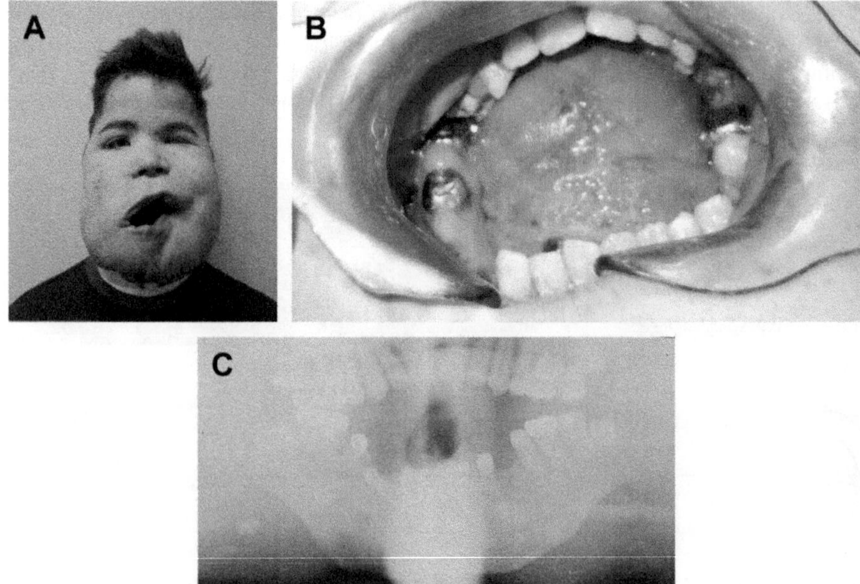


**Fig. 12.** Patient 3. (*A*) 17-year-old boy with bilateral cervicofacial LM and right flaccid facial paralysis. (*B*) Open bite deformity. (*C*) Panoramic radiograph.

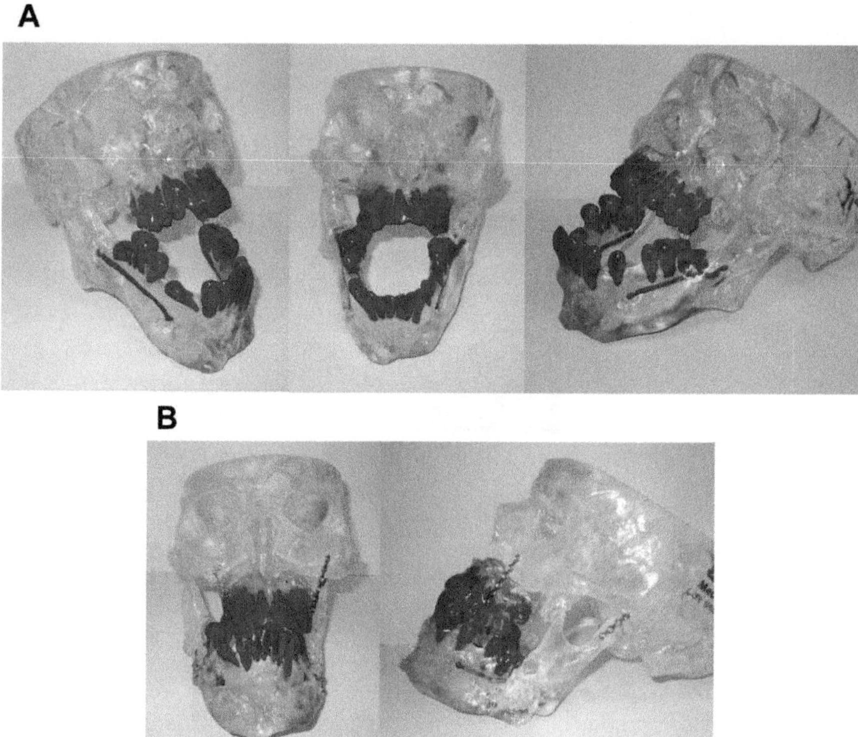


Fig. 13. Patient 3. (*A*) Stereolithic model views show class III occlusion, open bite, and abnormal eruption of dentition. (*B*) Planning osteotomies (Le Fort I with bone graft, bilateral sagittal split osteotomies, plates, and screws). 2.0 titanium plate with 7 mm screws.

postoperative elastic therapy as well as persistent soft tissue disease that was not fully treated on 1 side. He had a pre-existing unilateral flaccid facial paralysis since childhood deterring the family from agreeing to surgical debulking on the nonparalyzed side. Also, the main disfigurement was the mandible and not the

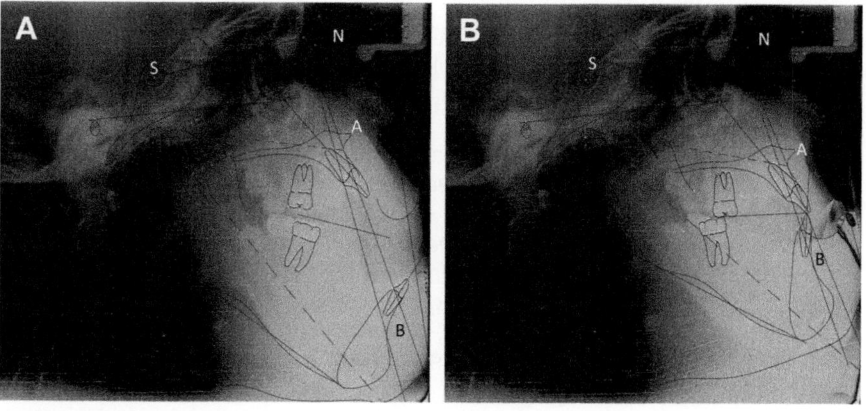


Fig. 14. Patient 3. Cephalometric measurements. (*A*) Class III and open bite. (*B*) Planned correction.

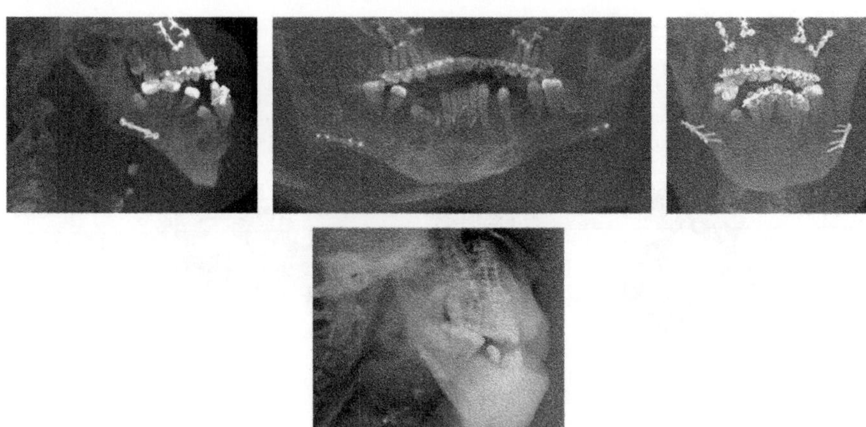

**Fig. 15.** Patient 3. Postoperative radiographs showing improvement in occlusion.

maxilla. This resulted in difficulty obtaining a stable result with the mandibular surgery. Intraoperatively, the cortex of the rams was noted to be exceptionally thinned and was not able to adequately seat the screws. Upon consideration, the anterior body of the mandible, may have been a better choice for osteotomies. This would have required mobilization of the inferior alveolar nerve. The excess bulk on the nonparalyzed side, may have also promoted the relapse.

In all cases, the reproducibility of the measurements was validated by retracing cephalometric landmarks by the senior oromaxillary facial surgeon (SS).

In summary, vascular malformations of all types may directly or indirectly involve the craniofacial skeletal. Open bite deformities and other orthognathic abnormalities lead to difficulties with speech, feeding, and social presentation. These issues can be addressed with a multidisciplinary team approach using careful planning, cephalometric studies, CT, and 3-dimensional medical and stereolithic modeling. Conventional osteotomies and orthognathic techniques may be used to correct these deformities, restore function, and improve appearance.

## REFERENCES

1. Aldridge E, Cunningham LL Jr, Gal TJ, et al. Intraosseous venous malformation of the mandible: a review on interdisciplinary differences in diagnostic nomenclature for vascular anomalies in bone and report of a case. J Oral Maxillofac Surg 2012;70(2):331–9.
2. O TM, Kwak R, Portnof JE, et al. Analysis of skeletal mandibular abnormalities associated with cervicofacial lymphatic malformations. Laryngoscope 2011; 121(1):91–101.
3. TM O. Mandible and dentition: site-specific considerations in vascular malformations. In: Perkins JA, BK. editors. Management of head and neck vascular anomalies. Springer International Publishing AG, in press.
4. Boyd JB, Mulliken JB, Kaban LB, et al. Skeletal changes associated with vascular malformations. Plast Reconstr Surg 1984;74(6):789–97.
5. Burke RM, Morin RJ, Perlyn CA, et al. Special considerations in vascular anomalies: operative management of craniofacial osseous lesions. Clin Plast Surg 2011;38(1):133–42.

6. Lee JW, Chung HY, Cerrati EW, et al. The natural history of soft tissue hypertrophy, bony hypertrophy, and nodule formation in patients with untreated head and neck capillary malformations. Dermatol Surg 2015;41(11):1241–5.
7. Yamaguchi K, Lonic D, Chen C, et al. Correction of facial deformity in Sturge-Weber Syndrome. Plast Reconstr Surg Glob Open 2016;4(8):e843.
8. Padwa BL, Hayward PG, Ferraro NF, et al. Cervicofacial lymphatic malformation: clinical course, surgical intervention, and pathogenesis of skeletal hypertrophy. Plast Reconstr Surg 1995;95(6):951–60.
9. Mulliken JB, Glowacki J. Hemangiomas and vascular malformations in infants and children: a classification based on endothelial characteristics. Plast Reconstr Surg 1982;69(3):412–22.
10. Kaban LB, Mulliken JB. Vascular anomalies of the maxillofacial region. J Oral Maxillofac Surg 1986;44(3):203–13.
11. Lemound J, Brachvogel P, Gotz F, et al. Treatment of mandibular high-flow vascular malformations: report of 2 cases. J Oral Maxillofac Surg 2011;69(7): 1956–66.
12. Hasnaoui N, Gerard E, Simon E, et al. Massive bleeding after a tooth extraction: diagnosis of unknown arteriovenous malformation of the mandible, a case report. Int J Surg Case Rep 2017;38:128–30.
13. Rashid M, Tamimy MS, Ehtesham-Ul-Haq, et al. Benign paediatric mandibular tumours: experience in reconstruction using vascularised fibula. J Plast Reconstr Aesthet Surg 2012;65(12):e325–31.
14. Osborne TE, Levin LS, Tilghman DM, et al. Surgical correction of mandibulofacial deformities secondary to large cervical cystic hygromas. J Oral Maxillofac Surg 1987;45(12):1015–21.

# Hereditary Hemorrhagic Telangiectasia

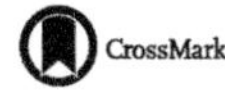

Thomas Kühnel, MD*, Kornelia Wirsching, MD, Walter Wohlgemuth, MD, Ajay Chavan, MD, Katja Evert, MD, Veronika Vielsmeier, MD

**KEYWORDS**

- Hereditary hemorrhagic telangiectasia • Dysplasias • Osler-Weber-Rendu syndrome
- Mucocutaneous lesions

**KEY POINTS**

- Hereditary hemorrhagic telangiectasia (HHT) describes the presenting manifestations of a disorder that is characterized by dilated blood vessels.
- HHT is inherited as an autosomal dominant trait with variable penetrance.
- The abnormal vascular structures (dysplasias) can affect all the organs in the human body.

## BASIC FACTS

Hereditary hemorrhagic telangiectasia (HHT) describes the presenting manifestations of a disorder that is characterized by dilated blood vessels. HHT is also known as Osler-Weber-Rendu syndrome (after the clinicians who first reported it) or as Osler's disease for short.

The characteristic defects in the vascular wall seen in HHT lead to a self-perpetuating process that results in the development of highly vulnerable lesions with extremely thin vessel walls.[1] Starting in the postcapillary vascular bed, the process escalates until it results ultimately in an arteriovenous shunt. HHT is inherited as an autosomal dominant trait with variable penetrance. The abnormal vascular structures (dysplasias) can affect all the organs in the human body. Almost all patients with HHT suffer from epistaxis; generally, this is the chief presenting symptom that prompts the initial diagnosis,[2] often commencing during the preschool years. The severity of epistaxis varies from just occasional minor bleeding to life-threatening blood loss necessitating repeated blood transfusions.

The development of nasal lesions and especially their tendency to bleed is triggered by the mechanical stresses generated by turbulent airflow.[3] The observation that

Disclosure Statement: T. Kühnel, K. Wirsching, W. Wohlgemuth, A. Chavan, and V. Vielsmeier have nothing they wish to disclose.
University of Regensburg, Franz-Josef-Strauss-Allee 11, D-93053 Regensburg, Germany
* Corresponding author. University of Regensburg, Department of ORL, Franz-Josef-Strauss-Allee 11, D-93053 Regensburg, Germany.
*E-mail address:* Thomas.Kuehnel@ukr.de

Otolaryngol Clin N Am 51 (2018) 237–254
https://doi.org/10.1016/j.otc.2017.09.017
oto.theclinics.com

mechanical trauma as well as ultraviolet light-generated stress can encourage the development of lesions raises important questions with regard to modern-day treatment options involving lasers and coagulation.[4,5] It is conceivable that the treatment itself may actually intensify the symptoms. Because 85% of patients report that their condition becomes more troublesome as they grow older, it is difficult to resolve these questions.[6] The methods of evidence-based medicine struggle to differentiate the natural course of HHT from iatrogenic factors related to treatment.

Mortality is higher in patients with organ manifestations,[7–10] but otherwise life expectancy is not reduced.[7,11,12] It has even been suggested that, owing to the changes in the angiogenic protein endoglin in patients with HHT, there may be survival benefits in terms of tumor progression in certain types of cancer. However, this has no effect on incidence.[13,14]

The quality of life of patients with HHT is routinely impaired to an appreciable degree.[15,16] The fact that HHT is a "rare disease" doubles the burden for patients. In most cases, the disorder is serious and patients almost invariably have to make the effort to seek out a specialist center to receive an appropriate diagnostic workup and therapy.[17] In many respects, orphan diseases such as HHT pose particular challenges to both patients and clinicians.

## *Prevalence*

The reported prevalence of HHT ranges between 1:5000 and 1:8000 in different regions.[2,3,18,19] HHT thus belongs in the category of rare diseases or orphan diseases; historically, these diseases have attracted only limited attention and they are still considered to be underdiagnosed compared with more common health problems. In more recent times, political and private initiatives have raised awareness levels, thereby promoting earlier diagnosis and more specific treatment.[18]

## *Etiology and Genetics*

HHT is inherited as an autosomal dominant trait. Currently, mutations of 5 different genes have been identified as causing the disease. Mutations in ENG (endoglin) on chromosome 9 encoding a defective endoglin lead to type 1 HHT (61%), and mutations in ACVRL1 (activin A receptor type II-like 1 gene) on chromosome 12 encoding ALK1 lead to type 2 HHT (37%). Both genes are membrane proteins that are important in modulating the signal pathway of transforming growth factor (TGF)-β. They are expressed on endothelial cells. A rarer condition is the combined form of juvenile polyposis with HHT in which there are mutations of MADH4 on chromosome 18 (2%). The gene responsible encodes proteins that modulate the signal pathway of the TGF-β superfamily and acts on vascular endothelial cells. It has been postulated that there are further genes located on chromosomes 5 and 7. The homozygous form of HHT leads to nonviable fetuses (homozygous lethality).[3] Subforms of primary pulmonary hypertension show a close genetic relationship with HHT.

Once a mutation has been identified in a family of patients with HHT, then specific screening for carriers of this trait can be performed among any children in the family who are still asymptomatic. This testing opens up the opportunity to diagnose clinically silent but complication-prone pulmonary arteriovenous malformations (pAVMs) and cerebral AVMs. In concrete terms, molecular genetic testing is carried out in a definitely confirmed case in the family. Screening is performed for the endoglin gene (ENG, HHT1), for activin A receptor type II–like 1 gene (ACVRL1, HHT2) and for mutations of the MADH4 gene on chromosome 18. Most patients have mutations of ENG or ACVRL1. However, further gene loci are known to exist and there is a high variability of mutations. The prevalence of SMAD4 mutations is approximately 20% in patients with juvenile polyposis and approximately 10% in patients with HHT. Overlap is observed in 2% of cases.[5,20] Even though this overlap syndrome occurs rarely in clinically diagnosed patients with HHT, it is of major importance. The risk of these patients developing bowel cancer should prompt appropriate diagnostic workup and therapy.

Two further gene loci have been identified on chromosomes 5 and 7. Nevertheless, one-fifth of families with HHT display none of the mutations responsible for the disease.[1]

All the proteins affected by these mutations modulate the signaling pathway of the TGF-β superfamily, and it is this pathway that regulates a number of cellular functions in angiogenesis (**Table 1**).[1]

### *Phenotype*

The lesions that result from the genetic mutations in HHT may range in size from very small (microvascular dilatations) to several centimeters in diameter (AVMs). They occur preferentially at certain locations in the circulation. Despite their different manifestations, telangiectases involving the nasal mucosa can be identified fairly reliably. A search for these lesions, therefore, constitutes a key element in the diagnostic workup. The endoscopic images in **Fig. 1** illustrate typical telangiectasias and their distribution in the nose.

**Table 1**
**Treatment regimens for HHT according to international guidelines**

| Clinical Manifestation | Frequency (%) | Other Symptoms | Measures |
|---|---|---|---|
| Epistaxis | 95 | Anemia, iron deficiency | Treatment of epistaxis: measures to humidify and protect the nasal mucosa, packing, laser therapy, coagulation, oral tranexamic acid, iron replacement, blood transfusions |
| Gastrointestinal bleeding | 20 | Anemia, iron deficiency | Argon plasma beam, embolization, blood transfusion, pharmacologic therapy |
| pAVMs | 50 | Right–left shunt, brain abscess, stroke, migraine | Embolization, prophylactic antibiotics during surgical and dental procedures, avoid scuba diving |
| Hepatic AVMs | 30 | Upper right quadrant pain postprandially, high-output cardiac failure, pulmonary hypertension, portal hypertension | Interventional therapy, surgery, with liver transplantation as a last resort |
| Central nervous AVMs (cerebral, spinal) | 10 | Headache, subarachnoid hemorrhage, stroke, gait abnormalities, and bladder dysfunction | Interventional or surgical therapy as agreed by a specialist interdisciplinary team |

*Abbreviations:* AVM, arteriovenous malformation; HHT, hereditary hemorrhagic telangiectasia; pAVM, pulmonary arteriovenous malformation.

*Data from* Faughnan ME, Palda VA, Garcia-Tsao G, et al. International guidelines for the diagnosis and management of hereditary haemorrhagic telangiectasia. J Med Genet 2011;48(2):73–87.

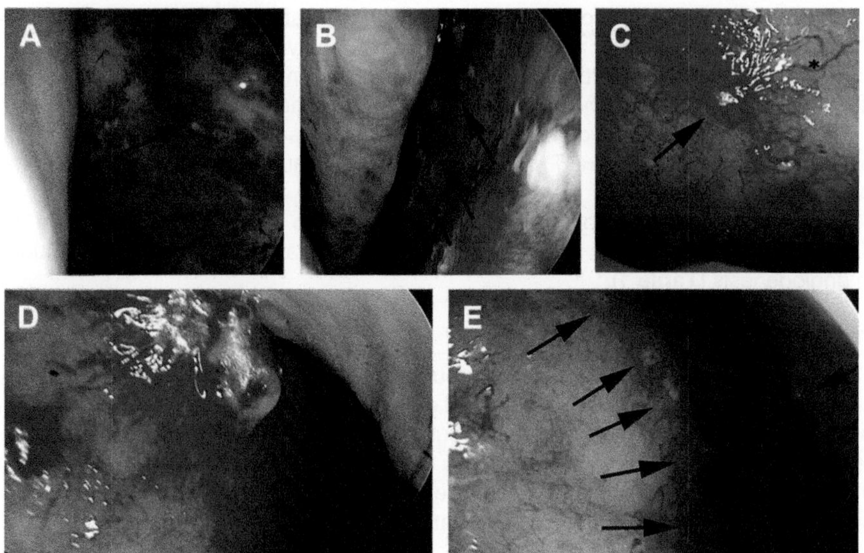


**Fig. 1.** Typical telangiectasias and their distribution in the nose. Arrows point to lesions of the nasal mucosa. (*A*) Septum at the level of the nasal valve. (*B*) Septum coresponding to the middle turbinate, inferior margin (*C*) Septum, Kiesselbach's region. (*D & E*) Lesions on opposite sites of the nasal valve, apex.

## DIAGNOSIS

Diagnosis is based primarily on clinical symptoms. Epistaxis; telangiectasias involving the perioral region, tongue, oral mucosa, and fingertips (**Figs. 2** and **3**); visceral involvement; and a positive family history are features that are straightforward to identify in adults. These findings permit a diagnosis to be made even without human genetic testing. The diagnostic criteria for HHT were named after the Consensus Conference in Curaçao (see **Table 1**). The diagnosis of HHT is definite if 3 or more criteria are satisfied. Where only 2 criteria are satisfied, there are grounds for suspecting HHT, even if the diagnosis cannot be made with certainty. In children, neither history taking nor physical examination necessarily yield conclusive evidence. A suspected diagnosis cannot, therefore, be discounted without exclusion on genetic

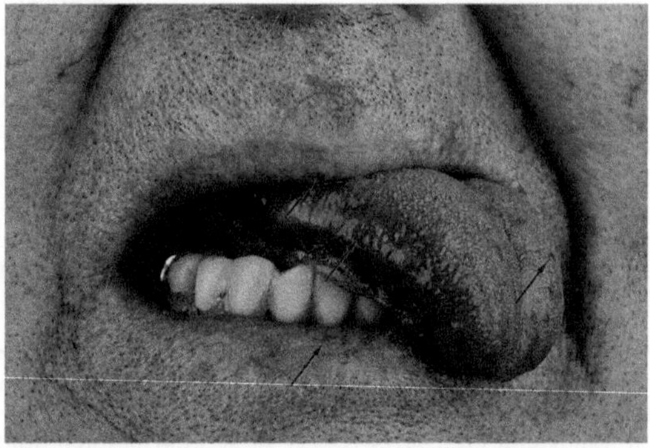

**Fig. 2.** Tongue epistaxis. Arrows point to Osler pits of the tongue and lips.

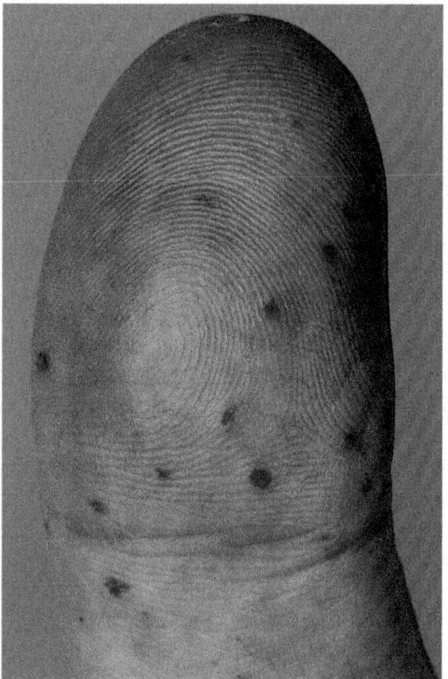

**Fig. 3.** Finger epistaxis.

grounds because further symptoms may emerge over the course of time.[2,21,22] The diagnosis should be regarded as "possible" if there is a positive family history.

Owing to the various manifestation sites including different organs, a multidisciplinary approach is necessary to detect all potentially dangerous manifestations and to achieve complete diagnosis and therapeutic interventions (**Table 2**).

Even today HHT is underdiagnosed and inadequate use is made of facilities for organ diagnosis in at-risk patients to exclude pulmonary, hepatic, and cerebral AVMs.[2]

HHT can occur with significant variation even within 1 family, with an uncomplicated clinical course in some family members alongside severe visceral complications in others.[23]

Hemorrhage is not an overt risk in the lungs and the liver where arteriovenous shunts are of major importance. Life-threatening complications (discussed elsewhere in this

**Table 2**
**Curaçao criteria for the diagnosis of HHT**

| | Symptom/Finding | Approximate Frequency (%) | Average Age at Onset (y) |
|---|---|---|---|
| 1 | Epistaxis, spontaneous and recurrent | 90–95 | 12 |
| 2 | Mucocutaneous telangiectasia: involving the fingertip pulps, lips, lingual or oral mucosa, nose | 90 | 30 |
| 3 | Visceral involvement (gastrointestinal, pulmonary, hepatic, central nervous system, spinal AVMs) | 20–80, 30–50, 32–48, 23 | ? |
| 4 | Positive family history in a first-degree relative | | |

If $\geq$3 are satisfied, the diagnosis of HHT may be considered definite; if 2 criteria are present, a suspected diagnosis of HHT must not be discounted.

*Abbreviations:* AVM, arteriovenous malformation; HHT, hereditary hemorrhagic telangiectasia.

article) occur and justify precautionary screening of the pulmonary, gastrointestinal, and central nervous systems. Even in cases where visceral manifestations remain asymptomatic, early diagnosis is the ideal and surveillance is indicated at the very least.

The patient should be recommended to undergo organ diagnosis ideally in facilities that are fully equipped to handle the special problems posed by HHT. Exclusion of pAVMs is a matter of paramount importance (**Table 3**).

## MUCOCUTANEOUS LESIONS OF THE NOSE AND EPISTAXIS

### *Diagnosis*

Epistaxis impairs patient quality of life in more than 90% of cases.[15,24] It is considered as the cardinal symptom of HHT and typically occurs earliest in life, often before puberty but almost always by the age of 40.[25] Telangiectasias increase from the third decade of life onward. Anterior rhinoscopy and endoscopy with a Hopkins telescope provide conclusive diagnostic evidence for the experienced examiner. A standard bleeding classification is key to promoting good communication between attending clinicians and also within the scientific community. The Epistaxis Severity Score proposed by Hoag and colleagues[26] has proved useful in this respect. Patients are recommended to keep a diary of nosebleeds to document the course of their condition and to adjust their treatment in light of any changes.

### *Therapy*

The modern therapy of epistaxis follows a stepped algorithm that takes individualized account of each patient's situation. Different treatment modalities are selected, depending on the severity of epistaxis and the impairment of lifestyle.[27]

#### *Care of nasal mucosa*

The first and most important step in therapy is for patients to care for their nasal mucosa. Protecting the nasal mucosa from drying out is the best way of preventing epistaxis. This measure can be achieved by daily application of creams, oils, splints, and hygroscopic sprays. Temporary nasal occlusion with adhesive plaster protects the nose against the mechanical trauma of airflow turbulence, and thus simulates the effect of Young's procedure.[28] In parallel, or if simple nasal mucosal care alone proves insufficient, tranexamic acid and *N*-acetylcysteine can be prescribed.

**Table 3**
**Cellular functions in angiogenesis**

| Type | Prevalence (%) | Mutation | Manifestations |
|---|---|---|---|
| 1 | 61 | Endoglin on chromosome 9 | Pulmonary and cerebral arteriovenous malformations (more common) |
| 2 | 37 | ACVRL1 on chromosome 12 | Hepatic arteriovenous malformations (more common) |
| Juvenile polyposis with hereditary hemorrhagic telangiectasia | 2 | MADH4 on chromosome 18 | |
| 3 and 4 | | 5q and 7p | |

#### *Pharmacologic management*

A reduction in epistaxis in patients with HHT was demonstrated in a randomized, double-blind, placebo-controlled, cross-over phase IIIB study conducted by Geisthoff and colleagues[29] to evaluate the efficacy of treatment with the antifibrinolytic agent tranexamic acid in an oral dose of 1 g 3 times daily. Tranexamic acid is currently the only medication approved specifically for use in HHT.[30] *N*-acetylcysteine 600 mg 3 times daily seems to reduce epistaxis, especially in male patients with type 1 HHT. This approach can be recommended because of the negligible adverse effect profile.[31]

#### *Lasers and coagulation*

The specialist literature describes numerous laser systems for coagulating nasal mucosal lesions with a minimum of inconvenience. There is unanimity that lasers designed primarily for cutting, such as focused $CO_2$ lasers, are unsuitable in this setting. The pulsed Nd:YAG laser (near infrared 1064 nm), the frequency-doubled Nd:YAG laser (potassium-titanyl-phosphate KTP, 532 nm), and diode lasers have proved particularly beneficial. Diode lasers cannot be pulsed and are, therefore, slightly less advantageous, but this drawback is offset by more ready availability owing to their low cost. High-flow shunts cannot be treated with lasers without causing mucosal damage. If it is evident that a lesion in the nose is more extensive than telangiectasia, we recommend coagulation with high-frequency alternating current, that is, bipolar radiofrequency.[28,32] The literature also contains reports concerning use of the argon plasma beam as a coagulation technique for lesions of the nasal mucosa.[33] This agent is an ionized noble gas that is used in visceral surgery to achieve hemostasis in parenchymal organs. Because argon plasma coagulation causes largely undefined surface sloughing of the nasal mucosa, the authors consider this technique to be unsuitable. Even if good hemostasis can be achieved, the mucosal damage seems in our opinion to be excessive. Lesions in the lateral nasal walls can assume large dimensions. Because the greater part of the malformation is not accessible from the nose and central ligation of a branch of the external carotid artery does not yield longer term success in such cases, open surgery may be indicated to resect the nidus. If these measures fail to produce success and the patient would be seriously harmed by the attendant blood loss and the number of banked blood transfusions required, treatment may be attempted with substances such as bevacizumab.

#### *Nasal packing*

Nasal packing is always necessary in cases where bleeding from the nose does not cease within a short time or if bleeding is so violent that a wait-and-see approach cannot be justified.[34] Given the wide range of packing materials available on the market, use should be restricted to those that, when removed, do not cause fresh damage to the sensitive vessels of the nasal mucosa. Smooth surface materials such as latex or polyethylene are available, and surface-treated nasal packings coated with hemostatic materials (eg, carboxymethyl cellulose) are a good option. We train our patients how to insert nasal packing themselves in an emergency. Pneumatic nasal packing has the advantage of applying pressure that is adapted to the individual anatomic situation.

### *Surgery and Invasive Measures*

Saunders' septal dermoplasty of the nose is a technique in which parts of the nasal septum showing the most numerous protruding HHT lesions are replaced with split skin (**Box 1**).[1] In Saunders' original description, anterior mucosal areas of the lateral

**Box 1**
**Surgery and invasive measures**

- Epistaxis is the most common symptom (>90%)
- Stepped treatment strategy
- Practice self-treatment
- Rule out other causes of epistaxis

nasal wall were also replaced by epidermis. Aside from surgical morbidity, the major disadvantages of the technique are its time-limited success in terms of bleeding and a tendency for the nose to become dry.[35–37]

In the case of branched high-flow lesions that seem to emanate from the lateral nasal wall and extend into the cheek, resection is the final option before surgical closure of the nose. Such lesions are poorly delineated and the nidus is virtually undefined.

Likewise, because of the risk of considerable pain, local necrosis and very limited duration of efficacy, ligation of the larger branches of the external carotid artery or embolization of the nasal vessels are not advisable treatment options and should be reserved for life-threatening emergencies.[38,39]

In terms of local measures involving the nose, permanent surgical closure of the external nasal cavities is the last resort.[40] This closure technique, known as Young's procedure, is simple to perform and does not inconvenience the patient. Even though this operation can be done under local anesthesia, we always opt for general anesthesia so that all options remain open if we need to respond to more major bleeding events.

After making a circumferential incision into the vestibular epidermis at the floor of the nose, the lateral nasal wall, and the columella, 3 epidermis flaps are mobilized from the inside outward and joined with absorbable interrupted mattress sutures.[27] We choose not to include the alar cartilage in the flaps so as not to compromise the outer shape of the nose. **Fig. 4** shows the 3 flaps and mattress sutures. Variations of Young's procedure have been reported and the success of treatment using a surgical technique involving just 2 flaps remains good with this simpler variant of the operation.[1,41]

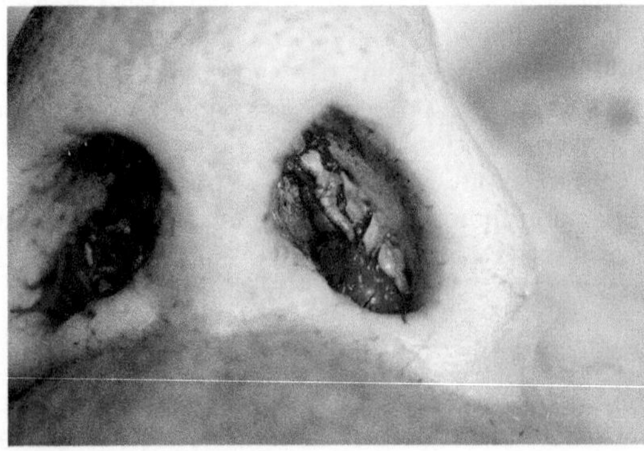

**Fig. 4.** Three flaps and mattress sutures.

## LESIONS OF THE GASTROINTESTINAL TRACT AND GASTROINTESTINAL BLEEDING

Gastrointestinal telangiectasias are found in some 80% of cases, and these lesions bleed in 15% to 30% of cases, predominantly in the second half of life (**Box 2**). Gastrointestinal symptoms reach their peak in the sixth decade of life.[2] Not uncommonly, repeated bleeding from the nose and gastrointestinal tract leads to anemia requiring blood transfusions. If discernible gastrointestinal bleeding occurs or if anemia cannot be accounted for by the severity of epistaxis, endoscopy is recommended. If lesions are detected in the stomach and duodenum, then further lesions can be assumed to be present in the more distal sections of the bowel. Lesions are coagulated with laser or the argon plasma beam, but the jejunum is not accessible to direct therapy. Where iron replacement and transfusions are insufficient to stabilize the patient's condition, recourse may be necessary to nonapproved medications such as bevacizumab. Patients with juvenile polyposis and HHT should undergo regular endoscopy because of the risk of malignant neoplastic disease.

## PULMONARY LESIONS

Pulmonary AVMs develop in 15% to 50% of patients with HHT during their lifetime (**Box 3**).[42–44] Their incidence is higher (85%) in type 1 patients with HHT. Dyspnea can be a prominent symptom in this setting, being noted in one-third of patients. The cause is generally a right–left shunt owing to pAVMs in the lung. The association of pAVMs and HHT is responsible for 80% to 90% of all cases of pAVMs. Pulmonary AVMs form a direct connection between the arterial and venous components of the pulmonary circulation. The shunt causes the capillary filter to be bypassed locally, with the result that emboli (paradoxic embolization) and septic particles may trigger a cerebral abscess (8%–19%) or stroke (10%–36%).[45] In advanced cases the shunt may lead to exertional dyspnea and cyanosis. In very rare cases rupture of the aneurysmal part of the pAVM can also result in massive bleeding. Consequently, pAVMs are the manifestations of HHT associated with the highest level of risk. Currently, the treatment of choice is transcatheter embolization, usually with coils or Amplatzer vascular plugs[46]. Pulmonary AVMs exceeding a certain size should be treated prophylactically to forestall intracerebral complications.[47] Pulmonary AVMs can be reliably occluded by embolization interventions. Cerebral abscesses can be avoided with good success in this way even though the risk cannot be eliminated entirely (**Fig. 5**).[47,48]

Pulmonary hypertension occurs more commonly in patients with HHT than random chance would dictate. Overlap has been identified between the genotype–phenotype of HHT and primary pulmonary hypertension.[49] Given the poor prognosis of pulmonary arterial hypertension, all patients with HHT should be screened by echocardiography.

**Box 2**
**Lesions of the gastrointestinal tract and gastrointestinal bleeding**

- Gastrointestinal bleeding starts late in life
- Often latent for long period
- If epistaxis insufficient to account for anemia, perform endoscopy of gastrointestinal tract
- Rule out juvenile polyposis syndrome

**Box 3**
**Pulmonary lesions**

- Most common dangerous complications
- Risk of septic emboli in brain and of stroke
- Good success possible with interventional therapy
- Rule out pulmonary arteriovenous malformations in asymptomatic children of parents with hereditary hemorrhagic telangiectasia

## HEPATIC LESIONS

Although symptomatic hepatic AVMs affect only a relatively small proportion of patients with HHT, their repercussions are generally very pronounced (**Box 4**, **Fig. 6**). The first clinical sign is usually upper right quadrant pain postprandially. Hepatic AVMs affect both hepatic lobes and are slowly progressive; they often also become hemodynamically relevant from the age of 40 to 50 years onward. Complications include biliary ischemia, portal vein hypertension, as well as fatal high-output cardiac failure. Routine investigations are performed using ultrasound examination; if liver laboratory variables are abnormal, then Doppler ultrasound imaging is also used. MRI and catheter angiography round off the diagnostic workup in cases where it is important to confirm the suspicion of clinically relevant shunts and to define the diagnosis more precisely. The treatment of choice consists of several staged sessions of interventional embolization therapy[50] (**Fig. 7**). In this alternative option to liver transplantation, branches of the right or left hepatic artery are embolized selectively. Improved treatment methods have brought marked reductions in complications.[51] However, liver transplantation does become necessary in isolated cases. The literature also contains increasing numbers of reports concerning the successful systemic administration of bevacizumab.[52,53]

## CEREBRAL AND SPINAL LESIONS

### *Cerebral Arteriovenous Malformations*

Endocranial manifestations occur as arteriovenous fistulas, small AVMs, micro-AVMs, capillary telangiectases, and cavernous malformations (**Box 5**). They are seen in 1% to 10% of patients with HHT irrespective of gender. Prevalence rates are apparently higher in patients with type 1 HHT (13.4%) than in those with type 2 HHT (2.4%). In 55.2% of cases, the AVMs were symptomatic.[54] Arteriovenous fistulas tend to be found exclusively in children. The risk of an arteriovenous fistula bleeding is extremely high.[55]

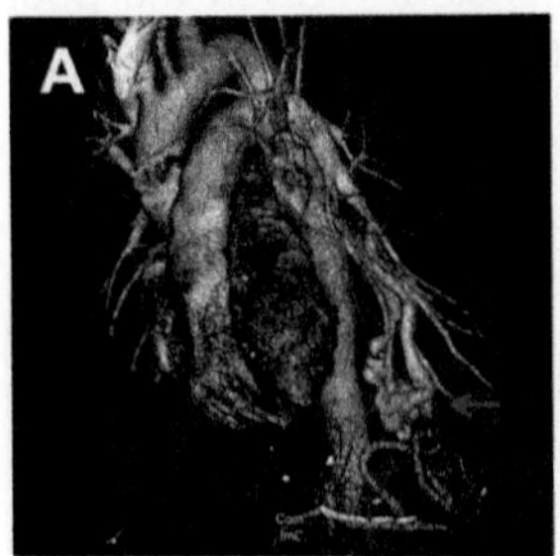

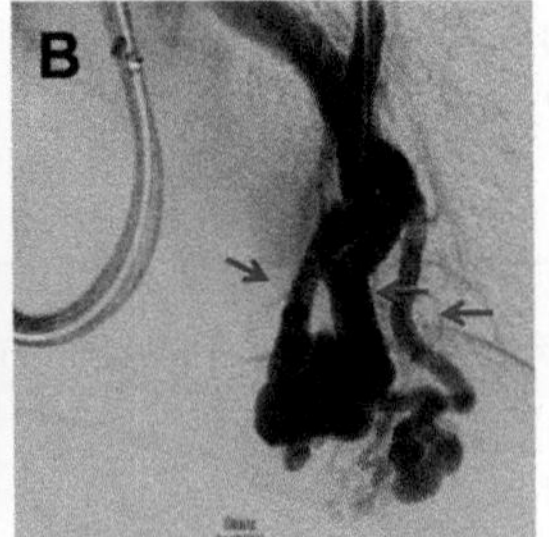

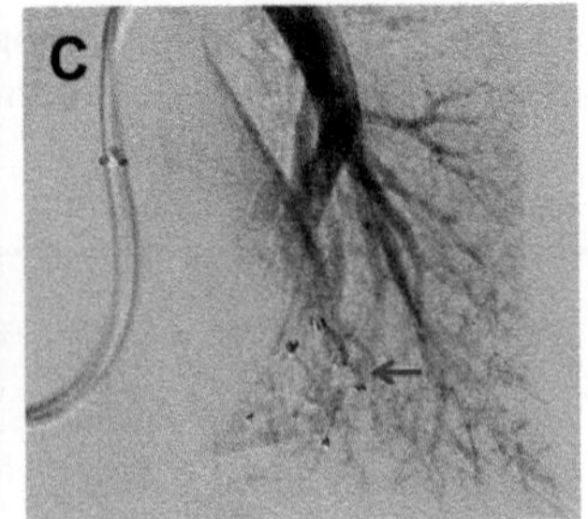


**Fig. 5.** Transcatheter embolization. (*A*) Arrow shows lesion in three dimensional aspect. (*B*) Angiographic detail of inflow and outflow of the lesion. (*C*) Postinterventional aspect. Arrow indicates embolization material.

**Box 4**
**Hepatic lesions**

- Postprandial upper right quadrant pain is often the first symptom
- Complications are rare
- Transcatheter embolization is the treatment of choice
- Liver transplantation is the last resort

Guidelines recommend cranial MRI to exclude cerebral AVMs.[2] When conducting informed consent discussions with patients, it should be borne in mind that both diagnostic catheter angiography and interventional therapy are associated with more than a minimal risk (6.5% event probability) and conversely that the probability of cerebral AVM bleeding (0.5% per year[56]) is low.[55]

### *Spinal Arteriovenous Malformations*

The sequelae of spinal AVMs are potentially serious. Such events are rare in the context of complications of HHT and manifest themselves as neurologic deficits such as paresis and paraplegia, stroke, or headache after subarachnoid hemorrhage. Treatment is currently endovascular in 80% of cases.[57]

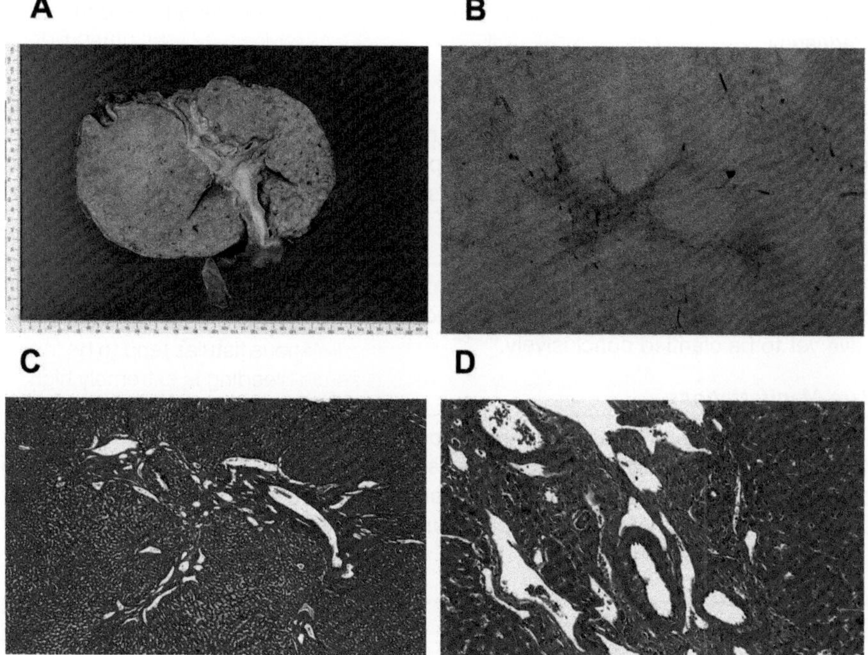


**Fig. 6.** Hepatic arteriovenous malformations. Liver of a patient suffering on HHT who underwent a liver transplantation. The liver shows dilatated vessels observable on cross sections (*A* and *B*). Corresponding slides show dilatated arteries and veins. (*A*) Organ specimen, overview. (*B*) low magnification. (*C*) (H&E, original magnification ×6.3) overview. (*D*) (H&E, original magnification ×26.9).

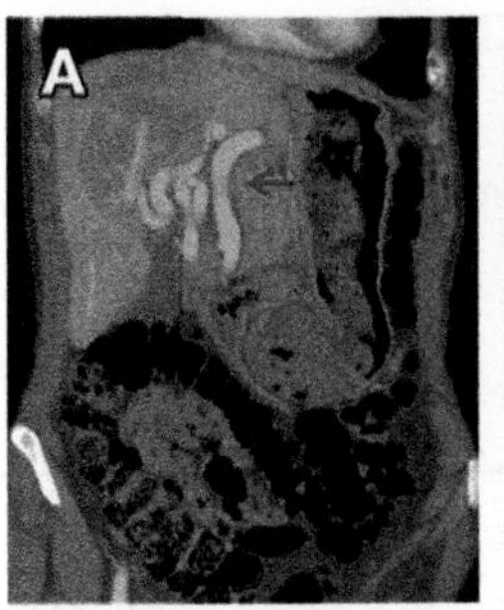

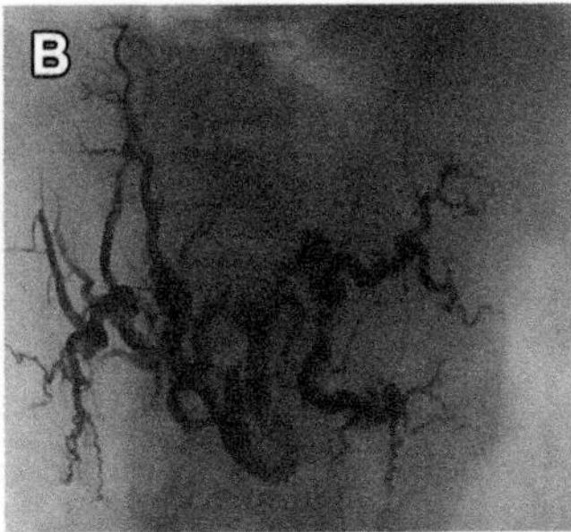

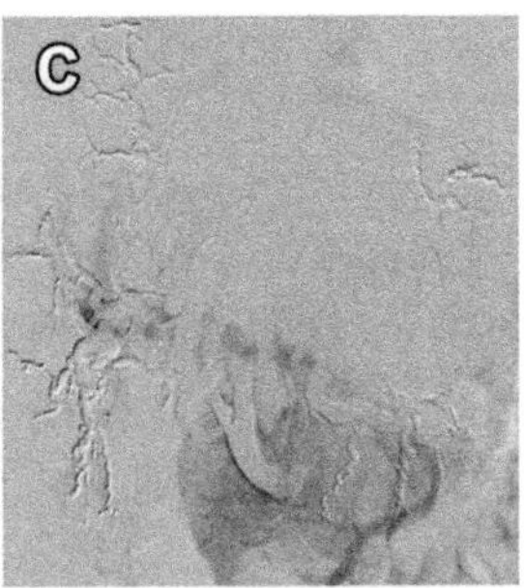


**Fig. 7.** Interventional embolization therapy. *(A)* Hepatic malformation, arrow points to high flow AV-shunt. *(B)* before embolization. *(C)* catheter angiography following therapy.

## OTHER ASPECTS OF DIAGNOSIS, COMPLICATIONS, AND RARE MANIFESTATIONS

### *Pregnancy*

Special caution is imperative in the management of pregnant women with HHT. Spinal AVMs must be excluded before giving epidural or spinal anesthesia. Miscarriages are reported in 20% of pregnancies, and the increased frequency of complications seems to be attributable to the hormonal changes occurring during pregnancy.[23,56] There seems to be an increased risk of complications during pregnancy, in particular of bleeding from pAVMs (1% of pregnancies), strokes (1.2% of pregnancies), and maternal death (1% of pregnancies).[58] Screening is, therefore, recommended before pregnancy.

### *Children*

Children in whom HHT has not yet become manifest as epistaxis may already be experiencing complications owing to high-flow pial arteriovenous fistulas and pAVMs. This circumstance justifies screening in at-risk settings.[59]

### *Immunodeficiency and Cancers*

Possible associations of HHT with elevated factor VIII levels, with immunologic deficiencies involving an increased tendency to infection, and with specific cancer types have yet to be clarified conclusively.[60–64]

### *Rare Manifestations*

Ocular manifestations occur very rarely in patients with HHT. In 1 study of 75 patients the prevalence of retinal telangiectasia was less than 1.3%.[65] An investigation in 106 patients with HHT demonstrated an increased prevalence of migraine (39.6%) compared with the control group (19.8%). Independent of the presence of pulmonary

**Box 5**
**Cerebral arteriovenous malformations**

- Diagnosis and therapy are topics of debate
- Complications of bleeding are usually catastrophic
- Diagnosis and treatment are the preserve of centers with specialist expertise

or cerebral shunts, it is speculated that dysfunction of TGF-β signal pathway and the resulting vascular changes contribute to the pathophysiology of increased migraine prevalence.[66] There have been occasional reports of hematuria that might be attributable to the presence of HHT.[67]

## CONTROVERSIES

### *Bevacizumab*

Pharmacologic therapy designed to inhibit angiogenesis is becoming increasingly important in HHT management, as evidenced by numerous publications and ongoing studies. The efficacy of systemic administration of bevacizumab as an antagonist of vascular endothelial growth factor has been confirmed for the treatment of HHT.[41,68,69]

Choosing the optimal dose has proved problematic and further investigations are required. One commonly used regimen uses 5 mg/kg bodyweight every 2 weeks for 6 courses.[53] It can be assumed that a dosage lower than that used for the approved indication in colon cancer displays adequate efficacy.[70] It should always be borne in mind that patients must be informed about off-label status and that the criteria for named patient use must be adhered to.

Topical therapy with bevacizumab offers the possibility of avoiding adverse effects while still acting on local plasma levels of vascular endothelial growth factor. Studies conducted to date do not justify any conclusive recommendation. Spray administration has not been effective.[71] Topical administration of bevacizumab, tranexamic acid, and estriol in comparison with placebo failed to demonstrate any efficacy for the selected bevacizumab dose and estriol.[41]

Encouraging results have been reported for submucosal injection. A retrospective analysis in 11 patients showed that intranasal submucosal injection of only 3.75 mg bevacizumab in conjunction with Nd:YAG laser therapy compared with laser therapy alone had a positive effect on patients' subjective experience and that hemoglobin levels also increased as an objective measure.[72]

### *Propranolol and Beta-Blockers*

Propranolol has become established as a therapeutic agent in the management of infantile hemangiomas and is now also being investigated in HHT because of its inhibitory effect on angiogenesis. It has been demonstrated in cell culture that cellular migration und tube formation are reduced in response to propranolol.[73] For beta-blockers, however, despite promising individual observations, there are no robust data concerning topical nasal application.[41,74]

### *Other Treatment Options*

Hormone therapy has a long tradition in the context of HHT therapy, with many case reports suggesting apparent efficacy for estradiol. However, high doses are required,[75] and adverse effects can be considerable. This form of treatment is not advocated for use in male patients in particular. Thalidomide may be effective but, owing to severe adverse effects, its use has not yet become widespread.

Patients also repeatedly inquire about alternative treatment methods. Even though these methods cannot be recommended on strict scientific grounds, they do carry a certain weight among self-help groups. Attempts are also being made to demonstrate their efficacy in clinical trials. One example is Ankaferd, a traditional mixture of various herbs from Anatolia that has been tested in the treatment of epistaxis and has demonstrated favorable efficacy in one particular study.[76] A similar situation applies with regard to recommendations on diet. No general rule can be inferred from the information available to date, but individual situations have been noted to improve in response to certain diets.

## UNRESOLVED QUESTIONS

Currently, it is not possible to define the topography of HHT lesions on mucous membranes with adequate precision. To document the fate of individual lesions over time would require millimeter accuracy.[77] Detailed mapping of individual lesions would establish whether a previously treated lesion in the nose or gut had recurred or whether the lesion in question was appearing for the first time.

The link between a physical stimulus and new lesion development has been established for mucosal trauma owing to nasal airflow turbulence, for ultraviolet exposure to the fingers, and for mechanical trauma to the dominant hand. The pressing question then is whether HHT treatment constitutes a stimulus that is sufficient to trigger new lesion development.

## REFERENCES

1. Rimmer J, Lund VJ. A modified technique for septodermoplasty in hereditary hemorrhagic telangiectasia. Laryngoscope 2014;124(1):67–9.
2. Faughnan ME, Palda VA, Garcia-Tsao G, et al. International guidelines for the diagnosis and management of hereditary haemorrhagic telangiectasia. J Med Genet 2011;48(2):73–87.
3. Govani FS, Shovlin CL. Hereditary haemorrhagic telangiectasia: a clinical and scientific review. Eur J Hum Genet 2009;17(7):860–71.
4. Geisthoff U, Maune S. Trauma can induce teleangiectases in patients with hereditary hemrhagic teleangiectasia. Hematol Rep 2011;3:s2.
5. Iyer NK, Burke CA, Leach BH, et al. SMAD4 mutation and the combined syndrome of juvenile polyposis syndrome and hereditary haemorrhagic telangiectasia. Thorax 2010;65(8):745–6.
6. Verkerk MM, Shovlin CL, Lund VJ. Silent threat? A retrospective study of screening practices for pulmonary arteriovenous malformations in patients with hereditary haemorrhagic telangiectasia. Rhinology 2012;50(3):277–83.
7. Kjeldsen AD, Vase P, Green A. Hereditary haemorrhagic telangiectasia: a population-based study of prevalence and mortality in Danish patients. J Intern Med 1999;245(1):31–9.
8. Moulinet T, Mohamed S, Deibener-Kaminsky J, et al. High prevalence of arterial aneurysms in hereditary hemorrhagic telangiectasia. Int J Cardiol 2014;176(3): 1414–6.
9. Trembath RC, Thomson JR, Machado RD, et al. Clinical and molecular genetic features of pulmonary hypertension in patients with hereditary hemorrhagic telangiectasia. N Engl J Med 2001;345(5):325–34.
10. Donaldson JW, McKeever TM, Hall IP, et al. Complications and mortality in hereditary hemorrhagic telangiectasia: a population-based study. Neurology 2015; 84(18):1886–93.
11. Rendu H. Èpistaxis répétées chez un sujet porteur de petits angiomes cutanés et muque. Gazettes des Hopitaux 1896;135:1322–3.
12. de Gussem EM, Edwards CP, Hosman AE, et al. Life expectancy of parents with hereditary haemorrhagic telangiectasia. Orphanet J Rare Dis 2016;11:46.
13. Duarte CW, Murray K, Lucas FL, et al. Improved survival outcomes in cancer patients with hereditary hemorrhagic telangiectasia. Cancer Epidemiol Biomarkers Prev 2014;23(1):117–25.

14. Duarte CW, Black AW, Lucas FL, et al. Cancer incidence in patients with hereditary hemorrhagic telangiectasia. J Cancer Res Clin Oncol 2017;143(2):209–14.
15. Lennox PA, Hitchings AE, Lund VJ, et al. The SF-36 health status questionnaire in assessing patients with epistaxis secondary to hereditary hemorrhagic telangiectasia. Am J Rhinol 2005;19(1):71–4.
16. Geisthoff UW, Heckmann K, D'Amelio R, et al. Health-related quality of life in hereditary hemorrhagic telangiectasia. Otolaryngol Head Neck Surg 2007;136(5): 726–33 [discussion: 34–5].
17. Kuehnel T. Morbus osler - erkrankung. Forum Sanitas 2014;(3):26ff.
18. Latino GA, Brown D, Glazier RH, et al. Targeting under-diagnosis in hereditary hemorrhagic telangiectasia: a model approach for rare diseases? Orphanet J Rare Dis 2014;9:115.
19. Donaldson JW, McKeever TM, Hall IP, et al. The UK prevalence of hereditary haemorrhagic telangiectasia and its association with sex, socioeconomic status and region of residence: a population-based study. Thorax 2014;69(2):161–7.
20. Gallione CJ, Repetto GM, Legius E, et al. A combined syndrome of juvenile polyposis and hereditary haemorrhagic telangiectasia associated with mutations in MADH4 (SMAD4). Lancet 2004;363(9412):852–9.
21. Shovlin CL, Guttmacher AE, Buscarini E, et al. Diagnostic criteria for hereditary hemorrhagic telangiectasia (Rendu-Osler-Weber syndrome). Am J Med Genet 2000;91(1):66–7.
22. Morgan T, McDonald J, Anderson C, et al. Intracranial hemorrhage in infants and children with hereditary hemorrhagic telangiectasia (Osler-Weber-Rendu syndrome). Pediatrics 2002;109(1):E12.
23. Shovlin CL, Winstock AR, Peters AM, et al. Medical complications of pregnancy in hereditary haemorrhagic telangiectasia. QJM 1995;88(12):879–87.
24. Geirdal AO, Dheyauldeen S, Bachmann-Harildstad G, et al. Quality of life in patients with hereditary hemorrhagic telangiectasia in Norway: a population based study. Am J Med Genet A 2012;158A(6):1269–78.
25. Begbie ME, Wallace GM, Shovlin CL. Hereditary haemorrhagic telangiectasia (Osler-Weber-Rendu syndrome): a view from the 21st century. Postgrad Med J 2003;79(927):18–24.
26. Hoag JB, Terry P, Mitchell S, et al. An epistaxis severity score for hereditary hemorrhagic telangiectasia. Laryngoscope 2010;120(4):838–43.
27. Lund VJ, Howard DJ. A treatment algorithm for the management of epistaxis in hereditary hemorrhagic telangiectasia. Am J Rhinol 1999;13(4):319–22.
28. Wirsching KE, Kuhnel TS. Update on clinical strategies in hereditary hemorrhagic telangiectasia from an ENT point of view. Clin Exp Otorhinolaryngol 2017;10(2): 153–7.
29. Geisthoff UW, Seyfert UT, Kubler M, et al. Treatment of epistaxis in hereditary hemorrhagic telangiectasia with tranexamic acid - a double-blind placebo-controlled cross-over phase IIIB study. Thromb Res 2014;134(3):565–71.
30. Gaillard S, Dupuis-Girod S, Boutitie F, et al. Tranexamic acid for epistaxis in hereditary hemorrhagic telangiectasia patients: a European cross-over controlled trial in a rare disease. J Thromb Haemost 2014;12(9):1494–502.
31. de Gussem EM, Snijder RJ, Disch FJ, et al. The effect of N-acetylcysteine on epistaxis and quality of life in patients with HHT: a pilot study. Rhinology 2009; 47(1):85–8.
32. Kühnel T, Wagner B, Schurr C, et al. Clinical strategy in hereditary hemorrhagic telangiectasia. Am J Rhinol 2005;19(5):508–13.

33. Pagella F, Matti E, Chu F, et al. Argon plasma coagulation is an effective treatment for hereditary hemorrhagic telangiectasia patients with severe nosebleeds. Acta Otolaryngol 2013;133(2):174–80.
34. Sautter NB, Smith TL. Treatment of hereditary hemorrhagic telangiectasia-related epistaxis. Otolaryngol Clin North Am 2016;49(3):639–54.
35. Levine CG, Ross DA, Henderson KJ, et al. Long-term complications of septal dermoplasty in patients with hereditary hemorrhagic telangiectasia. Otolaryngol Head Neck Surg 2008;138(6):721–4.
36. Fiorella ML, Ross D, Henderson KJ, et al. Outcome of septal dermoplasty in patients with hereditary hemorrhagic telangiectasia. Laryngoscope 2005;115(2): 301–5.
37. Saunders WH. Hereditary hemorrhagic telangiectasia. control of nosebleeds by septal dermoplasty. JAMA 1960;174:1972–4.
38. Fischer M, Dietrich U, Labisch C, et al. Critical evaluation of vascular embolization in patients with Rendu-Osler disease. Laryngorhinootologie 1997;76(8):490–4 [in German].
39. Elden L, Montanera W, Terbrugge K, et al. Angiographic embolization for the treatment of epistaxis: a review of 108 cases. Otolaryngol Head Neck Surg 1994;111(1):44–50.
40. Lund VJ, Howard DJ. Closure of the nasal cavities in the treatment of refractory hereditary haemorrhagic teleangiectasia. J Laryngol Otol 1996;(111):30–3.
41. Arthur H, Geisthoff U, Gossage JR, et al. Executive summary of the 11th HHT international scientific conference. Angiogenesis 2015;18(4):511–24.
42. van Gent MW, Post MC, Snijder RJ, et al. Real prevalence of pulmonary right-to-left shunt according to genotype in patients with hereditary hemorrhagic telangiectasia: a transthoracic contrast echocardiography study. Chest 2010;138(4): 833–9.
43. Blivet S, Cobarzan D, Beauchet A, et al. Impact of pulmonary arteriovenous malformations on respiratory-related quality of life in patients with hereditary haemorrhagic telangiectasia. PLoS One 2014;9(3):e90937.
44. Shovlin CL, Chamali B, Santhirapala V, et al. Ischaemic strokes in patients with pulmonary arteriovenous malformations and hereditary hemorrhagic telangiectasia: associations with iron deficiency and platelets. PLoS One 2014;9(2):e88812.
45. Faughnan ME, Granton JT, Young LH. The pulmonary vascular complications of hereditary haemorrhagic telangiectasia. Eur Respir J 2009;33(5):1186–94.
46. Tau N, Atar E, Mei-Zahav M, et al. Amplatzer vascular plugs versus coils for embolization of pulmonary arteriovenous malformations in patients with hereditary hemorrhagic telangiectasia. Cardiovasc Intervent Radiol 2016;39(8):1110–4.
47. Gallitelli M, Lepore V, Pasculli G, et al. Brain abscess: a need to screen for pulmonary arteriovenous malformations. Neuroepidemiology 2005;24(1–2):76–8.
48. Shovlin CL, Letarte M. Hereditary haemorrhagic telangiectasia and pulmonary arteriovenous malformations: issues in clinical management and review of pathogenic mechanisms. Thorax 1999;54(8):714–29.
49. Vorselaars VM, Velthuis S, Snijder RJ, et al. Pulmonary hypertension in hereditary haemorrhagic telangiectasia. World J Cardiol 2015;7(5):230–7.
50. Chavan A, Caselitz M, Gratz KF, et al. Hepatic artery embolization for treatment of patients with hereditary hemorrhagic telangiectasia and symptomatic hepatic vascular malformations. Eur Radiol 2004;14(11):2079–85.
51. Chavan A, Luthe L, Gebel M, et al. Complications and clinical outcome of hepatic artery embolisation in patients with hereditary haemorrhagic telangiectasia. Eur Radiol 2013;23(4):951–7.

52. Chavan A, Schumann-Binarsch S, Luthe L, et al. Systemic therapy with bevacizumab in patients with hereditary hemorrhagic telangiectasia (HHT). VASA Z Gefasskrankheiten 2013;42(2):106–10.
53. Dupuis-Girod S, Ginon I, Saurin JC, et al. Bevacizumab in patients with hereditary hemorrhagic telangiectasia and severe hepatic vascular malformations and high cardiac output. JAMA 2012;307(9):948–55.
54. Brinjikji W, Iyer VN, Wood CP, et al. Prevalence and characteristics of brain arteriovenous malformations in hereditary hemorrhagic telangiectasia: a systematic review and meta-analysis. J Neurosurg 2017;127(2):302–10.
55. Krings T, Chng SM, Ozanne A, et al. Hereditary hemorrhagic telangiectasia in children: endovascular treatment of neurovascular malformations: results in 31 patients. Neuroradiology 2005;47(12):946–54.
56. de Gussem EM, Lausman AY, Beder AJ, et al. Outcomes of pregnancy in women with hereditary hemorrhagic telangiectasia. Obstet Gynecol 2014;123(3):514–20.
57. Brinjikji W, Nasr DM, Cloft HJ, et al. Spinal arteriovenous fistulae in patients with hereditary hemorrhagic telangiectasia: a case report and systematic review of the literature. Interv Neuroradiol 2016;22(3):354–61.
58. Shovlin CL, Sodhi V, McCarthy A, et al. Estimates of maternal risks of pregnancy for women with hereditary haemorrhagic telangiectasia (Osler-Weber-Rendu syndrome): suggested approach for obstetric services. BJOG 2008;115(9):1108–15.
59. Mont'Alverne F, Musacchio M, Tolentino V, et al. Giant spinal perimedullary fistula in hereditary haemorrhagic telangiectasia: diagnosis, endovascular treatment and review of the literature. Neuroradiology 2003;45(11):830–6.
60. Shovlin CL, Sulaiman NL, Govani FS, et al. Elevated factor VIII in hereditary haemorrhagic telangiectasia (HHT): association with venous thromboembolism. Thromb Haemost 2007;98(5):1031–9.
61. Cirulli A, Loria MP, Dambra P, et al. Patients with hereditary hemorrhagic telangectasia (HHT) exhibit a deficit of polymorphonuclear cell and monocyte oxidative burst and phagocytosis: a possible correlation with altered adaptive immune responsiveness in HHT. Curr Pharm Des 2006;12(10):1209–15.
62. Dupuis-Girod S, Giraud S, Decullier E, et al. Hemorrhagic hereditary telangiectasia (Rendu-Osler disease) and infectious diseases: an underestimated association. Clin Infect Dis 2007;44(6):841–5.
63. Guilhem A, Malcus C, Clarivet B, et al. Immunological abnormalities associated with hereditary haemorrhagic telangiectasia. J Intern Med 2013;274(4):351–62.
64. Hosman AE, Devlin HL, Silva BM, et al. Specific cancer rates may differ in patients with hereditary haemorrhagic telangiectasia compared to controls. Orphanet J Rare Dis 2013;8:195.
65. Geisthoff UW, Hille K, Ruprecht KW, et al. Prevalence of ocular manifestations in hereditary hemorrhagic telangiectasia. Graefes Arch Clin Exp Ophthalmol 2007; 245(8):1141–4.
66. Marziniak M, Jung A, Guralnik V, et al. An association of migraine with hereditary haemorrhagic telangiectasia independently of pulmonary right-to-left shunts. Cephalalgia 2009;29(1):76–81.
67. Di Gennaro L, Ramunni A, Suppressa P, et al. Asymptomatic microhematuria: an indication of hereditary hemorrhagic telangiectasia? J Urol 2005;173(1):106–9.
68. Ou G, Galorport C, Enns R. Bevacizumab and gastrointestinal bleeding in hereditary hemorrhagic telangiectasia. World J Gastrointest Surg 2016;8(12):792–5.
69. Arizmendez NP, Rudmik L, Poetker DM. Intravenous bevacizumab for complications of hereditary hemorrhagic telangiectasia: a review of the literature. Int Forum Allergy Rhinol 2015;5(11):1042–7.

70. Wee JW, Jeon YW, Eun JY, et al. Hereditary hemorrhagic telangiectasia treated with low dose intravenous bevacizumab. Blood Res 2014;49(3):192–5.
71. Riss D, Burian M, Wolf A, et al. Intranasal submucosal bevacizumab for epistaxis in hereditary hemorrhagic telangiectasia: a double-blind, randomized, placebo-controlled trial. Head Neck 2015;37(6):783–7.
72. Rohrmeier C, Sachs HG, Kuehnel TS. A retrospective analysis of low dose, intranasal injected bevacizumab (Avastin) in hereditary haemorrhagic telangiectasia. Eur Arch Otorhinolaryngol 2012;269(2):531–6.
73. Albinana V, Recio-Poveda L, Zarrabeitia R, et al. Propranolol as antiangiogenic candidate for the therapy of hereditary haemorrhagic telangiectasia. Thromb Haemost 2012;108(1):41–53.
74. Ichimura K, Kikuchi H, Imayoshi S, et al. Topical application of timolol decreases the severity and frequency of epistaxis in patients who have previously undergone nasal dermoplasty for hereditary hemorrhagic telangiectasia. Auris Nasus Larynx 2016;43(4):429–32.
75. Jameson JJ, Cave DR. Hormonal and antihormonal therapy for epistaxis in hereditary hemorrhagic telangiectasia. Laryngoscope 2004;114(4):705–9.
76. Beyazit Y, Kurt M, Kekilli M, et al. Evaluation of hemostatic effects of Ankaferd as an alternative medicine. Altern Med Rev 2010;15(4):329–36.
77. Mahoney EJ, Shapshay SM. New classification of nasal vasculature patterns in hereditary hemorrhagic telangiectasia. Am J Rhinol 2006;20(1):87–90.

# Acquired Vascular Tumors of the Head and Neck

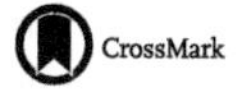

Mark Persky, MD, Theresa Tran, MD*

**KEYWORDS**

- Paraganglioma • Carotid body tumor • Glomus jugulare tumor • Glomus vagale
- Juvenile nasopharyngeal angiofibroma • Hemangiopericytoma

**KEY POINTS**

- Acquired head and neck vascular tumors are rare and account for less than 5% of head and neck neoplasms.
- Management of head and neck paragangliomas has evolved from primarily surgical to more conservative treatment consisting of observation and nonsurgical therapy.
- The mainstay treatment of juvenile nasopharyngeal angiofibroma and hemangiopericytoma is surgery, with radiation reserved for adjuvant therapy and recurrent tumors.

## INTRODUCTION

Vascular tumors of the head and neck consist of a diverse group of both benign and malignant neoplasms, many of which arise in close association with blood vessels or tissues. Head and neck vascular tumors are exceedingly rare, with each type accounting for no more than 0.5% of head and neck neoplasms. Although varying greatly in biologic behavior, with exceptions of a few, most of these tumors are similar in their indolent growth and tendency for local recurrence.

Vascular neoplasms of the head and neck present with a wide spectrum of signs and symptoms. Patients usually complain of nonspecific symptoms, which often have been present for a prolonged period of time. Diagnosis, therefore, requires a high index of suspicion and is usually made after these tumors are large enough to be visually apparent or cause symptoms. This article discusses the most common acquired benign and malignant vascular tumors, with an emphasis on their evaluation and treatment.

## PARAGANGLIOMA

### *Natural History and Physical Findings*

Paragangliomas are vascular neoplasms that arise from the extraadrenal paraganglia derived from the neural crest and most commonly occur in the head and neck region.

Disclosure: The authors have nothing to disclose.

Department of Otolaryngology–Head and Neck Surgery, NYU School of Medicine, New York, NY, USA
* Corresponding author.
*E-mail address:* Theresa.Tran@nyumc.org

Otolaryngol Clin N Am 51 (2018) 255–274
https://doi.org/10.1016/j.otc.2017.09.015
0030-6665/18/

These tumors are closely associated with either blood vessels (carotid artery, jugular bulb) or nerves (vagus, tympanic plexus). Paragangliomas are usually slow-growing tumors with an average growth rate of 1 to 2 mm per year and a median doubling time of 4.2 years. Their growth pattern may be described as biphasic because very small and very large paragangliomas have a lower growth rate when compared with that of intermediate-sized tumors.[1]

Although all paragangliomas have the potential of releasing vasoactive substances, such as catecholamines and dopamine,[2] only 1% to 3% of paragangliomas produce the associated clinical findings.[2,3] Secreting paragangliomas release norepinephrine, and a 4-fold to 5-fold elevation of serum norepinephrine is necessary to produce symptoms,[4] such as excessive sweating, hypertension, tachycardia, nervousness and weight loss.[2] Urinary laboratory screening tests, including 24-hour urinary metanephrine (normal <1.3 mg) and vanillylmandelic acid levels (normal range is 1.8–7.0 mg), are frequently elevated 10 to 15 times normal in patients with actively secreting tumors.[2] Serum catecholamine levels, including norepinephrine and epinephrine, are also of value in the evaluation of the patient.

### *Multicentric and hereditary paragangliomas*

A familial history of paragangliomas may be present and there is a significant incidence of multicentric tumors in both familial and sporadic cases. Familial or hereditary paragangliomas have been previously reported to account for 5% to 10%[5,6] of all cases of head and neck paragangliomas but it seems that these estimates were low due to the complex mode of inheritance and variable phenotypic expression.[7] It may, in fact, account for up to 25% to 50% of cases.[8,9] Most (90%) cases of hereditary paragangliomas involve the carotid body.[10] If a familial history is present, there is a 78% to 87% possibility of multiple paragangliomas.[6,11] Bilateral carotid body paragangliomas occur more frequently with familial cases (31.8%) than nonfamilial cases (4.4%).[5]

The potential to develop multicentric tumors has important clinical implications. The presence of bilateral carotid paragangliomas poses a difficult challenge in management because excision of these tumors results in loss of baroreceptive function and subsequent refractory hypertension. Multiple tumors, including vagal or jugular paragangliomas, present problems concerning significant morbidity of multiple lower cranial nerve (CN) dysfunction, perhaps bilaterally, resulting from direct tumor involvement or surgical resection. Because multicentric tumors may be metachronous, routine follow-up MRI, $^{111}$indium pentetreotide (Octreoscan) or fluorine-18-labeled dihydroxyphenylalanine ($^{18}$F-DOPA) PET imaging is indicated.

### *Malignant variant*

Malignant paragangliomas are uncommon and their diagnosis can only be confirmed by metastatic disease, usually within regional lymph nodes, because histologic examination of the primary tumor is unreliable for establishing a malignant diagnosis. The prevalence of malignancy depends on site of the primary tumor and there has been considerable variability in the reported frequency. Although malignant carotid body tumor has been reported in up to 20% of patients, most reports indicate a rate of 3% to 6% of cases.[12,13] Malignancy is generally less common in familial paragangliomas compared with sporadic cases.[5] The jugulotympanic paraganglioma malignancy rate ranges widely from less than 1% to 25% but is most often reported to be approximately 5%.[13,14] Vagal paragangliomas probably represent the highest rate of malignancy (16%–19%) of the more common types of head and neck paragangliomas.[13]

### *Carotid body tumor*

The carotid body is located in the adventitia of the posterior medial aspect of the carotid artery bifurcation. As the tumor grows, it tends to splay the carotid bifurcation and progressively involves the carotid adventitia. Typically, the internal carotid artery (ICA) is displaced posteriorly and laterally (**Fig. 1**).[15] With continued growth, the tumor extends superiorly along the internal carotid to the skull base and may affect adjacent CNs, most commonly the vagal and hypoglossal nerves. Occasionally, the sympathetic chain is involved. The median age of presentation for carotid body tumors is 45 to 54 years, with a range of 12 to 78 years.[16–18] Most series report a female predominance of approximately 2 to 1.[16–18] The most common presenting symptom of a carotid body tumor is a neck mass located at or superior to the carotid bifurcation and deep to the carotid bifurcation and deep to the sternocleidomastoid muscle.[15,16]

### *Jugular and tympanic paragangliomas*

Tympanic paragangliomas arise from the paraganglia associated with Jacobson's or Arnold's nerves. They may fill the middle ear cavity and extend posteriorly into the mastoid air cells or inferiorly to the jugular bulb. Tympanic paragangliomas occur most commonly during the sixth decade of life, have a marked female preponderance, and usually present with a conductive hearing loss, pulsatile tinnitus, and a mass behind the tympanic membrane.[19] Within the middle ear, ossicular involvement by tympanic paraganglioma may result in conductive hearing loss. Continued growth with vestibular involvement produces sensorineural hearing loss; vertigo; and, occasionally, pain from the associated inflammatory response.

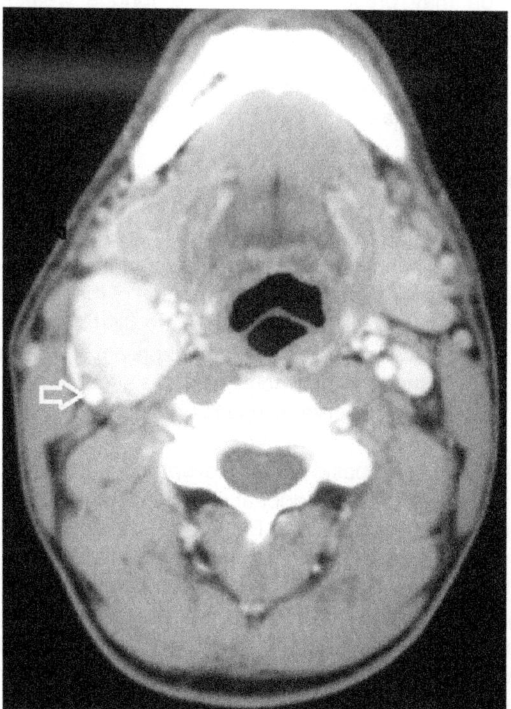

**Fig. 1.** Axial CT scan with contrast showing posterolateral displacement of the ICA (*arrow*) by carotid body tumor.

Jugular paragangliomas tend to spread along the paths of least resistance in multiple directions and gain access to various portions of the temporal bone and base of skull neurovascular foramina. Intracranial extension can occur via several pathways: posterior extension directly through the petrous bone, extension into and through the internal auditory canal, or infralabyrinthine extension.[20,21] There is early intraluminal jugular extension into the sigmoid sinus and internal jugular vein (IJV) with possible growth into the inferior petrosal sinus. Tumor can invade into the middle ear cleft, the petrous apex, or into the mastoid and retrofacial air cells. Inferiorly, jugular paragangliomas may extend into the infratemporal fossa and poststyloid parapharyngeal space into the neck. Jugular paragangliomas that invade the middle ear will result in signs and symptoms similar to that of a tympanic paraganglioma. However, a computed tomography (CT) scan evaluation usually can distinguish the 2 by the presence or absence of erosion of the bony plate at the lateral aspect of the jugular fossa.

Jugular paragangliomas most commonly occur in the fifth and sixth decades of life,[22] and demonstrate a female to male ratio of 4:1 to 6:1.[19,23] They often demonstrate early skull-base involvement with extension into the middle ear and IJV. Superior extension into the middle ear results in symptoms similar to tympanic paragangliomas and may result in a conductive or sensorineural hearing loss, depending on the extent of vestibular involvement.[24,25] Hearing loss (55%–77%) and tinnitus (56%–72%) are the most common presenting symptoms.[19,26–28] Symptoms related to lower CN deficits (VII-XII) are also common. Tumor can invade into the middle ear cleft, the petrous apex, or into the mastoid and retrofacial air cells with a resulting facial nerve paralysis. Tumors of the skull base without extensive middle ear extension may present with isolated tongue weakness, hoarseness, dysphagia, or shoulder drop, or with symptoms of multiple CN dysfunction. The jugular foramen syndrome (CNs IX, X, XI palsy or Vernet syndrome) is occasionally encountered, and CN IX-XII palsy (Collet-Sicard syndrome) occurs in approximately 10% of jugular paragangliomas.

### *Vagal paragangliomas*

Vagal paragangliomas are uncommon and account for up to 5% of all head and neck paragangliomas.[10,11] Although they most commonly arise from the nodose (inferior) ganglion, vagal paragangliomas may also originate from the middle and superior ganglia and, less frequently, anywhere along the course of the vagus nerve. Compared with the discrete carotid body, vagal paraganglia are distributed diffusely within the nerve or perineurium. Vagus nerve fibers fan out or splay over the surface of the vagal paraganglioma or, early in their development, enter the substance of the tumor; therefore, preservation of the vagus nerve is usually not possible with complete tumor resection.[11,29–31]

Vagal paragangliomas have 3 basic patterns of spread.[11] Because most vagal paragangliomas originate at the inferior (nodose) ganglion, they tend to spread inferiorly into the poststyloid parapharyngeal area. Extension superiorly toward the skull base in the area of the jugular foramen results in early involvement of the IJV and adjacent CNs (IX, XI, XII). The tumor causes early anterior displacement of the ICA.

Vagal paragangliomas most commonly present as an asymptomatic mass of the upper neck, typically more cephalad than carotid body tumors. Vagal paragangliomas are slow-growing with a female to male preponderance of 2:1 to 3:1 and a mean duration of 2 to 3 years of before presentation.[10,11,19,32] As the tumor enlarges, it encroaches on the lower CNs and the adjacent sympathetic chain. Signs and symptoms of cranial neuropathy include unilateral vocal cord paralysis, hoarseness, dysphagia, nasal regurgitation, atrophy of the hemitongue, shoulder weakness, and Horner syndrome. Hearing loss and pulsatile tinnitus usually indicate temporal bone extension.

### *Diagnostic Evaluation*

A CT scan and MRI usually establish the diagnosis of paraganglioma. MRI is often the morphologic imaging modality of choice because it offers multiplanar imaging with better contrast resolution than CT scan and does not use ionizing radiation. A variety of radionuclide imaging techniques, such as $^{111}$indium pentetreotide (Octreoscan),18F-DOPA PET, fluorine-18-labeled fluorodeoxy-D-glucose ($^{18}$F-FDG) PET, or $^{123}$I- metaiodobenzylguanidine (MIBG) scintigraphy, can also be used to evaluate paragangliomas, define multiple tumors, and detect the possible presence of metastatic disease.[33,34] Angiography (CT or magnetic resonance angiography) defines the vascular supply, visualizes vessel involvement (invasion), and paves the way for preoperative embolization, which is important if surgery is contemplated.

### *Treatment*

The approach to treatment of paragangliomas is in evolution. Traditionally, surgical resection has been the mainstay of treatment of paragangliomas, especially with development of more sophisticated skull base approaches, safer embolization protocols, and advanced vascular bypass procedures.[24,26] However, the anticipation of postoperative CN dysfunction requiring extensive rehabilitation efforts, along with improved understanding of the natural history of these tumors, has increasingly shifted emphasis to observation and nonsurgical therapy for many patients with paragangliomas.[35–37]

#### *Observation*

Observation has been shown to have acceptable outcomes for selected patients with paragangliomas in several short-term and long-term studies,[35,36] given their low incidence of malignancy and indolent growth with slowly progressive cranial neuropathy, which allows for adequate physiologic compensation. Some paragangliomas, especially very small ones, have been shown not to be progressive, and a wait and scan management may be advisable.[1] Regardless of size, vagal paragangliomas often require vagus nerve sacrifice for adequate resection, which may result in significant vocal and deglutition dysfunction.[38] This is especially significant in the older patients who do not adapt well to acute neural deficits that may define their postoperative course.[29] Even with preexisting CN dysfunction, patients may not easily tolerate postoperative total nerve paralysis with absolute loss of function, especially in the setting of multiple nerve deficits or patient's advanced age. Relative contraindications to surgery include extensive skull base or intracranial involvement, advanced age of the patient, medical comorbidities, and bilateral or multiple paragangliomas for which surgery may result in the unacceptable postoperative morbidity of bilateral lower CN palsies.

#### *Preoperative embolization*

If surgery is the chosen treatment course, preoperative embolization of paragangliomas is often considered and has been a useful adjunct in the treatment protocol at many institutions. However, experience has allowed successful surgical resections of selective paragangliomas without preoperative embolization. When embolization is deemed appropriate, it should be performed 24 to 48 hours before surgery to minimize revascularization and local edema or inflammation.[25]

Postembolization paragangliomas often manifest a reduction in tumor size by as much as 25% as a result of diminished blood flow to the tumor. Embolization of tumor vasculature reduces blood loss during dissection of the neoplasm.[15,39–41] Reduced bleeding during surgery improves exposure, better defines the planes of dissection, and reduces the need for transfusion.[42–44] The decision to embolize preoperatively should depend on the location and extent of the tumor, as well as the experience of the surgeon and the interventional radiologist. If embolization is elected, surgery is performed within 2 days of angiography and embolization to avoid recruitment of collateral tumor blood supply, and before the onset of significant postinflammatory effect.[25] Short-term steroids are administered if there is concern about tumor edema that may compromise tumor dissection.

### *Surgery*

**Carotid body tumors** Adequate carotid body tumor removal requires a subadventitial dissection of the carotid artery; therefore, it is important to obtain proximal and distal control of the common, internal, and external carotid arteries. Mobilization of the ICA is the initial step of tumor dissection. Occasionally, the tumor must be dissected through and split to remove the ICA from its encasement. Once the ICA is free, any tumor that extends inferior to the bifurcation should be dissected off the common carotid artery. The external carotid artery (ECA) and its branches may then be dissected, although difficulty with this part of the procedure may warrant sacrifice of the ECA, if necessary, for adequate tumor excision. The last step is freeing the tumor from the carotid bifurcation where there is most intimate involvement of the artery because the tumor originates in the carotid body (**Fig. 2**).

Nerves adherent to, but not infiltrated by, carotid body tumors can usually be mobilized in an intact fashion, including the vagus; hypoglossal; and, occasionally, glossopharyngeal nerves. These nerves are at risk for postoperative dysfunction, especially with larger tumors.[10,25] The sympathetic chain and the superior laryngeal nerve are often adherent to the tumor, especially those with medial extension into the parapharyngeal space.

Surgical resection is considered the treatment of choice for smaller carotid body tumors (<5 cm), especially in younger and healthy patients. Other factors, such as pain, possibility of malignancy, and rapid growth, also support surgical intervention of carotid body tumors. On the other hand, patient's advanced age and medical comorbidities make surgery less advisable.[37]

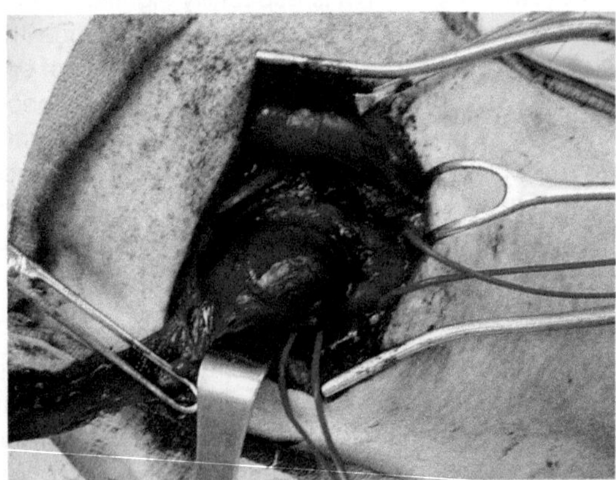

**Fig. 2.** Mobilization of a carotid body tumor with vessel loops around the common and internal carotid arteries.

**Jugulotympanic paragangliomas** Tympanic paragangliomas confined to the middle ear (Glasscock-Jackson type I, Fisch class A) can be approached through a transcanal approach.[45] These small tumors do not require preoperative embolization. If the margins of the tumor are not easily discernible but the bone over the jugular bulb and the carotid canal is intact (Glasscock-Jackson type II-III, Fisch class B), a postauricular, transmastoid extended facial recess approach provides excellent exposure for tumor resection.[4,45] A tympanoplasty can be performed at that time if necessary.

For glomus jugulare tumors, involvement of the jugular bulb requires a combined transmastoid and transcervical approach.[46] If there is limited involvement of the jugular bulb without carotid artery involvement, a complete mastoidectomy and extended facial recess approach are performed. The sigmoid sinus is exposed and traced to the jugular bulb. Isolation and control of the IJV and ICA are performed, and CNs IX through XII are dissected to the skull base. The IJV is ligated. Mobilization of the distal facial nerve at the second genu with the stylomastoid periosteum provides excellent exposure of the jugular bulb area. The superior sigmoid sinus is occluded, and the inferior sigmoid sinus is opened with mobilization of the tumor. Bleeding from the inferior petrosal sinus is controlled. Inadvertent trauma in this area risks damage to CNs IX through XII in their courses through the jugular canal.

More extensive involvement of the jugular bulb or involvement of the intrapetrous ICA requires an infratemporal fossa approach as developed by Fisch and Mattox.[47] A wide mastoidectomy approach is performed. The facial nerve is mobilized from the geniculate ganglion to the stylomastoid foramen with anterior translocation of the nerve. The ICA, IJV, and CNs IX through XII are dissected to the skull base with ligation of the IJV and control of the ICA. The mandibular condyle is retracted anteriorly. The ICA is followed through its intrapetrous course with transection of the Eustachian tube. The sigmoid sinus, jugular bulb, and IJV are resected with the tumor. The tumor is meticulously dissected off the ICA. Additional exposure into the infratemporal fossa can be accomplished with resection of the mandibular condyle and zygomatic arch. Through this approach, there is access to the posterior, middle, and anterior cranial fossae; if necessary, continued tumor resection is accomplished through a neurosurgical, intracranial approach. A pedicled temporalis, temporal-parietal, or sternomastoid flap is used for reconstruction and obliteration of the defect.

Until 20 years ago, radical resection was considered standard of care for jugular paragangliomas. More recently, however, subtotal resection and radiosurgery (see later discussion of radiation therapy) have been advocated in the treatment of jugular paragangliomas to reduce neurologic morbidity in patients, especially those with advanced age or limited life expectancy.[36,48] The investigators[1,36,49] advocate initial observation, followed by radiosurgery if tumor growth is observed.

**Vagal paragangliomas** Vagal paragangliomas may vary in the extent of skull base or intracranial involvement. A combined cervical-mastoid approach to the skull base is best for safe and wide exposure, and anterior displacement of the mandible will facilitate exposure of the parapharyngeal space.[29] The carotid sheath structures and CNs IX-XII are dissected up to the skull base with careful dissection of the ICA off the vagal paraganglioma. Control of the ICA is obtained. Paragangliomas without skull base involvement can be safely resected with this approach. If the tumor extends into the jugular canal, then a mastoidectomy with facial nerve mobilization and transposition will allow exposure of the jugular bulb. The sigmoid sinus can be packed off or ligated with subsequent removal of the sigmoid, jugular bulb, and IJV complex. The carotid canal is dissected superiorly, and the ICA is carefully separated off the tumor. The tumor can then be excised, and this almost always involves sacrifice of the vagus nerve and additional CNs according to tumor size and local involvement.[11] Closure is achieved by obliterating the mastoid cavity with a fat graft. More extensive defects would require a temporoparietal fascia flap[50] or a sternocleidomastoid muscle flap.

Surgery is currently less commonly recommended for vagal paragangliomas due to the associated speech and swallowing morbidity following resection. Thus, for most patients with vagal paragangliomas, especially the elderly and those with bilateral tumors, observation is more frequently being considered, with radiation therapy offered to patients with tumor progression.[37]

#### *Radiation therapy*

Radiotherapy has traditionally been the treatment of choice for unresectable paragangliomas or those tumors in the medically infirm and elderly. However, for the past several decades, radiotherapy has been proven to be an effective therapeutic option and, therefore, should be considered as a form of primary treatment. Moreover, a combined approach (surgery and radiation) does not seem to improve local control compared with radiotherapy alone. Kim and colleagues[51] also emphasized that there is no obvious benefit of a debulking subtotal resection in conjunction with definitive radiotherapy. When treating with radiation, both conventionally fractionated radiotherapy (45 Gy over 5 weeks) and stereotactic radiosurgery (SRS) have been used.

SRS offers the possibility of a single, highly focused small field treatment with a steep dose gradient to maximally spare the surrounding normal tissue. Multiple series have reported success using this approach to treat primarily jugular paragangliomas with high local control.[52–55] SRS is suitable for skull base paragangliomas that are less than 3 cm in maximum diameter.[56]

## JUVENILE NASOPHARYNGEAL ANGIOFIBROMA

### *Natural History and Physical Findings*

Juvenile nasopharyngeal angiofibroma (JNA) is a highly vascular, histologically benign but locally aggressive and destructive tumor that exclusively affects adolescent boys. It accounts for approximately 0.5% of all head and neck neoplasms.[57,58] The etiologic factors and pathogenesis of the disease remain to be elucidated. The tumor seems to originate in the posterior nasal cavity instead of the nasopharynx, specifically in the posterolateral wall of the superior aspect of the nasal cavity, at the junction of the sphenoid process of the palatine bone, the horizontal ala of the vomer, and the root of the pterygoid process of the sphenoid bone, near the superior margin of the sphenopalatine foramen.[59] These tumors are unencapsulated and consist of proliferating, irregular vascular spaces lined by a single endothelial layer. These channels lack a complete muscular layer between the endothelial cells and stromal cells and are, therefore, subject to severe bleeding.[57]

At diagnosis, most angiofibromas have extended beyond the nasal cavity and nasopharynx. Extension into the nasal cavity is followed by anterolateral erosion of the posterior wall of the maxillary sinus and lateral growth into the pterygomaxillary fossa. Extension into the pterygomaxillary fossa can erode the pterygoid process of the sphenoid bone. Further lateral extension via the pterygomaxillary fissure can fill the infratemporal fossa and produce the classic bulging cheek. Tumor can extend under the zygomatic arch and cause swelling above the arch. From the pterygomaxillary fossa, the angiofibroma can erode the greater wing of the sphenoid bone and into the middle cranial fossa and invade both inferior and superior orbital fissures. Posterior extension into the sphenoid sinus through the floor or ostium fills the sinus, pushes upward and back to displace the pituitary, and then can fill the sella turcica. Tumor in the sella or orbit can cause loss of vision.[59] These tumors typically grow by centrifugal expansion and not by invasion; therefore, they may be intracranial but usually extradural. The cavernous sinus may be compressed but not invaded. CN palsies are rare even with large tumors. However, particularly aggressive angiofibromas may invade the cavernous sinus and threaten multiple CNs, ICA, hypophysis, and optic chiasm.[59,60]

Several classification systems were established to describe JNA based on tumor extent. The commonly used systems are Fisch, Chandler, and Radowski's adaptation of the Sessions classification.[61] Despite its tendency to be invasive, the rate of growth of JNA, although not known, is thought to be slow. Because the tumor is rarely seen in young adults, it is thought to spontaneously regress. However, because regression cannot be assumed, these tumors should be treated.[59] The prognosis for patients with JNA is good with early diagnosis[62]; unfortunately, diagnosis most often occurs during later stages of the disease due to the nonspecific and innocuous presenting symptoms of JNA.[63,64]

JNA is typically found in adolescent males, ranging from 7 to 29 years of age, with a median age of 15 years at diagnosis.[65] Patients typically present with the triad of unilateral nasal obstruction, recurrent severe epistaxis, and nasopharyngeal mass.[66] Other common but nonspecific symptoms are purulent nasal discharge due to infection secondary to obstruction, hyponasal speech, and anosmia. Nasal obstruction and epistaxis occur in more than 80% of the patients. Symptoms may be present for months to years before the diagnosis is made. Delay in presentation and/or diagnosis can be attributed to the tendency to associate the indolent symptoms of JNA with the more common entities, such as rhinitis, sinusitis, and nasal polyposis.[67]

### *Diagnostic Evaluation*

The radiographic findings of angiofibroma are characteristic. On CT scan, there is anterior bowing of the posterior wall of the maxillary sinus, known as the Holman-Miller sign, and enlargement of the superior orbital fissure, which are considered diagnostic for JNA (**Fig. 3**).[65] CT scan is also ideal for tumor localization and useful in the delineation of the extent of the tumor. MRI is indicated in patients with intracranial extension. Angiography is not necessary in most patients but is useful in patients whose diagnosis remains in question, usually for those in whom previous treatment has failed. It also is necessary for embolization, especially when surgery is anticipated.

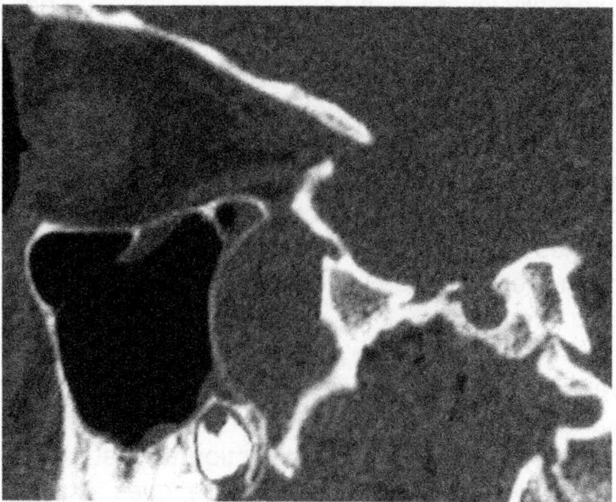

**Fig. 3.** Sagittal CT scan displaying the anterior bowing of the posterior wall of the maxillary sinus, known as the Holman-Miller sign diagnostic for JNA.

## TREATMENT

The mainstay treatment of JNA is surgery, especially for the early-stage disease process. Previously, the various surgical approaches were: transpalatal, transnasal, transantral, transmandibular, transzygomatic, combined craniotomy and rhinotomy, lateral rhinotomy, and midface degloving. With increasing experience using endoscopic nasal techniques, excellent results have been achieved with this more minimally invasive approach. Ultimately, the approach chosen is determined by tumor location, extent of the tumor, and the surgeon's expertise.

### *Preoperative Embolization*

Preoperative embolization of JNA may greatly reduce intraoperative blood loss, a major source of morbidity. Most commonly, the ipsilateral internal maxillary artery is the major arterial supply to these neoplasms. However, some tumors receive their blood supply from the contralateral external carotid system, and some receive branches from both the ipsilateral and the contralateral internal carotid systems, especially from the inferolateral branches off the cavernous carotid artery. The potential but small risk of embolization is outweighed by the overall surgical safety as the result of the ability to decrease the ipsilateral, as well as the contralateral, blood supply. Several investigators[68,69] reported a 60% to 68% reduction in intraoperative blood loss in patients who received preoperative embolization when compared with those who did not.

### *Surgery*

Selection of a surgical approach is based on extent of the tumor and the surgeon's expertise and experience.

**Endoscopic endonasal** The endoscopic approach was previously reserved for tumors limited to the nasal cavity; however, as endoscopic instrumentation and skills of endoscopic surgeons improved, these techniques were adopted to expand the boundaries of minimally invasive skull base surgery. Endoscopic excision is promoted as the preferred approach for JNA for several reasons. The tumor can often be pulled into the nasal cavity with minimal dissection. Additionally, endoscopic techniques provide excellent access to feeding vessels, as well as enhance the surgeon's ability to explore sites that are prone to residual tumor and, thus, recurrence.[69]

Besides being minimally invasive, the endoscopic approach has several other potential advantages, including decreased intraoperative blood loss, complication rates, hospital stay, and recurrence rates.[69] Pryor and colleagues[69] reported an average blood loss of 225 mL in subjects who undergo an endoscopic procedure compared with 1250 mL loss in subjects undergoing excision via the lateral rhinotomy approach. They attributed this decreased loss to the careful attention to hemostasis, which is crucial to the outcome of endoscopic procedures, and claim that much of the blood loss in open approaches results from the incisions and osteotomies in providing tumor access. Endoscopic surgery is becoming the method of choice and eventually may be replaced with robotic surgery.[70]

Recurrence rates are reported in the range of 6% to 39.5% in JNA surgery. Pryor and colleagues[69] reported a recurrence rate of 24% in subjects treated by a standard surgical approach and 0% in endoscopic excisions. This decreased recurrence, however, is perhaps more a result of subjects selection than an advantage of the technique. In the series reported by Pryor and colleagues,[69] none of the subjects chosen to undergo the endoscopic approach had intracranial extension, whereas 36% of the subjects who underwent an open procedure had intracranial extension.

This is consistent with findings published by other investigators, reporting a 10% to 20% incidence of intracranial extension, with a rate of 50% recurrence.[69,71–73]

**Transpalatal and combined transpalatal and transzygomatic** The transpalatal technique may be used for tumors limited to the nasopharynx, nasal cavity, and the sphenoid sinus. Lateral exposure is very limited,[74] thus the approach has fallen out of favor due to poor exposure of large tumors, resulting in greater incidence of recurrence.[75,76]

The combined transzygomatic and transpalatal approach can be used to remove large tumors with limited intracranial, extradural extension. The tumor is removed via an extended palatobuccal incision; a bicoronal incision in the transzygomatic approach allows for safe mobilization of the superior extent of the tumor.[77,78]

**Medial maxillectomy** Medial maxillectomy allows access to tumors in the nasopharynx, orbit, ethmoid sinus, sphenoid sinus, pterygopalatine fossa, infratemporal fossa, and medial aspect of the cavernous sinus. The medial maxillectomy may be performed through a lateral rhinotomy incision, or through Weber-Ferguson or midfacial degloving approaches (**Fig. 4**). The use of midfacial degloving approach is preferred over the lateral rhinotomy due to lack of facial scars.[79] Additionally, the midfacial degloving approach provides the exposure necessary to gain access to a wide field of possible tumor involvement extending from the nasal cavity, maxillary sinus, nasopharynx, pterygomaxillary fossa, and infratemporal fossa.

**Infratemporal fossa approach** The infratemporal fossa approach is used for tumors with involvement of the middle cranial fossa and lateral aspect of the cavernous sinus. Visualization of the contralateral nasopharynx is achieved by partial tumor removal or by removal of the outer cortex of the infratemporal skull base at the base of the pterygoid plates. It does not provide a direct view of the medial aspect of the cavernous sinus. This approach limits blood loss by allowing for ligation of the internal maxillary artery early in the dissection, as well as facilitating exposure of the ICA for proximal control.[80,81]

**Craniofacial approach** Craniofacial approaches have allowed for surgical resections of advanced JNAs with minimal postoperative complications.[60] This approach consists of a combination of transfacial and infratemporal fossa approaches, and permits access to the sphenoid sinus, cavernous sinus, anterior skull base, and nasopharynx.

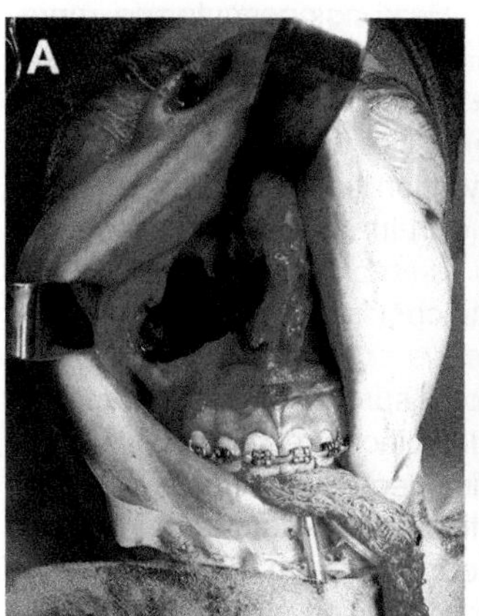


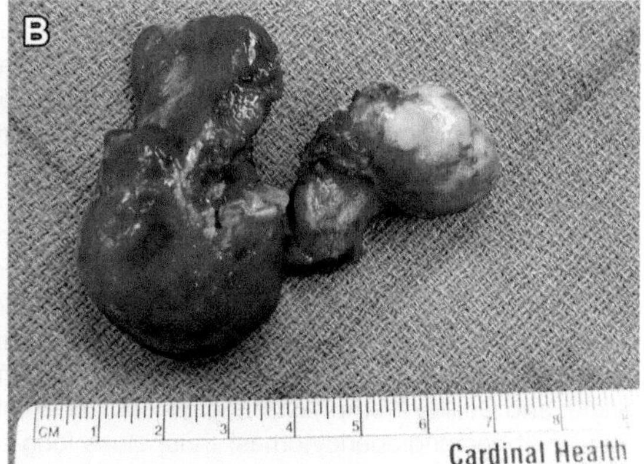


**Fig. 4.** (*A, B*) Excision of JNA via a sublabial hemifacial degloving approach.

An infratemporal fossa approach is used to dissect the tumor from the sphenoid sinus, superior orbital fissure, middle cranial fossa, and the lateral cavernous sinus, and a standard facial translocation (ie, Weber-Ferguson) incision provides anterior exposure and tumor mobilization from the nasopharynx, paranasal sinuses, pterygopalatine fossa, infratemporal fossa, and medial cavernous sinus.[60]

**Combined open and endoscopic surgery** The open approach when used in combination with endoscopic techniques is advocated by some investigators, allowing for meticulous inspection of the surgical cavity facilitated by an endoscopic examination, thereby potentially decreasing the likelihood of tumor recurrence[82] and facilitating intraoperative repair of cerebrospinal fluid leak created during surgery.[83]

***Radiation therapy***

Although surgery is considered to be the treatment of choice for JNA, controversy arises regarding the best treatment of the more locally advanced disease or disease with intracranial involvement that may necessitate a combination of treatment modalities, including surgery and postoperative radiation. Radiotherapy is often considered an appropriate option for treatment of recurrent angiofibromas. Lee and colleagues[84] reported on 27 subjects with extensive tumors who received radiation as the primary mode of treatment with minimal complications and, perhaps, less risk of significant morbidity and mortality associated with surgical intervention. Recurrence rates of 20% to 30% can be expected with radiation treatment alone.[70] Long-term complications of radiation consist of osteoradionecrosis, growth retardation, panhypopituitarism, temporal lobe necrosis, cataracts, and radiation keratopathy.[84]

New techniques in radiotherapy, such as conformal intensity-modulated radiotherapy (IMRT) and gamma knife SRS, may have enormous potential for the management of JNA. Good results were reported with 3-dimensional IMRT and gamma knife SRS,[85] as well as image-guided, robotic radiotherapy (Cyberknife).[86]

## HEMANGIOPERICYTOMA

### *Natural History and Physical Findings*

Hemangiopericytoma of the head and neck is a rare neoplasm that originates from the pericytes or cells of Zimmerman surrounding normal vascular channels.[87] It is considered by some to be a lesion with low risk of malignant potential and by others a malignant lesion of high metastatic potential.[87,88] Thus, it is known as a tumor that varies greatly in appearance and biologic behavior.[89] Hemangiopericytomas represent 3% to 5% of all soft-tissue sarcomas[90] and 1% of all vascular tumors.[91] Approximately 10% to 25% of hemangiopericytoma occur in the head and neck; of these, 5% occur within the sinonasal cavity (**Fig. 5**).[89,92–95] It is thought that sinonasal hemangiopericytomas behave less aggressively than those occurring in other parts of the body; the 5-year survival rate for patients with tumors in this location approaches 88%.[96,97]

In the head and neck, the clinical behavior of hemangiopericytoma may vary from a slowly enlarging rubbery mass to an infiltrating aggressive neoplasm. Distant metastasis to lung, liver, and bone may occur; however, regional spread to lymph nodes has not been observed. The rate of metastasis varies significantly from 10% to 60%[98] and is consistent with the observation that this tumor varies greatly in biologic behavior. Gengler and Guillou[99] emphasize the difficulty of predicting the prognosis and clinical behavior of hemangiopericytomas; thus, close long-term follow-up is crucial for patients with hemangiopericytomas because of the high incidence of local recurrence and potentially metastasizing course.[100,101]

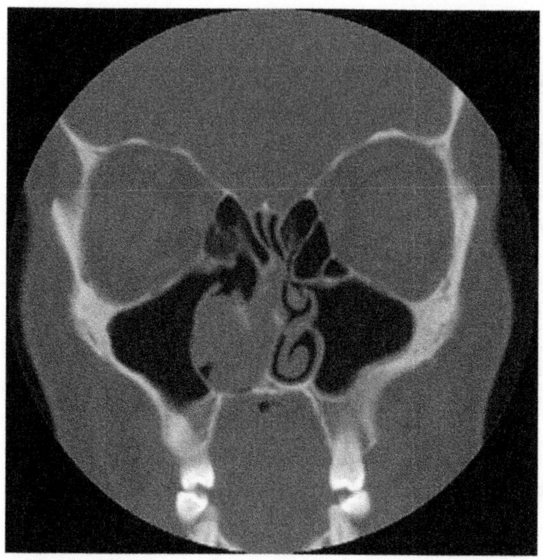

**Fig. 5.** Coronal CT scan showing hemangiopericytoma within right nasal cavity.

Hemangiopericytomas occur most commonly in the sixth and seventh decades of life and have no sex predilection.[87] Many of these tumors may have been present for a long time before they are diagnosed, and patients typically present with a slowly growing mass that occasionally reaches a considerable size.[98] Symptoms include facial pain; occasionally, facial swelling; epistaxis; sinusitis; visual changes; and nasal obstruction, depending on the anatomic site of involvement. Facial skin overlying tumor may be warm to touch due to the rich vascularity of the hemangiopericytoma.[102] In the oral cavity, its clinical appearance is a firm, usually well-circumscribed swelling of the mucosa. In the nose, it is usually described as soft, rubbery, pale gray or tan polypoid mass. Despite the pale avascular appearance, these tumors bleed vigorously when biopsied. Because of their benign clinical appearance, they can be misdiagnosed as benign tumors or nasal polyps.[89,93,103]

### *Diagnostic Evaluation*

Diagnosis of hemangiopericytoma depends on accurate pathologic assessment of the biopsied specimen.[101] Radiographic imaging assists in the diagnosis. Hemangiopericytomas appear as rounded, sharply outlined or well-circumscribed, homogenous masses that often displace neighboring structures on CT scan.[98] CT scan can clearly demonstrate bone destruction within the nasal cavity, paranasal sinuses, and adjacent intracranial structures.[104] Angiography shows a richly vascularized mass, dilated arteries, and diffuse capillary blush. Occasionally, early visualization of the veins suggests arteriovenous shunting. MRI reveals several characteristic features suggesting the diagnosis of a solitary fibrous tumor-isointense on T1-weighted imaging and isointense to hypointense on T2-weighted imaging.[98,105]

### *Treatment*

The preferred treatment of hemangiopericytomas is wide surgical excision, usually performed via 1 of the following approaches: lateral rhinotomy (**Fig. 6**), midface degloving, craniofacial resection, or endoscopic resection. Many investigators

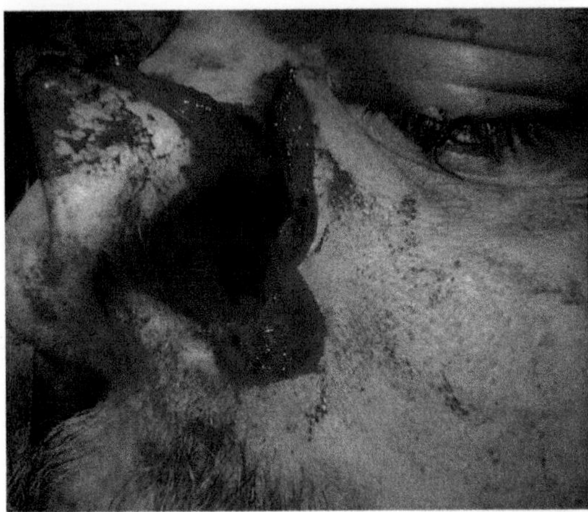

**Fig. 6.** Excision of hemangiopericytoma via lateral rhinotomy approach.

advocate a craniofacial approach for tumors with cribriform plate or base of skull involvement.[105] Many investigators have demonstrated that endoscopic approaches can provide excellent visualization and tumor resection while avoiding external facial incisions and complications associated with the open techniques. They report successful resection of tumors with skull base erosion, thereby avoiding open approaches.[87]

***Preoperative embolization***

Perioperative embolization has been suggested as an adjuvant for decreasing tumor vascularity and size preoperatively,[106,107] although most head and neck hemangiopericytomas are relatively small in size and amenable to en bloc resection without embolization.[101] Several investigators encourage the use of routine angiography and preoperative embolization to delineate the extent of these tumors and their feeding vessels, and to reduce intraoperative hemorrhage.[101,107] Of course, the experienced interventional vascular radiology team can perform these procedures with an acceptable rate of morbidity and mortality.

***Adjuvant therapy***

The role of adjuvant radiotherapy remains to be clarified. Radiation therapy may decrease the size of the tumor, but cure is rare with radiation alone. Radiation therapy has been advocated as adjuvant treatment of hemangiopericytoma to reduce the rate of local recurrence.[108–110] Some investigators recommend adjuvant radiotherapy for patients with hemangiopericytoma greater than 5 cm in size or when the resection margins are inadequate.[111,112] However, it is not clear whether the addition of radiotherapy improves survival.[91,97] The role of adjuvant or palliative chemotherapy is not well defined for patients with hemangiopericytomas, even for advanced or unresectable disease.[113]

Follow-up of patients with hemangiopericytoma should include regular clinical and radiological examinations, especially in patients with deep-seated tumors or in patients with suspicion of tumor recurrence and/or metastasis. Long-term follow-up of patients with these tumors should be maintained because some hemangiopericytomas, including histologic low-grade tumors, display late recurrence and metastasis, even beyond 5 years after treatment.[101,111]

**Summary points**

*Paraganglioma summary points*

- Vascular neoplasms
- Closely associated with blood vessels and nerves
- Slow growing
- Significant rate of multiple tumors, especially with hereditary forms
- Carotid body tumors are most common type
- Tumors are radiosensitive
- Low rate of malignancy; highest in vagal paragangliomas
- Preoperative embolization for extensive skull base paragangliomas

*JNA summary points*

- Occurs in adolescent boys
- Tumor originates near sphenopalatine foramen
- Slow growing
- Symptoms: unilateral nasal obstruction, recurrent sever epistaxis
- Preoperative embolization indicated
- Most treated with transnasal endoscopic approach

*Hemangiopericytoma summary points*

- Varies in biological behavior
- Treatment is surgical resection
- If metastatic disease, usually systemic (eg, lungs, liver)
- High incidence of postoperative local recurrence

## REFERENCES

1. Jansen JC, van den Berg R, Kuiper A, et al. Estimation of growth rate in patients with head and neck paragangliomas influences the treatment proposal. Cancer 2000;88:2811–6.
2. Schwaber MK, Glasscock ME, Nissen AJ, et al. Diagnosis and management of catecholamine secreting glomus tumors. Laryngoscope 1984;94:1008–15.
3. Zak F. The paraganglionic chemorector system. New York: Springer-Verlag; 1982.
4. Gulya AJ. The glomus tumor and its biology. Laryngoscope 1993;103:7–15.
5. Grufferman S, Gillman MW, Pasternak LR, et al. Familial carotid body tumors: case report and epidemiologic review. Cancer 1980;46:2116–22.
6. Netterville JL, Reilly KM, Robertson D, et al. Carotid body tumors: a review of 30 patients with 46 tumors. Laryngoscope 1995;105:115–26.
7. Oosterwijk JC, Jansen JC, van Schothorst EM, et al. First experiences with genetic counselling based on predictive DNA diagnosis in hereditary glomus tumours (paragangliomas). J Med Genet 1996;33:379–83.
8. van der Mey AG, Maaswinkel-Mooy PD, Cornelisse CJ, et al. Genomic imprinting in hereditary glomus tumours: evidence for new genetic theory. Lancet 1989;2:1291–4.

9. Drovdlic CM, Myers EN, Peters JA, et al. Proportion of heritable paraganglioma cases and associated clinical characteristics. Laryngoscope 2001;111:1822–7.
10. Lawson W. Glomus bodies and tumors. N Y State J Med 1980;80:1567–75.
11. Netterville JL, Jackson CG, Miller FR, et al. Vagal paraganglioma: a review of 46 patients treated during a 20-year period. Arch Otolaryngol Head Neck Surg 1998;124:1133–40.
12. Shamblin WR, ReMine WH, Sheps SG, et al. Carotid body tumor (chemodectoma). Clinicopathologic analysis of ninety cases. Am J Surg 1971;122:732–9.
13. Thirlwall AS, Bailey CM, Ramsay AD, et al. Laryngeal paraganglioma in a five-year-old child–the youngest case ever recorded. J Laryngol Otol 1999;113:62–4.
14. Manolidis S, Shohet JA, Jackson CG, et al. Malignant glomus tumors. Laryngoscope 1999;109:30–4.
15. Wax MK, Briant TD. Carotid body tumors: a review. J Otolaryngol 1992;21:277–85.
16. Williams MD, Phillips MJ, Nelson WR, et al. Carotid body tumor. Arch Surg 1992;127:963–7 [discussion: 967–8].
17. Gaylis H, Davidge-Pitts K, Pantanowitz D. Carotid body tumours. A review of 52 cases. S Afr Med J 1987;72:493–6.
18. Dickinson PH, Griffin SM, Guy AJ, et al. Carotid body tumour: 30 years experience. Br J Surg 1986;73:14–6.
19. Jackson CG, Harris PF, Glasscock ME 3rd, et al. Diagnosis and management of paragangliomas of the skull base. Am J Surg 1990;159:389–93.
20. Swartz JD, Harnsberger HR, Mukherji SK. The temporal bone. Contemporary diagnostic dilemmas. Radiol Clin North Am 1998;36:819–53, vi.
21. Valavanis A, Schubiger O, Oguz M. High-resolution CT investigation of nonchromaffin paragangliomas of the temporal bone. AJNR Am J Neuroradiol 1983;4:516–9.
22. Bishop GB Jr, Urist MM, el Gammal T, et al. Paragangliomas of the neck. Arch Surg 1992;127:1441–5.
23. Alford BR, Guilford FR. A comprehensive study of tumors of the glomus jugulare. Laryngoscope 1962;72:765–805.
24. Jackson CG. Neurotologic skull base surgery for glomus tumors. Diagnosis for treatment planning and treatment options. Laryngoscope 1993;103:17–22.
25. Persky MS, Setton A, Niimi Y, et al. Combined endovascular and surgical treatment of head and neck paragangliomas–a team approach. Head Neck 2002;24:423–31.
26. Wenig B. Part III pathology of head and neck cancer. Philadelphia: Lippincott-Raven; 1999.
27. Ogura JH, Spector GJ, Gado M. Glomus jugulare and vagale. Ann Otol Rhinol Laryngol 1978;87:622–9.
28. Gardner G, Cocke EW Jr, Robertson JH, et al. Skull base surgery for glomus jugulare tumors. Am J Otol 1985;(Suppl):126–34.
29. Glenner G, Grimley P. Tumors of the extra-adrenal paraganglion system (including chemorecetors). Washington, DC: Armed Forces Institute of Pathology; 1974.
30. Biller HF, Lawson W, Som P, et al. Glomus vagale tumors. Ann Otol Rhinol Laryngol 1989;98:21–6.
31. Urquhart AC, Johnson JT, Myers EN, et al. Glomus vagale: paraganglioma of the vagus nerve. Laryngoscope 1994;104:440–5.

32. Moore G, Yarington CT Jr, Mangham CA Jr. Vagal body tumors: diagnosis and treatment. Laryngoscope 1986;96:533–6.
33. Venkataramana NK, Kolluri VR, Kumar DV, et al. Paraganglioma of the orbit with extension to the middle cranial fossa: case report. Neurosurgery 1989;24:762–4.
34. Brink I, Hoegerle S, Klisch J, et al. Imaging of pheochromocytoma and paraganglioma. Fam Cancer 2005;4:61–8.
35. Langerman A, Athavale SM, Rangarajan SV, et al. Natural history of cervical paragangliomas: outcomes of observation of 43 patients. Arch Otolaryngol Head Neck Surg 2012;138:341–5.
36. Carlson ML, Sweeney AD, Wanna GB, et al. Natural history of glomus jugulare: a review of 16 tumors managed with primary observation. Otolaryngol Head Neck Surg 2015;152:98–105.
37. Moore MG, Netterville JL, Mendenhall WM, et al. Head and neck paragangliomas: an update on evaluation and management. Otolaryngol Head Neck Surg 2016;154:597–605.
38. Heath D, Smith P. The pathology of the carotid body and sinus, vol. 17. Baltimore (MD): Edward Arnold Publishers Ltd; 1985.
39. Gardner P, Dalsing M, Weisberger E, et al. Carotid body tumors, inheritance, and a high incidence of associated cervical paragangliomas. Am J Surg 1996;172:196–9.
40. Murphy TP, Brackmann DE. Effects of preoperative embolization on glomus jugulare tumors. Laryngoscope 1989;99:1244–7.
41. Robison JG, Shagets FW, Beckett WC Jr, et al. A multidisciplinary approach to reducing morbidity and operative blood loss during resection of carotid body tumor. Surg Gynecol Obstet 1989;168:166–70.
42. Muhm M, Polterauer P, Gstottner W, et al. Diagnostic and therapeutic approaches to carotid body tumors. Review of 24 patients. Arch Surg 1997;132:279–84.
43. LaMuraglia GM, Fabian RL, Brewster DC, et al. The current surgical management of carotid body paragangliomas. J Vasc Surg 1992;15:1038–44 [discussion: 1044–5].
44. Ward PH, Liu C, Vinuela F, et al. Embolization: an adjunctive measure for removal of carotid body tumors. Laryngoscope 1988;98:1287–91.
45. House WF, Glasscock ME 3rd. Glomus tympanicum tumors. Arch Otolaryngol 1968;87:550–4.
46. Brackmann DE, Arriaga M. Surgery for glomus tumors. Philadelphia: WB Saunders; 1994.
47. Fisch F, Mattox D. Microsurgery of the skull base. New York: Thieme Medical Publishers; 1988.
48. Wanna GB, Sweeney AD, Carlson ML, et al. Subtotal resection for management of large jugular paragangliomas with functional lower cranial nerves. Otolaryngol Head Neck Surg 2014;151:991–5.
49. Prasad SC, Mimoune HA, D'Orazio F, et al. The role of wait-and-scan and the efficacy of radiotherapy in the treatment of temporal bone paragangliomas. Otol Neurotol 2014;35:922–31.
50. Netterville JL, Civantos FJ. Defect reconstruction following neurotologic skull base surgery. Laryngoscope 1993;103:55–63.
51. Kim JA, Elkon D, Lim ML, et al. Optimum dose of radiotherapy for chemodectomas of the middle ear. Int J Radiat Oncol Biol Phys 1980;6:815–9.
52. Jordan JA, Roland PS, McManus C, et al. Stereotastic radiosurgery for glomus jugulare tumors. Laryngoscope 2000;110:35–8.

53. Feigenberg SJ, Mendenhall WM, Hinerman RW, et al. Radiosurgery for paraganglioma of the temporal bone. Head Neck 2002;24:384–9.
54. Liscak R, Vladyka V, Simonova G, et al. Leksell gamma knife radiosurgery of the tumor glomus jugulare and tympanicum. Stereotact Funct Neurosurg 1998; 70(Suppl 1):152–60.
55. Foote RL, Pollock BE, Gorman DA, et al. Glomus jugulare tumor: tumor control and complications after stereotactic radiosurgery. Head Neck 2002;24:332–8 [discussion: 338–9].
56. Mendenhall WM, J AR. Radiotherapy for head and neck paragangliomas. Oper Tech Otolaryngol 2016;27:55–7.
57. Batsakis JG. Paragangliomas of the head and neck. Baltimore (MD): Williams and Wilkins; 1979.
58. Gullane PJ, Davidson J, O'Dwyer T, et al. Juvenile angiofibroma: a review of the literature and a case series report. Laryngoscope 1992;102:928–33.
59. Cody DT II, DeSanto LW. Neoplasms of the nasal cavity, vol. 2. St Louis (MO): Mosby-Year Book, Inc; 1998.
60. Bales C, Kotapka M, Loevner LA, et al. Craniofacial resection of advanced juvenile nasopharyngeal angiofibroma. Arch Otolaryngol Head Neck Surg 2002;128: 1071–8.
61. Sessions RB, Bryan RN, Naclerio RM, et al. Radiographic staging of juvenile angiofibroma. Head Neck Surg 1981;3:279–83.
62. Coutinho-Camillo CM, Brentani MM, Nagai MA. Genetic alterations in juvenile nasopharyngeal angiofibromas. Head Neck 2008;30:390–400.
63. Ungkanont K, Byers RM, Weber RS, et al. Juvenile nasopharyngeal angiofibroma: an update of therapeutic management. Head Neck 1996;18:60–6.
64. Hollander VP. Hormonally responsive tumors. New York: Academic Press; 1985.
65. Neel HB, Fee WE. Benign and malignant tumors of the nasopharynx, vol. 2. St Louis (MO): Mosby-Year Book, Inc; 1998.
66. Enepekides DJ. Recent advances in the treatment of juvenile angiofibroma. Curr Opin Otolaryngol Head Neck Surg 2004;12:495–9.
67. Bremer JW, Neel HB 3rd, DeSanto LW, et al. Angiofibroma: treatment trends in 150 patients during 40 years. Laryngoscope 1986;96:1321–9.
68. Antonelli AR, Cappiello J, Di Lorenzo D, et al. Diagnosis, staging, and treatment of juvenile nasopharyngeal angiofibroma (JNA). Laryngoscope 1987;97: 1319–25.
69. Pryor SG, Moore EJ, Kasperbauer JL. Endoscopic versus traditional approaches for excision of juvenile nasopharyngeal angiofibroma. Laryngoscope 2005;115:1201–7.
70. Hodges JM, McDevitt AS, El-Sayed Ali AI, et al. Juvenile nasopharyngeal angiofibroma: current treatment modalities and future considerations. Indian J Otolaryngol Head Neck Surg 2010;62:236–47.
71. Jafek BW, Krekorian EA, Kirsch WM, et al. Juvenile nasopharyngeal angiofibroma: management of intracranial extension. Head Neck Surg 1979;2:119–28.
72. Standefer J, Holt GR, Brown WE Jr, et al. Combined intracranial and extracranial excision of nasopharyngeal angiofibroma. Laryngoscope 1983;93:772–9.
73. Krekorian EA, Kato RH. Surgical management of nasopharyngeal angiofibroma with intracranial extension. Laryngoscope 1977;87:154–64.
74. Fagan JJ, Snyderman CH, Carrau RL, et al. Nasopharyngeal angiofibromas: selecting a surgical approach. Head Neck 1997;19:391–9.
75. Mann WJ, Jecker P, Amedee RG. Juvenile angiofibromas: changing surgical concept over the last 20 years. Laryngoscope 2004;114:291–3.

76. Marshall AH, Bradley PJ. Management dilemmas in the treatment and follow-up of advanced juvenile nasopharyngeal angiofibroma. ORL J Otorhinolaryngol Relat Spec 2006;68:273–8.
77. Haines SJ, Duvall AJ. Transzygomatic and transpaletal excison of juvenile nasopharyngeal angiofibroma with intracranial extension. New York: Raven Press; 1993.
78. Browne JD, Jacob SL. Temporal approach for resection of juvenile nasopharyngeal angiofibromas. Laryngoscope 2000;110:1287–93.
79. Danesi G, Panizza B, Mazzoni A, et al. Anterior approaches in juvenile nasopharyngeal angiofibromas with intracranial extension. Otolaryngol Head Neck Surg 2000;122:277–83.
80. Fisch U. The infratemporal fossa approach for nasopharyngeal tumors. Laryngoscope 1983;93:36–44.
81. Zhang M, Garvis W, Linder T, et al. Update on the infratemporal fossa approaches to nasopharyngeal angiofibroma. Laryngoscope 1998;108:1717–23.
82. Roger G, Tran Ba Huy P, Froehlich P, et al. Exclusively endoscopic removal of juvenile nasopharyngeal angiofibroma: trends and limits. Arch Otolaryngol Head Neck Surg 2002;128:928–35.
83. El-Banhawy OA, Shehab El-Dien Ael H, Amer T. Endoscopic-assisted midfacial degloving approach for type III juvenile angiofibroma. Int J Pediatr Otorhinolaryngol 2004;68:21–8.
84. Lee JT, Chen P, Safa A, et al. The role of radiation in the treatment of advanced juvenile angiofibroma. Laryngoscope 2002;112:1213–20.
85. Dare AO, Gibbons KJ, Proulx GM, et al. Resection followed by radiosurgery for advanced juvenile nasopharyngeal angiofibroma: report of two cases. Neurosurgery 2003;52:1207–11 [discussion: 1211].
86. Deguchi K, Fukuiwa T, Saito K, et al. Application of cyberknife for the treatment of juvenile nasopharyngeal angiofibroma: a case report. Auris Nasus Larynx 2002;29:395–400.
87. Schlosser RJ, Woodworth BA, Gillespie MB, et al. Endoscopic resection of sinonasal hemangiomas and hemangiopericytomas. ORL J Otorhinolaryngol Relat Spec 2006;68:69–72.
88. Ceylan A, Kagan Degerliyurt M, Celenk F, et al. Haemangiopericytoma of the hard palate. Dentomaxillofac Radiol 2008;37:58–61.
89. Batsakis JG, Jacobs JB, Templeton AC. Hemangiopericytoma of the nasal cavity: electron-optic study and clinical correlations. J Laryngol Otol 1983;97:361–8.
90. Hekkenberg RJ, Davidson J, Kapusta L, et al. Hemangiopericytoma of the sinonasal tract. J Otolaryngol 1997;26:277–80.
91. Bhattacharyya N, Shapiro NL, Metson R. Endoscopic resection of a recurrent sinonasal hemangiopericytoma. Am J Otolaryngol 1997;18:341–4.
92. Auguste LJ, Razack MS, Sako K. Hemangiopericytoma. J Surg Oncol 1982;20: 260–4.
93. Daniels RL, Haller JR, Harnsberger HR. Hemangiopericytoma of the masticator space. Ann Otol Rhinol Laryngol 1996;105:162–5.
94. Pitluk HC, Conn J Jr. Hemangiopericytoma. Literature review and clinical presentations. Am J Surg 1979;137:413–6.
95. Sutbeyaz Y, Selimoglu E, Karasen M, et al. Haemangiopericytoma of the middle ear: case report and literature review. J Laryngol Otol 1995;109:977–9.
96. Thompson LD, Miettinen M, Wenig BM. Sinonasal-type hemangiopericytoma: a clinicopathologic and immunophenotypic analysis of 104 cases showing perivascular myoid differentiation. Am J Surg Pathol 2003;27:737–49.

97. Herve S, Abd Alsamad I, Beautru R, et al. Management of sinonasal hemangiopericytomas. Rhinology 1999;37:153–8.
98. Koch M, Nielsen GP, Yoon SS. Malignant tumors of blood vessels: angiosarcomas, hemangioendotheliomas, and hemangioperictyomas. J Surg Oncol 2008;97:321–9.
99. Gengler C, Guillou L. Solitary fibrous tumour and haemangiopericytoma: evolution of a concept. Histopathology 2006;48:63–74.
100. Fletcher CD. Distinctive soft tissue tumors of the head and neck. Mod Pathol 2002;15:324–30.
101. Billings KR, Fu YS, Calcaterra TC, et al. Hemangiopericytoma of the head and neck. Am J Otolaryngol 2000;21:238–43.
102. Weiss SW, Goldblum JR. Malignant vascular tumors. St Louis (MO): Mosby; 2001.
103. Volpe AG, Sullivan JG, Chong FK. Aggressive malignant hemangiopericytoma in the neck. J Surg Oncol 1991;47:136–8.
104. Morrison DA, Bibby K. Sellar and suprasellar hemangiopericytoma mimicking pituitary adenoma. Arch Ophthalmol 1997;115:1201–3.
105. Palacios E, Restrepo S, Mastrogiovanni L, et al. Sinonasal hemangiopericytomas: clinicopathologic and imaging findings. Ear Nose Throat J 2005;84:99–102.
106. Abdel-Fattah HM, Adams GL, Wick MR. Hemangiopericytoma of the maxillary sinus and skull base. Head Neck 1990;12:77–83.
107. Craven JP, Quigley TM, Bolen JW, et al. Current management and clinical outcome of hemangiopericytomas. Am J Surg 1992;163:490–3.
108. Pisters PW, Harrison LB, Woodruff JM, et al. A prospective randomized trial of adjuvant brachytherapy in the management of low-grade soft tissue sarcomas of the extremity and superficial trunk. J Clin Oncol 1994;12:1150–5.
109. Yang JC, Chang AE, Baker AR, et al. Randomized prospective study of the benefit of adjuvant radiation therapy in the treatment of soft tissue sarcomas of the extremity. J Clin Oncol 1998;16:197–203.
110. Duval M, Hwang E, Kilty SJ. Systematic review of treatment and prognosis of sinonasal hemangiopericytoma. Head Neck 2013;35:1205–10.
111. Spitz FR, Bouvet M, Pisters PW, et al. Hemangiopericytoma: a 20-year single-institution experience. Ann Surg Oncol 1998;5:350–5.
112. Robb PJ, Singh S, Hartley RB, et al. Malignant hemangiopericytoma of the parapharyngeal space. Head Neck Surg 1987;9:179–83.
113. Delsupehe KG, Jorissen M, Sciot R, et al. Hemangiopericytoma of the head and neck: a report of four cases and a literature review. Acta Otorhinolaryngol Belg 1992;46:421–7.

Printed and bound by CPI Group (UK) Ltd, Croydon, CR0 4YY

07/10/2024

01040505-0005